BRADY

Emergency Vehicle Operations

Jeffrey Lindsey

Richard Patrick

PEARSON
Prentice
Hall

Upper Saddle River,

Library of Congress Cataloging-in-Publication Data

Patrick, Richard.
   Emergency vehicle operations / Jeffrey Lindsey, Richard Patrick.
      p. cm.
   ISBN 0-13-118155-6
    1.   Ambulance driving. I. Title.

TL152.5.P377 2007
362.18′8—dc22

2006049452

Publisher: Julie Levin Alexander
Publisher's Assistant: Regina Bruno
Executive Editor: Mariene McHugh Pratt
Senior Acquisitions Editor: Stephen Smith
Associate Editor: Monica Moosang
Director of Marketing: Karen Allman
Executive Marketing Manager:
   Katrin Beacom
Marketing Coordinator: Michael Sirinides
Marketing Assistant: Wayne Celia, Jr.
Managing Production Editor: Patrick Walsh
Production Liaison: Julie Li
Production Editor: Lisa Garboski, bookworks
Media Product Manager: John Jordan
Manager of Media Production: Amy Peltier
New Media Project Manager: Tina Rudowski
Manufacturing Manager: Ilene Sanford

Manufacturing Buyer: Pat Brown
Senior Design Coordinator:
   Christopher Weigand
Cover Designer: Christopher Weigand
Cover Photos: Getty Images
Director, Image Resource Center:
   Melinda Reo
Manager, Rights and Permissions:
   Zina Arabia
Manager, Visual Research: Beth Brenzel
**Manager, Cover Visual Research
   and Permissions:** Cathy Mazzucca
Image Permission Coordinator:
   Annette Linder
Composition: Techbooks
Printing and Binding: Bind Rite Graphics
Cover Printer: Phoenix Color Corporation

Pearson Education Ltd.
Pearson Education Singapore, Pte. Ltd.
Pearson Education Canada, Ltd.
Pearson Education—Japan
Pearson Education Australia Pty. Limited

Pearson Education North Asia Ltd.
Pearson Educación de Mexico, S.A. de C.V.
Pearson Education Malaysia, Pte. Ltd.
Pearson Education, Inc., Upper Saddle River,
   New Jersey

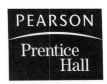

10 9 8 7 6 5 4 3 2 1
ISBN 0-13-118155-6

This book is dedicated to my wife and best friend, Kandace, for her love and support in everything I do. In addition I want to dedicate this to my three wonderful children—my daughters, Natasha and Melissa, and my son, Matthew. Also, my gratitude to my parents, Thomas and Janet Lindsey, for always encouraging me in everything I do. I need to give the most credit to God for allowing me the opportunities and bestowing on me the many blessings I have had in my career and life. Thank you.

Jeffrey Lindsey

This book is dedicated to my wife and best friend, Linda, for her love and support in everything I do. In addition, I want to dedicate this to my two wonderful sons, Ryan and Nathan. A special thanks goes to all the emergency service personnel I have had the opportunity to work with over the past 29 years. The lessons shared have been invaluable. Thank you.

Richard Patrick

Contents

Foreword

We are a country at war. To date, the loss of U.S. soldiers, sailors, and airmen in the Global War on Terrorism exceeds 2,000 souls. Since that fateful day in our country's history on September 11, 2001, many more lives have been lost in motor vehicle crashes in the United States. In fact, the National Highway Traffic Safety Administration's annual statistics show that over 40,000 citizens are killed *per year* in traffic crashes in the United States. Some of those responsible for these deaths are the very people our citizens call when they need help.

Law enforcement officers, firefighters, emergency medical technicians, park rangers, security officers, first responders, tow truck drivers, and anyone else who drives an emergency vehicle serve the people of our country and all who visit. Although some may not agree or use their emergency vehicles for the purposes listed, to others the vehicle is a tool—a mode of getting from one place to another, a barrier to block traffic, a warning sign, a "room" where more waking hours are spent than any other, a place to sleep while posted on a street corner, a dining room where meals are eaten, a computer station, an intensive care unit, a power supply, a lighting system, an elevated platform, a water system with pumps, and even a restroom for those with camping or incinerator toilets. The one factor common to almost all of these platforms is that they move from one place to another on wheels.

Sir Isaac Newton wrote some laws that pertain to emergency vehicles. His first law states that "objects will remain in their state of motion unless a force acts to change the motion," describing the concept of inertia. If we break through an intersection without regard for those around us and hit another vehicle or vehicles, the vehicles change direction due to the forces exerted by each moving object, including the people in the vehicles. The second law, the law of conservation, deals with outside forces, stating that "the mass of an object times the acceleration (or velocity) equals the net force on an object." This applies only to outside forces. In our emergency vehicles, this equates to "speed kills." The third law, known to most as the law of symmetry, states, "for every external force that acts on an object, there is a force of equal magnitude but opposite direction that acts back on the object that exerted that external force." Once again, if we operate our emergency vehicles without regard to safety standards, laws of the road, and those around us, this law shows how people die from the symmetry of forces exerted on vehicles, bodies, and internal organs.

Most of us are touched in some way by the Global War on Terrorism after 9-11. Air travel, deployment of family members and friends to combat zones, loss of employees to deployments, federal dollar allocations, and other ways too numerous to mention have impacted everyone to a certain extent. Our hunt for terrorists continues. Every one of us driving or riding in emergency vehicles has a huge responsibility to train intently and operate these vehicles with the utmost professionalism and safety. We, too, feel the impact of citizens and public servants killed when an emergency vehicle is involved in a fatal crash. It is imperative that we operate our vehicles with the attitude of "privilege" rather than the attitude of "entitlement" or "it's my right."

The authors have written this book to provide us with a guideline, a tool, and a standard for safe, professional, prudent emergency vehicle operations. It is my hope that you use it and share it with your charges. It is a privilege to serve our citizens as public servants, as emergency responders, and as soldiers. Thank you, Rick and Jeff, for sharing your knowledge so that others may live. May God bless you and BE SAFE!

Ben Chlapek
Deputy Fire Chief—Paramedic
Lieutenant Colonel, U.S. Army

Preface

According to the 2000 Census, 300,000,000 people live in the United States. It is estimated that approximately 90,000,000 may drive motor vehicles. Each American alone drives hundreds of millions of miles. The National Highway Traffic Safety Administration's 2000 Economic Cost of Motor Vehicle Traffic Collisions data show a nationwide cost of $230,568 billion. Most driving habits are learned at very early ages from habits of parents, siblings, and other family drivers. Most drivers at the age of 16 learn formally what to do when approached by an emergency vehicle. It may be safe to assume that moments after obtaining the driver's license most of these drivers forget what they are to do when approached by an emergency vehicle. The United States Fire Administration estimates that there are approximately 1,000,000 firefighters, of which 400,000 are emergency vehicle drivers. In addition, add in the thousands of private and third-service emergency medical ambulance drivers. Emergency vehicles spend many hours on the highways, often in less than optimal conditions. The major question at hand is, which is easier to educate, the citizen or the emergency vehicle driver?

Driving is not as simple a process as many motorists are schooled to believe. According to the National Highway Traffic Safety Administration, the United States averages 48,000 highway fatalities each year and tens of thousands more people are injured.[1] Canada averages 2,500 annual fatalities and tens of thousands of injuries each year. Driving is often viewed solely as a skilled task. This belief can lead to somewhat effective but inefficient operation of the vehicle. The process of driving involves the knowledge behind the skilled task, which is frequently a critical missing component for the safest operation of the vehicle. According to 2004 data from the National Highway Traffic Safety Administration's *Passenger Vehicle Occupant Fatalities,* out of all the recorded vehicle collisions, 17,575 were unrestrained, and 10,553 were vehicle rollovers.

Many motorists develop driving habits long before obtaining a learner's permit. The driving habits of family and friends are passed generation to generation with little if any consideration. When the time approaches to obtain a learner's permit, the prospective driver has already gained habits, many of which are inappropriate. Many of these inappropriate driving habits become part of the new driver's common practices. Such habits are carried throughout the driving experience and become more challenging to deal with as time passes. This often results in experienced drivers who have become very effective at doing the right thing the wrong way. Over time, this frequency of practice often breeds severity in resulting collisions.

Coupled with the common driving practices of citizen motorists is the issue of emergency vehicles being granted special response provisions by many state and provincial laws. These provisions often permit emergency vehicle drivers the ability to function irrespective of the common driving practices. Such provisions can cause additional undue confusion with terrifying results.

Understanding human aspects and the history of roadway driving and safety is paramount to implementing an effective and efficient emergency services driving program. According to the United States Fire Administration (USFA), emergency personnel often carry a sense of invulnerability and invincibility. The belief by many emergency service providers that "it can't happen to me" is known as the Magic Box Syndrome.[2] This syndrome may also contribute to many collisions involving emergency vehicles. Emergency service managers must be intuitively aware of the scope of issues and factors encompassing driving in order to confront them with success.

The driving and operation of an emergency vehicle may be the single most important aspect of an emergency responder's responsibilities. No greater challenge exists than to provide the safest transportation of personnel and equipment to and from incidents. There is no difference for career versus volunteer responders. The vehicles and their applicable dynamics do not discriminate. State laws and local regulations may vary, and individuals should follow their specific state and municipality rules, regulations, and laws.

Little, if anything, outweighs the heightened level of responsibility that must be carried on the shoulders of every emergency vehicle driver. Simply put, an emergency vehicle driver must be keenly aware of his or her surroundings at all times and anticipate the unexpected actions and reactions of citizen drivers. No single aspect of emergency services carries a greater potential for liability.

Every year some 250 persons die and thousands are injured as a result of emergency vehicle–related collisions. The numbers are staggering, and statistics point to annual increases even against the efforts of many industry-related organizations and associations. Emergency vehicles are four times more likely to be in a collision than the average driver on the roadway. Statistics tell us when, where, why, and even how emergency vehicle collisions occur. So what is the problem?

Every emergency responder should receive formal driver training when entering the profession. Driver training is a comprehensive, ongoing process throughout the emergency responder's career. Initial training must include classroom, hands-on competencies, written testing, driver testing, and actual roadway evaluation.

This text explores the extent of the situations surrounding emergency vehicle driving and offers solutions to confronting the challenges. An opportunity exists to excel far beyond many of the issues confronting emergency services in relation to the driving and operation of respective vehicles.

What do these three things have in common?

Tires
Window blinds
Vehicles

Answer: Lawsuits and deaths

Think about this:

Tires—Firestone	150 deaths in 3 years (50/year) = Recall
Window blinds	130 children in 5 years (26/year) = Recall

Vehicles—Fire/EMS   25 firefighters/year
                        Unknown EMS personnel = NOTHING
                        5,000 Injuries
                        Number of civilians killed?

= No driver education and training, no license recall. Who is accountable?

OVERVIEW CASE STUDY

Scenario-based case studies enhance the educational experience by providing practical application of the core content. Each chapter provides a case study. This scenario-based review concentrates on the specific chapter content. The content of each subsequent chapter addresses various issues encompassing the scenario and related rationale. Case and content review questions follow every chapter.

---

[1]National Highway Traffic Safety Administration.
[2]USFA, "EMS Safety—Techniques and Applications," FEMA, April 1994, p. 8.

Acknowledgments

Katrin Beacom from Brady for giving us the opportunity to write this text. Stephen Smith for his encouragement and guidance and Monica Moosang for all her assistance and guidance during the process.

Richard Patrick, co-author and my closest friend, for always being there when I need someone to bounce things off, but most of all for being my critic to make me a better individual.

Jeff Lindsey, co-author and closest friend, for always being there when I need someone to discuss ideas with or just simply chat.

Jeffrey Lindsey
Richard Patrick

Reviewers

David W. Goldblum, Ex-Chief
Stewart Manor Fire Department
Stewart Manor, New York

Mark G. Hopkins, Chief
Greater Philadelphia Search and Rescue
Philadelphia, Pennsylvania

Jeff Och
Carver Fire and Rescue Department
Carver, Minnesota

Brenda Skipworth
Morrow County EMS
Cardington, Ohio

Jeff Travers
Great Oaks Institute
Cincinnati, Ohio

About the Authors

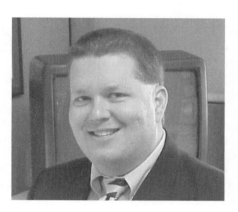

Dr. Jeffrey Lindsey has served in a variety of roles in the fire and EMS arena since 1979. He started his career in the profession as Junior Firefighter in Carlisle, Pennsylvania. He has held positions of firefighter, paramedic, dispatcher, educator, coordinator, deputy chief, and chief. He has also worked in the insurance industry in education and risk control. Dr. Lindsey serves on various advisory boards and state and national committees. He is the education chair for the Florida Fire Service Association EMS section, is a board member for the National Association of EMS Educators, and serves on the state advisory board for education in Florida. He is also a member of the American Society of Training and Development, Florida Society of Fire Service Instructors, and International Society of Fire Service Instructors.

He is currently the Fire Chief for Estero Fire Rescue. In 1985 he pioneered the first advanced life support service in Cumberland County, Pennsylvania. Dr. Lindsey has experience in various environments from the Philadelphia Fire Department to hospitals, third-service organizations, and currently Estero Fire Rescue.

He holds an associate degree in Para-medicine from Harrisburg Area Community College, a bachelor degree in Fire and Safety from the University of Cincinnati, a master degree in Safety from Kennedy-Western University, and a master degree in Instructional Technology from the University of South Florida. He has earned a Ph.D. in Instructional Technology/Adult Education from the University of South Florida. Dr. Lindsey is completing the Executive Fire Officer Program at the National Fire Academy.

He has designed and developed various courses in fire and EMS. Dr. Lindsey is accredited with the Chief Fire Officer Designation. He also is a certified Fire Officer II, Fire Instructor III, and paramedic in the state of Florida. He holds a paramedic certificate from the state of Pennsylvania. He is also a certified instructor in a variety of courses. Dr. Lindsey has taught courses throughout the country and has been a speaker at many national and state conferences including Fire Rescue Med, Fire Rescue East, NAEMSE Symposium, Colorado EMS conference, Fire Rescue International, JEMS Technology conference, and many others.

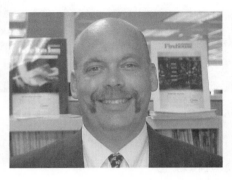

Mr. Richard Patrick is the Division Chief of Health, Safety & Training for Estero Fire Rescue in Estero, Florida. He is the past Director of EMS Programs and Emergency Service Initiatives for VFIS, a division of Glatfelter Insurance Group, York, PA, and remains as a consultant to the education, training and consulting division. Rick is a nationally known leader, educator, lecturer, author, speaker, and consultant in emergency services. He is a former Chief of EMS in the City of Lebanon, PA.

Rick is a certified Paramedic/Firefighter and holds a Bachelor of Science Degree in Engineering Safety with a concentration in Emergency Services, and a Masters Degree in Public Safety Administration from Saint Joseph's University in Philadelphia. He is also a small business entrepreneur, involved in local politics, and an alumnus of the Lebanon Valley Chamber of Commerce-Leadership Lebanon Valley program.

Rick has over twenty-eight years of diverse experience in Emergency Services. He was recently appointed Chairman of the Congressional Fire Services Institute (CFSI) National Advisory Board and is chairperson of the NAEMT Health & Safety Task Group. He is a Principal Member of the Technical Committee on EMS for the National Fire Protection Association. Rick also serves on the ICHIEFS Health and Safety Committee. He is an Adjunct Faculty Member for Paramedic Education-Allied Health and the Public Safety Center at Harrisburg Area Community College, Harrisburg Area Community College Paramedic Advisory Council and served as Regional Faculty for the American Heart Association in Advanced Cardiac Life Support. Rick is a reviewer for the Continuing Education Coordinating Board for EMS (CECBEMS), and is a certified Emergency Medical Dispatcher. Rick is a member of the IAFC, IAFC-EMS Section, National Association of EMS Educators (NAEMSE), International Society of Fire Service Instructors (ISFSI), NFPA, NAEMT, a Fellow with the National Academy of Emergency Dispatch, National of EMS Physicians, and the Fire Department Safety Officers Association.

Rick is a past Chief Executive Officer of the Annville Fire Department, Annville, Lebanon County, PA, and served as the Annville Township Fire Marshal. His career has scaled the ranks as a Firefighter, Lieutenant, Captain, EMT, Paramedic, Flight Medic, Administrator, and EMS Chief. He served on one of the first Quick Response Medical Units in Pennsylvania and worked his way to "Chief of Operations" at one of the largest EMS Fire Systems in South Central PA. Rick was responsible for conceptualizing and implementing the first Advanced Life Support Service for Eastern Lebanon County and the City of Lebanon, PA. He also served on his local municipality planning commission.

Mr. Patrick has had the privilege to travel throughout the United States and abroad consulting, educating and speaking on a variety of business, industrial and public safety topics.

Leadership and Management

Objectives

After completing this chapter, you should be able to:

- Describe the characteristic differences between Theory X and Y leaders.
- List the core components for effective management.
- Identify critical emergency service topics that require the attention of leadership based on the Firefighter Life Safety Summit.

Case Study

A fire truck responding to an automatic fire alarm fails to stop at a red traffic light and strikes a minivan broadside, injuring five in the van and two of the firefighters. During the investigation it is alleged that the fire truck operator was not required to complete a driver training program. The plaintiff's attorney alleged that the fire department failed as the employer to establish policy and train its vehicle operators to operate department vehicles safely. In fact, the department did have a policy in place and records indicate that the driver in question did not attend a prescribed driving course.

◆ INTRODUCTION

The process of emergency vehicle operations is comprehensive and entails dozens of administrative and operational factors to accomplish the emergency response mission safely. Emergency service injuries and fatalities associated with emergency vehicle collisions are tragic. Compounding this tragedy are the injuries, deaths, and accompanying litigation that can occur when civilians are involved. Yet with sound department policy, proper driver training, public education programs, and emergency vehicle response procedures, many of these collisions can be avoided. It is not only time but also a necessity for a cultural change to occur in every **emergency service organization (ESO)**. The change needed is for the ESO leadership to place and promote safe driving practices second to nothing in the operation of its organization. Leadership must understand that if something is predictable, it is preventable. Incidents surrounding safe vehicle operation are predictable.

Simply put, ESOs must address this subject with a top-down approach. A cultural change at the top can positively affect a behavioral change in the ranks. Leaders and providers alike must understand that just because someone has a driver's license and possibly attends an Emergency Vehicle Operator Course (**EVOC**) does not qualify him or her to operate an emergency vehicle. To imply such beliefs is an open invitation for things to go wrong. The goal is clear: Create a culture within the ESO that positively demands a high standard of driving behavior of all personnel.

◆ LEADERSHIP

Lao Tzu was a sixth-century B.C. philosopher credited with writing *Tao Te Ching,* one of China's best-loved books of wisdom. Lao Tzu has been referenced by A. J. Heightman, editor in chief of the *Journal of Emergency Medical Services (JEMS),* and Chief Dennis Compton, Mesa, Arizona (retired), in emergency service leadership seminars across North America.

Tao Te Ching (pronounced "dow duh jing") was originally directed to the wise political and governmental leaders of ancient China. It was supposedly a response to social, political, and philosophical conditions of life two and half millennia ago in China.

Leadership has been described as an art, a science, and a style. It is a third dimension. Leadership goes beyond doing "things the old way." Leaders know the value of the bottom line, but a leader looks beyond the numbers and sets the direction of the organization. A leader not only values the financial survival of an organization but also integrates the significance of the bottom line with the how's, why's, and when's of the business.

According to Heightman (2005), some scholars believe Lao Tzu was a slightly older contemporary of Confucius. Other scholars purport that *Tao Te Ching* is really a compilation of paradoxical poems written by several Taoists using the pen name Lao Tzu. Regardless, *Tao Te Ching* is a classic of world literature that unites the leader's leadership skills and way of life: "Our work is our path."

In regard to the risk management activities of an organization, the leader promotes, supports, and provides valuable guidance and resources to the loss control effort. Often the leader may not do the actual inspection, crunch the numbers, or write the policies, though he or she could if the organization were small. The leader should know how a good risk control program provides the tools to achieve organizational success. Leaders establish the safety culture, set the vision, and guide the process through directing and empowering their people to translate the vision into reality. Leadership focuses on mainly behavioral issues regarding organizational growth. Evidence of effective leadership is seen when

- Leadership writes a policy statement regarding a risk control program.
- Leadership and management establish safety goals and standards.
- Management and supervision develop a risk control program.
- Leadership, management, and supervision perform to standard and hold volunteers/employees accountable for standards.
- Leadership, management, and supervision demonstrate knowledge of the company safety program through monitoring, evaluation, and feedback (Figure 1.1).

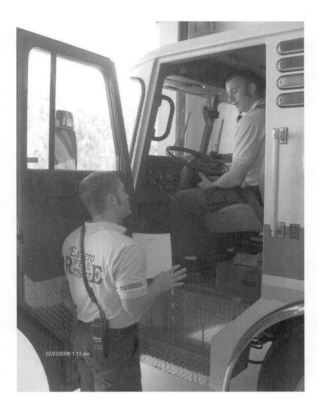

FIGURE 1.1 ◆ Emergency services officer speaking with emergency vehicle driver regarding the importance of safe operations.

Successful leaders must understand several core components of effective management. They must know how to

- Have foresight.
- Get people to do things that the organization needs done.
- Lead by example.
- Supervise, inspire, and train personnel.
- Create self-initiative.
- Support the team.
- Get staff to follow the leader.
- Get things done.

To be effective, leaders must:

- Have integrity.
- Display initiative.
- Be authoritative.
- Have insight.
- Maintain interest.
- Accept responsibility.
- Not show favoritism.
- Sustain staff intensity.
- Access and share information.

Management styles vary and one of the most prominent style divisions is that of **Theory X and Y**. According to McGregor (1960), Theory X and Y management styles

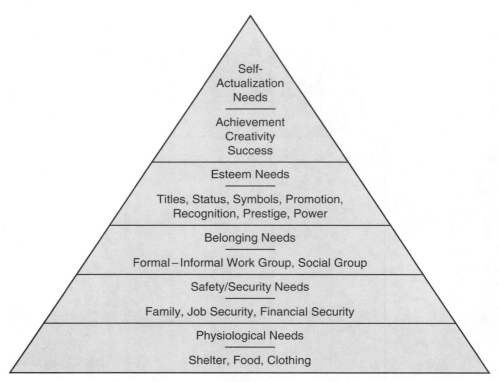

FIGURE 1.2 ◆ Maslow's hierarchy of basic human needs.

have assumptions that differentiate the X leader from the Y leader. The Theory X manager believes that people are inherently lazy, need to be told what to do, and will work only when threatened. Assumptions also include that people want to receive direction and don't like responsibility. The Theory X leader uses authoritative and hard techniques to punish or threaten employees or offer rewards for compliance with following company directives. A Theory Y manager tends to believe that providing people with a positive work environment in which the employee accepts responsibility also has the employee seeking additional responsibilities. McGregor believes that employees are self-motivated to perform work that is satisfying to them and that their ingenuity and creativity will stand out and enhance the overall performance of the organization. The Theory Y manager leads with a participatory and soft style. Through a good environment, the employee can be successful, learn new things, and everyone succeeds.

Abraham Maslow, a well-known researcher on human needs, determined that individuals would achieve success only if certain basic needs were met (Figure 1.2). One of the first basic needs is that of safety. It is foolish for any leader, manager, or supervisor to believe that his or her personnel will excel in reaching organizational goals if they feel unsafe. Participating in a formal program helps establish the concept that safety is important in every function, and any organization can reach its goals by shifting the priority from "production and revenue" to controlling losses and managing risk. This is a leadership and management responsibility.

◆ **MANAGEMENT CULTURE**

Every organization has a culture but what kind of culture is the issue. An ESO may need a culture change! That's right, a culture change in the way the ESO views and addresses the subject of driving: not only emergency driving but also all work-related characteristics of driving knowledge, habits, and skills. It all starts with the ESO's commitment to safety and the action-oriented process of leading by example.

Management and leadership are unique, according to VFIS. The manager concerns him- or herself with maintaining a quick response time, keeping adequate equipment levels, paying for incurred costs, and billing for services. The manager focuses on what needs to be accomplished, how to accomplish it, when, and by whom. Because of this action-oriented belief, one theory for the cause of collisions suggests that management share in the responsibility for collisions. This is not to say that management is to blame for collisions. If management fails to exercise its planning, organizing, directing, and controlling functions effectively, then the environment created will eventually lead to collisions. Managers can become so focused on "production" that they lose sight of the vision. As a result, risk control activities become secondary and the financial impact can be disastrous. Typically, management focuses on behavioral as well as nonbehavioral growth issues.

Supervisors deal with people, ideas, and plans. They hear, see, and feel the activities of the personnel. Supervisors balance personnel needs with the ESO vision. The responsibility of supervisors is to ensure the completion of the assigned work. They realize that the patient, hospital, and general public are all integral players in the delivery of emergency and related services. The supervisor, in this capacity, must support the risk control efforts through development, education, training, reinforcing, and encouragement of personnel. The supervisor's actions continue to show the continuity of the vision and function of the mission from leadership to emergency responder. Supervisors focus their energies on mostly nonbehavioral issues.

◆ **COMBINED EFFORTS**

Although the overall results of a risk control program depend on the combined efforts of all levels, the key to affecting a safe culture and controlling losses rests with the leadership. Leadership and management must support the philosophical view of any safety program and incorporate safety into the policies and procedures of the ESO. The supervisor must carry out the technical aspects of the program and safely plan, organize, direct, and control the work activities for which he or she has direct responsibility.

◆ **DRIVING AND LEADERSHIP**

Emergency vehicle crashes are the leading cause of liability claims against emergency service organizations (Figure 1.3). Preventing them must be one of the highest priorities for every emergency service. The experts agree that risk management, loss control specialists, chief officers, system administrators, and fleet managers should play a combined role in this process.

FIGURE 1.3 ◆ Ambulance involved in collision. (*Courtesy of PhotoEdit Inc.*)

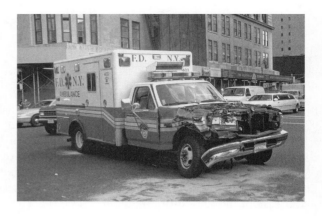

Emergency vehicle operations is a responsible position in the emergency medical and ambulance transportation industry. Whether your service is chartered as a volunteer fire department or municipally based, not-for-profit, or commercial, the responsibilities of and the penalties for not properly training your emergency and nonemergency vehicle operators are tremendous. Civil, criminal, and punitive damages and charges may become a part of your vocabulary if one of your vehicles is involved in a crash that injures or kills one of your staff members, a patient, or a civilian vehicle operator or pedestrian. However, emergency vehicle operation is more than the physical aspects of driving. Being able to understand the emotional aspect is just as important. Several **EMTs**, paramedics, and firefighters across this nation have learned what happens when they are involved in an emergency vehicle crash. Many have been charged with criminal charges as a result of the crash. Several have been sentenced to and served prison time because of their guilty convictions. The emotional aspect of this program is often not covered by other emergency vehicle driver safety programs.

Education versus training has long been discussed in the emergency service profession. It has been said that the difference between education and training is the understanding of why we do what we do. Technicians (i.e., EMT, firefighter, first responder) can be trained to perform a skill, like emergency driving but through higher education, we understand why that specific skill is performed. Many **EMS** educators would like to see more in-depth anatomy, physiology, and didactic reasoning added to programs. Still others have their own agendas on topics from pediatrics to geriatrics and from public education to injury prevention, to name a few.

For more than two decades, EVOC training has been evolving as a training and education tool to increase operator awareness of such matters as physical and dynamic forces, legal issues, preventive maintenance, and standard operating procedures. Programs have ranged in length from two to twelve hours. Many programs offered obstacle courses for the hands-on portion, but some did not require the actual application of driving in any form.

◆ LEADERSHIP AND MANAGEMENT'S MAJOR GOALS FOR DRIVING TOPICS

1. A safe and timely response to the scene
2. Safe transportation to the most appropriate medical facility, in accordance with state and local laws governing ambulance operation
3. Smooth and comfortable transportation with attention focused on the needs of the patients, and ensuring that medical procedures can be performed without unnecessary interruption

4. Driving performed with due regard for the safety of the public while operating under all circumstances
5. Maintaining a safe driving environment by complying with all company polices, protocols, standards of care, laws, statutes, rules, and regulations

◆ OBSERVATION AND ENFORCEMENT

It is important to monitor emergency vehicle drivers regularly to ensure they are following proper safe driving procedures in all components of the response. This may be undertaken by the officer in charge on the apparatus, the driver's partner, the operator of a second vehicle, or a designated responder. Emergency vehicle drivers should be made keenly aware that their on-road performance must mirror the ESO's operating policies. Violators need to be disciplined and counseled so that errors and violations are kept to a minimum.

First and foremost, administration should look at the driver selection process. An individual's attitude, past driving record, and driving habits are generally indicative of how this person will operate an organization's vehicles. Realizing that this may not be as easy as one may think, organizations must develop and enforce sound standard operating procedures and guidelines.

◆ TRAINING AND EDUCATION

Among the keys to preventing collisions are repetition during training exercises and other forms of continuing education (Figure 1.4). The ESO's standard operating procedures/standard operating guidelines (**SOP/SOGs**) should also be a key component of the training. Consider this: A responsible officer wouldn't dream of explaining the use of self-contained breathing apparatus (**SCBA**) gear one time and then consider the training complete. Instead, the lesson is repeated over and over until the trainee can literally "do it in the dark." The "how" and "when" to use SCBA is also part of the training. That same level of care and attention is needed in other facets of emergency service. Emergency and related vehicle driving practices is certainly one of them.

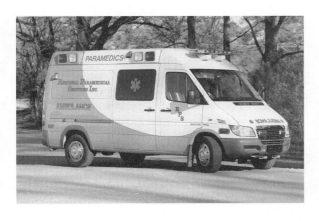

FIGURE 1.4 ◆ Emergency vehicle on driving course. (*Courtesy of Ken Kerr*).

◆ FIREFIGHTER LIFE SAFETY INITIATIVES

The Firefighter Life Safety Summit held in Tampa, Florida, in March 2004, produced 16 major initiatives that give the fire service a blueprint for making changes. Many of these initiatives impact components of driving. Even though these initiatives are fire based, EMS agencies should consider them as applicable to any emergency service operation.

1. Define and advocate the need for a cultural change within the fire service relating to safety, incorporating leadership, management, supervision, accountability, and personal responsibility.
2. Enhance the personal and organizational accountability for health and safety throughout the fire service.
3. Focus greater attention on the integration of risk management with incident management at all levels, including strategic, tactical, and planning responsibilities.
4. Empower all firefighters to stop unsafe practices.
5. Develop and implement national standards for training, qualifications, and certification (including regular recertification) that are equally applicable to all firefighters, based on the duties they are expected to perform.
6. Develop and implement national medical and physical fitness standards that are equally applicable to all firefighters, based on the duties they are expected to perform.
7. Create a national research agenda and data collection system that relate to the initiatives.
8. Utilize available technology wherever it can produce higher levels of health and safety.
9. Thoroughly investigate all firefighter fatalities, injuries, and near misses.
10. Ensure that grant programs support the implementation of safe practices and/or mandate safe practices as an eligibility requirement.
11. Develop and champion national standards for emergency response policies and procedures.
12. Develop and champion national protocols for response to violent incidents.
13. Provide firefighters and their families access to counseling and psychological support.
14. Provide public education more resources and champion it as a critical fire and life safety program.
15. Strengthen advocacy for the enforcement of codes and the installation of home fire sprinklers.
16. Make safety a primary consideration in the design of apparatus and equipment.

◆ CASE STUDY RECAP

Risk management experts say that if a situation is predictable it is preventable. Many emergency vehicle–related incidents are predictable. Although not all collisions can be prevented, the severity of many collisions can be reduced. If the fire truck in the case study would have stopped at the intersection and proceeded after obtaining eye contact with the other vehicle operators on the roadway, the incident might not have happened. If a collision still occurred, it might have been less severe. In addition, the decision to respond with lights and siren to automatic fire alarms should be reviewed.

The case discussed in this chapter resulted in needless injury and damage to property. Every ESO must develop and implement practical, realistic policy on safe driving response practices; deliver proper driver education and training; provide well-maintained vehicles to do the job safely; and enforce the policies.

The ability to lead trumps all components of an organization. Understanding the roles and responsibilities of leadership, management, and supervision is paramount to the success of any organization. Nothing is more important than the personnel in your ESO. Therefore, personnel safety must not take a backseat to anything—NOTHING! The ESO culture must not only promote but also breathe the concept of safety in every facet of the organization. Proper selection of drivers, sound policy with supporting doable procedures, quality education and training, competency-based testing, and continuing education are the minimum components for any safe driving program. Most importantly, organizational leadership must take, and thus make, the subject of safe driving the number-one priority of the ESO. The culture must be created at the top, promoted and maintained by line officers, and then it will be sustained by the ranks.

As part of the management and leadership in your organization, you must strive to reduce the risk of property damage and injury to civilians and emergency response personnel. Your personnel should be vigilant in their recognition of all hazards and exposures associated with negotiating intersections, particularly those with negative right-of-way. Drivers must constantly monitor and reduce the amount of risk and exposure to potential losses during each and every response. Safe arrival at the emergency should be, and must always remain, the first priority of all emergency vehicle drivers. Provide the ESO team with the tools to do the job, train them how to do the job, lead them over the right path, and let them do the job.

Review Questions

1. How important is the leadership culture in an emergency service organization?
2. List five of the core components of an effective leader.
3. What is a key difference between the Theory X and Y leaders?
4. How does a supervisor fit into the realm of safety in the ESO?
5. Why are policies and procedures important as they pertain to driving?

References

Battalion Chief John Salka, FDNY. April 8, 2005. Seminar on leadership for the Executive MBA Program at St. Joseph's University. Philadelphia, Pennsylvania.

Heightman, A. J. 2005. *The components of EMS leadership—Lessons from the 6th century.* Presented at EMS TODAY, Philadelphia, Pennsylvania.

NHTSA. 1994. *Emergency vehicle operators course (ambulance)—National standard curriculum.* Module 8.

Retrieved December 18, 2005, from http://www.itstime.com/mar2003.htm

Retrieved December 18, 2005, from http://www.valuebasedmanagement.net/methods_mcgregor_theory_X_Y.html

Patrick, R. W. Spring 2004. "Don't become a statistic." *Carolina Fire Rescue EMS Journal.*

Patrick, R. W. July 2004. "Driver training, a cultural perspective." *EMS Magazine.*

VFIS. 1997. *Emergency Vehicle Driver Training Program.* York, Pennsylvania.

Williams, D. July 2004. "Develop leaders by teaching the value of the head, hand and heart." *The Managers Toolbox.*

CHAPTER 2

Choosing the Right People

Objectives

After completing this chapter, you should be able to:

- Recognize that selecting the right personnel is the first step in developing an effective emergency vehicle driver program.
- Define the human aspects of selecting the emergency vehicle operator.
- Identify the important components in the driver selection process.
- List the abilities necessary for driving emergency vehicles that must be acquired.
- Relate the importance of maintaining emergency vehicle driving proficiency through an ongoing recertification program.
- Recognize the importance of maintaining accurate and complete personnel records for the protection of both the emergency service organization and the individual driver.

Case Study

The pager went off and the text message on the pager requested the Chief to call dispatch ASAP. The Chief knew there were not many times that the dispatch center called with an urgent message in the middle of the night. After hanging up from the dispatch center, she left to go immediately to the station to begin dealing with the issue no Chief likes to face.

The next morning the headlines in the local newspaper read "Emergency Vehicle Operator Is Arrested for DUI." The Chief knew last evening after the phone call informing her of the events that it was going to be a long day, a long week for that matter. How would she handle the media calls? What would this mean for the organization? What should be done with the driver accused of the charges? Could this have been prevented before it ever happened?

◆ INTRODUCTION

Through attitude and behavior, organization leaders must reflect the importance of safety in all aspects dealing with vehicles. It is vital to infuse this attitude in all organizational policies and training. Department commitment to driver competency and

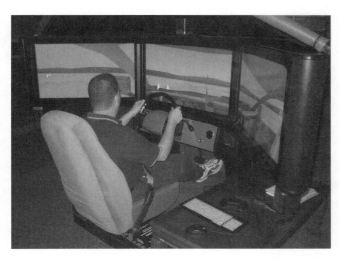

Figure 2.1 ◆ Driving simulators are being integrated into driving programs.

accountability can have a profound effect on reducing **crashes**, injuries, and fatalities. This begins with the factors used to select the driver candidate.

Training is the foundation of all safe practices (see Figure 2.1). The type of course, integration of classroom and applied practice, and instructor qualifications all contribute to the effectiveness of any training. This chapter reviews factors to consider in selecting driver candidates, practices, and programs related to several aspects of training (including initial basic driving courses); determining the use and value of a driving simulator in basic, remedial, and continuing training; and developing driver requirements.

Points to Ponder

What does it take to become a good emergency vehicle driver? If you wanted to become a star football player or world class pianist, how much training and practice time would you plan on? Serious players would expect to train with professional coaches and practice for years to get anywhere near the top of their field.

For the average emergency vehicle driver, it generally takes 8 to 24 hours of actual behind-the-wheel experience to be able to deal with the basic maneuvering of an emergency vehicle. There is no real test to measure ability once the emergency vehicle driver is released to drive in an emergency situation, so many people can fool themselves into believing they are very good drivers simply because they have not been involved in a crash.

Emergency vehicle drivers should understand that driving is a complex set of mental, social, emotional, and physical skills and processes. They need to be able to recognize and evaluate their own driving patterns and evaluate problem driving behaviors and attitudes.

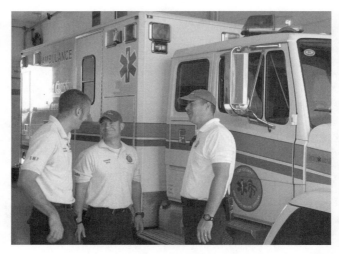

FIGURE 2.2 ◆ Selecting the appropriate personnel is a key component of a successful driving program.

◆ IMPORTANCE OF DRIVER SELECTION

In real estate the realtor states the three most important aspects are location, location, location. Emergency driving is very similar. The three most important aspects in emergency driving are personnel, personnel, personnel (see Figure 2.2). Without the right personnel, the organization is subjected to a variety of issues surrounding the operation of the organization. Selecting a driver and keeping a qualified driver behind the wheel are essential to the safe and efficient operation of the vehicle.

In emergency vehicle driving the three principles of safe operation are driver selection, driver training, and driver proficiency. Initial attention should be directed to effective driver selection.

A comprehensive approach to the selection of emergency vehicle drivers is the key element to developing and maintaining safe emergency vehicle operations. The major considerations of such a program are

- Human aspects
- Acquired abilities
- Vehicle characteristics
- Personnel records

◆ HUMAN ASPECTS

Whereas human attitude and activity can, with appropriate training, be altered, human nature is impossible to change. The various human aspects identified herein are factors that can promote a change in human activity to produce the safest possible emergency vehicle driver.

Four categories of human factors contribute to vehicle crashes: knowledge base, skills, ability, and attitude. Drivers may lack knowledge of traffic laws, knowledge of

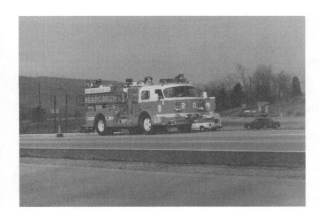

FIGURE 2.3 ◆ Emergency vehicle drivers need to position their vehicles in a safe manner on streets and highways. These areas are very dangerous to responders.

physical laws that govern the vehicle operation, or the awareness of potential dangers (see Figure 2.3). Inadequate skills in handling vehicles may be the result of insufficient training, lack of hands-on training, inexperience, slowed or improper reaction, or poor judgment. Attitude plays a major role in safe vehicle operations. Failure to obey laws or take proper precautions; improper use of the roads; and allowing excitement to lead to impulsive actions, dangerous shortcuts, and irresponsible or reckless behavior all contribute to emergency vehicle crashes and fatalities. Other factors include inattentiveness, failure to concentrate on driving tasks, and the emotional sense of power and urgency when running lights and siren. This sense can block out reason and prudence, leading to the reckless operation of the emergency vehicle.

A review of the *USFA Firefighter Fatalities in the United States* reports (FEMA, 2004) suggests that age (both young and older) appears to be a factor in both fire apparatus and ambulance crashes. Many who enter the emergency services field have only two to three years of normal driving experience. The older driver may have slowed responses. The suggested minimum age of 21 has been established for emergency vehicle drivers. In some cases, the organization's insurance company may determine this.

Another factor that contributes to emergency vehicle crashes is improper or no background checks of the potential drivers. According to an article in the *Detroit News* (Canan, 2000), 41 percent of ambulance drivers involved in fatal accidents had prior citations on their driving records (see Figure 2.4).

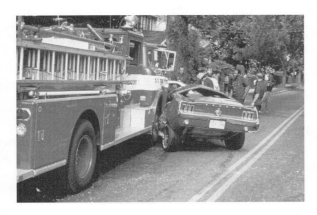

FIGURE 2.4 ◆ Emergency vehicles are not exempt from being in accidents. (*Courtesy of Pearson Education/PH College*)

DRIVING CHECKS

Prior to employment or volunteering, the department should verify driving records by having the applicant sign a consent form to allow the department to check records with the state. The applicant's driving record should be reviewed for the number of moving violations over the past 36 months, any driving under the influence (DUI) convictions, reckless driving citations, license suspensions, and so on. Evaluation of driver education certificates, specialized driving licenses (e.g., CDL), and physical qualifications (e.g., vision and hearing) can also help reduce the number of vehicular incidents that occur each year.

State Motor Vehicle Record Check. A review of state motor vehicle records for the previous three years should be conducted when a driver is first hired or begins to drive voluntarily for an organization. This review must include checking for any speeding, careless or reckless driving, driving under the influence of alcohol or other mind-altering substances, or moving violations. Many organizations do an annual motor vehicle record check on all their personnel.

Motor Vehicle Accident Check. The driving record should be checked for any accidents the driver has had in the previous five years.

License Check. The driver's license should be checked to make sure that the driver is licensed and qualified to operate the class of vehicle the driver will be operating.

ATTITUDE

Having a good attitude is the best influence on doing a good job. The driver's mental fitness may be affected by a lack of concentration or the use of alcohol or drugs. If drivers are worried about a sick family member, money problems, or problems concerning children, they may be distracted and not perform at their best. It is better for drivers not to drive until they are better able to concentrate.

Drivers can be distracted when they are angry about something. If drivers are angry, they may lose patience and take risks they normally wouldn't consider. Drivers should calm down before driving. It is illegal to drink and drive. Drinking should be prohibited for all emergency personnel. Many organizations designate a set amount of time, such as 12 hours, that personnel should not consume any alcoholic beverages before driving an emergency vehicle. Likewise, illegal drugs are never acceptable, under any circumstances, and should never be used while on or off duty. Drivers need to consider their physical and mental condition every time they respond to an incident to ensure personal safety and the safety of the crew and patients in transport units.

Attitude is the individual's disposition toward driving. Some identified types of unwanted attitude include the following:

Immature: Cares only about one's own safety.
Brazen/show-off: Is more concerned about image than reality.
Laid-back: Is so much so that reaction may be hours or days late.
Comic: Doesn't panic, sees humor in everything, even dangerous situations.

KNOWLEDGE

This is an individual's clear perception of truth, fact, or a series of issues relating to a specific subject:

> **An emergency vehicle driver's knowledge is vital concerning the vehicle, its features, behavior, and operational characteristics.**

In addition to obtaining knowledge, a potential emergency vehicle driver must not have wrong information or misconceptions regarding emergency vehicle driving.

MENTAL FITNESS

> ### Point to Ponder
>
> The state of mind about driving:
>
> **Does the individual understand and respect the responsibility of driving an emergency vehicle under all conditions? If he or she does, is this translated into driving characteristics that reflect attentiveness and caution when driving the vehicle?**

PHYSICAL FITNESS

Driving is a psychomotor skill that requires learning a certain set of skills and then being sure to practice, practice, practice until the motions become almost automatic. Although these skills are sometimes called "instinctive" reactions, they're not instinctive at all; they are learned responses.

New emergency vehicle drivers must split their attention between basic vehicle control (i.e., steering, braking, shifting gears) and the attention and concentration needed for the social and decision-making aspects of driving. Inexperienced drivers need to recognize that their ability to react effectively to traffic situations and avoid crashes will be limited until they master these vehicle-handling skills.

Physical and Mental Fitness. Drivers' physical and mental condition affects the daily performance of their job. Drivers are expected to be physically and mentally fit for every response (see Figure 2.5). Drivers' physical fitness may be affected by their health and the amount of rest they are getting. For example:

- Drivers who have the flu may not be alert and at their best.
- Shoulder injuries may affect drivers' ability to maneuver their vehicles.
- Over-the-counter medications may make drivers sleepy.
- Lack of sleep can make drivers' response time slower.

If the driver is not in good physical condition, it is better not to drive.

> ### Point to Ponder
>
> Regarding physical fitness policy, are annual physicals required? How do drivers report to their supervisor when they are not in condition to drive?

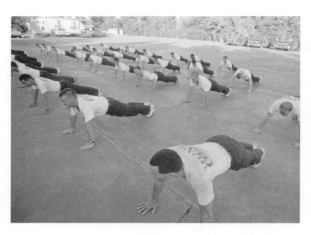

FIGURE 2.5 ◆ A driver's physical fitness impacts job performance. (*Courtesy of Corbis/Bettman*)

PERSONAL APPEARANCE AND HYGIENE

Although not exactly a part of physical and mental fitness, drivers' physical appearance and hygiene have a lot to do with how well they perform the job duties. First, a professional physical appearance builds confidence in the community that the driver may need to direct. The driver's professional bearing will be a credit to the organization. Second, personal hygiene and precautions in handling medical patients are required to prevent the spread of infection. If drivers get sick, they will not be of much use to their organizations.

Professional appearance relates not only to the person but also to the equipment. Clean, properly stowed equipment makes the task—driving the emergency vehicle and, when driving an ambulance, transporting patients—safer and easier, and makes the results more positive (see Figure 2.6).

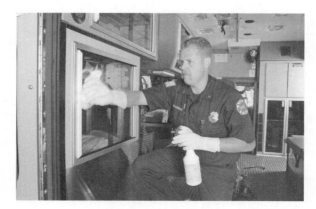

FIGURE 2.6 ◆ The emergency vehicle should be properly cleaned with all equipment properly secured. (*Courtesy of Pearson Education/PH College*)

JUDGMENT

Judgment is the ability to make good decisions:

Is the individual decisive? If decisive, does the individual typically assume an offensive or defensive posture? Many times the judgment of an individual is reflected in the personnel file. Excessive aggressiveness may be documented in the form of counseling sessions or disciplinary action.

Some traits that should be considered when evaluating a potential driver's judgment might include

Excitability: Becoming overly excited or agitated in a critical situation.
Maturity: The ability to keep emotions in check while driving.

TRAFFIC PSYCHOLOGY

Developed by Dr. Leon James at the University of Hawaii (2004), traffic psychology refers to how a driver learns to modify his or her own style of conduct in traffic situations and to monitor the impact of one's own driving behavior on other road users. The benefits of this idea include perfecting the American character by teaching interpersonal skills that encourage the following:

1. Chivalry (being polite to strangers)
2. Charity (caring for the feelings of other road users)
3. Freedom (showing self-responsibility)
4. Family values (being nice to your passengers)
5. Citizenship and respect for law and order (obeying traffic ordinances)
6. Spirituality (recognizing subtle connectedness among traffic users)
7. Morality and rationality (respecting people's rights in public places)
8. Empathy and sympathy (showing solidarity with other traffic users)
9. National unity and integration (identifying with positive symbols)
10. Creative driving practices (multitasking, recreation, artistic expression)

COORDINATION

The coordination of a variety of motor skills is critical in order to accomplish an intended action. Drivers must make split second decisions in reaction to traffic situations and execute those decisions smoothly. For instance, if a child runs into the road, the driver will have to simultaneously steer and brake (and perhaps clutch and shift gears), while watching for other potential hazards on the road, such as oncoming traffic, bystanders, or parked cars.

PHYSICAL CONDITION

Medical Check. A licensed physician determines whether someone is physically able to perform the job of driver under all conditions. The medical exam should reveal no medical or physical condition that would prove detrimental to operating an emergency vehicle.

The examination identifies drivers who may be impaired by

- Loss of consciousness
- Cardiovascular disease
- Neurological/neurovascular disorder

- Mental illness
- Substance abuse/dependency
- Insulin-dependent diabetes
- Rheumatic, arthritic, orthopedic, muscular, neuromuscular, or vascular disease that interferes with the ability to control and operate a motor vehicle

The presence of a medical condition alone may not indicate an impaired operator. However, it can identify an area to consider when determining a person's medical fitness to operate an emergency vehicle.

Emergency vehicle drivers' physical condition will substantially impact their ability to drive competently. Good drivers will be aware of their own physical limitations and will compensate appropriately (i.e., wearing corrective lenses) or will avoid driving entirely when fatigued. Being physically fit is an important aspect of driving an emergency vehicle. The following checklist is a guideline to assist in determining physical fitness in driving an emergency vehicle.

- You have trouble looking over your shoulder to change lanes or looking left and right to check traffic at intersections.
- You have trouble moving your foot from the gas to the brake pedal or turning the steering wheel.
- You have fallen down—not counting a trip or stumble—once or more in the previous year.
- You walk less than one block per day.
- You can't raise your arms above your shoulders.
- You feel pain in your knees, legs, or ankles when going up or down a flight of ten stairs.

There are a number of things drivers can do to improve their physical ability.

1. With your doctor's approval, do some stretching exercises and start a walking program. Walk around the block or in a mall. Also, check health clubs, YMCAs, and colleges for fitness programs.
2. Undergo a doctor's examination if you have pain or swelling in your feet. If you have pain or stiffness in your arms, legs, or neck, your doctor may prescribe medication and/or physical therapy.
3. Eliminate your driver's side blind spot by re-aiming your side mirror. First, lean your head against the window, then adjust your mirror outward so that when you look at the inside edge you can barely see the side of your vehicle. If you use a wide-angle mirror, get lots of practice judging distances to other cars before using it in traffic.
4. Keep alert to sounds outside your vehicle. Limit passenger conversation and background noises from the radio and stereo.
5. Sit at least ten inches from the steering wheel to reduce the chances of an injury from the air bag (see Figure 2.7). Remember always to wear your seat belt.

DRIVER READINESS

An emergency vehicle driver's effectiveness is controlled by a number of factors including fatigue, health, and personal problems.

Fatigue. Both mental and physical fatigue can influence the ability of an emergency vehicle driver. Some examples include a lack of sleep and a sudden awakening from a deep sleep. Although evidence is limited or inferential, chronic predisposing factors

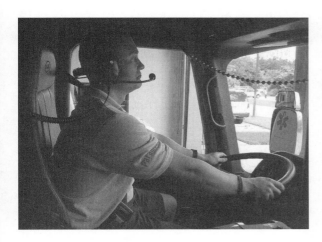

FIGURE 2.7 ◆ The emergency vehicle driver needs to be in the proper position with the appropriate safety equipment including seat belts and headsets.

and acute situational factors recognized as increasing the risk of drowsy driving and related crashes include the following.

- *Sleep loss*
- *Driving patterns,* including driving between midnight and 6 A.M.; driving a substantial number of miles each year and/or a substantial number of hours each day; driving in the midafternoon hours (especially for older persons); and driving for longer times without taking a break
- *Use of sedating medications,* especially prescribed anxiolytic hypnotics, tricyclic antidepressants, and some antihistamines
- *Untreated or unrecognized sleep disorders,* especially sleep apnea syndrome (SAS) and narcolepsy

These factors have cumulative effects; a combination of them substantially increases crash risk.

Shift Workers: Night shift workers typically get 1.5 fewer hours of sleep per 24 hours as compared with day workers. The midnight to 8 A.M. shift carries the greatest risk of sleep disruption because it requires workers to contradict circadian patterns in order to sleep during the day.

A study of hospital nurses reached conclusions based on real-world experiences. Rotating shifts (working four or more day or evening shifts and four night shifts or more within a month) caused the most severe sleep disruptions of any work schedule. Nurses on rotating schedules reported more "accidents" (including auto crashes, on-the-job errors, and on-the-job personal injuries due to sleepiness) and more near-miss crashes than did nurses on other schedules (National Sleep Foundation [NSF], 2000). About 95 percent of night nurses working 12-hour shifts reported having had an automobile accident or near-miss accident while driving home from night work (NSF, 2000).

Hospital interns and residents routinely lose sleep during on-call periods, which may last 24 hours or more. A survey of house staff at a large urban medical school found that respondents averaged 3 hours of sleep during 33-hour on-call shifts, much of which was fragmented by frequent interruptions (NSF, 2000). About 25 percent reported that they had been involved in a motor vehicle crash, 40 percent of which occurred while driving home from work after an on-call night. Others reported frequently falling asleep at the wheel without crashing, for example, while stopped at a traffic light.

Although this evidence does not demonstrate a conclusive association between shift work and crashes, it is believed that shift workers' increased risks for sleepiness are likely to translate into an increased risk for automobile crashes. Competing demands from family, second jobs, and recreation often further restrict the hours available for sleep and further disrupt the sleep schedule.

Employee Behavioral Steps: Shift workers themselves can take steps to reduce their risks of drowsy driving by planning time and creating an environment for uninterrupted, restorative sleep (good sleep hygiene) (NSF, 2000). Shift workers who completed a four-month physical training program reported sleeping longer and feeling less fatigue than did matched controls who did not participate in the program. However, individual response to the stresses of shift work varies (NSF, 2000), and the background factors or coping strategies that enable some workers to adapt successfully to this situation are not well defined.

Nurses working the night shift reported using white noise, telephone answering machines, and light-darkening shades to improve the quality and quantity of daytime sleep (NSF, 2000).

Educate Shift Workers About the Risks of Drowsy Driving and How to Reduce Them: Although many shift workers are not in a position to change or affect their fundamental work situation, they and their families may benefit from information on their risks for drowsy driving and effective countermeasures. Here are eight ways to maximize the chances of achieving quality sleep during the day.

1. Minimize light or wear a sleep mask.
2. Use "white noise" such as a fan to block out disruptive noises, turn off the phone, and turn the answering machine volume all the way down.
3. Lower room temperature.
4. Create an association with sleep by maintaining bedtime routines and using the bedroom for sleep only.
5. Post a "day sleeper" sign on the door.
6. Exercise moderately every day (but not within three hours of sleep).
7. Do not drink caffeine within five hours of bedtime.
8. Get the support of family and friends.

The following is a simple truth, according to the National Sleep Foundation (NSF, 2000): The average adult requires seven to nine hours of good-quality sleep per night. A few people can sleep less, sometimes as little as five hours per night, without a problem. Whatever your actual sleep needs are, regularly overextending yourself isn't wise. It'll catch up with you eventually. Acute and chronic illness, chronic pain, irritability, poor judgment, and diminished decision-making abilities are evidence of a sleep-deprived lifestyle. These are not ingredients for a healthful, enjoyable life (or consistently compassionate prehospital care). It may even be postulated that our collectively sleep-deprived population can count this phenomenon as an underlying reason for many of society's ills.

Clearly, this topic holds important consequences for both the emergency care world and the people we serve. For example, a very frightening and all too evident problem related to sleep deprivation is what the NSF (2000) calls "drowsy driving." A 1999 National Sleep Foundation poll found 62 percent of drivers admitted driving a vehicle while feeling drowsy in the past year. The U.S. National Highway Traffic Safety Administration (2004) estimates that 100,000 crashes per year involve drowsiness or fatigue as principal causes. NHTSA estimates conservatively that drowsy driving may cause 4 percent of all traffic crash fatalities. Emergency providers could possibly help prevent some of these fatal incidents by teaching people—especially themselves—not to drive drowsy. Here's a sampling of what you need to know:

- Drowsy drivers are susceptible to a phenomenon called "miscrosleep," which is a brief episode of unintentional sleep experienced by those who are so tired that they cannot resist. Microsleep may last from a split second to 20 or 30 seconds—certainly long enough to cause harm or death when driving, especially at high speed.
- Know the high-risk groups: shift workers (e.g., us!), commercial drivers, youths, people with undiagnosed sleep disorders, and business travelers.
- Sleepy times of day, according to research: 0000–0600 and 1300–1600 hours.
- Research shows that opening windows, playing loud radios or CD players, chewing gum, and other "tricks" fail to keep sleepy drivers alert.
- Caffeine works (1) only on people who don't drink it constantly and (2) not until about 30 minutes after ingestion.
- The only *safe* short-term solution to driving drowsy is to pull over and take a nap (being careful to stop in a safe location).
- The only long-term solution to driving drowsy is prevention (such as a good night's sleep ahead of a drive).

People who are tired and trying to drive are a hazard to both self and others. One study funded by the American Automobile Association Foundation for Traffic Safety took an in-depth look at the driving habits of 1,400 people (FEMA, 2004). It found that "drivers that sleep six hours or less are far more likely to be involved in sleep and fatigue crashes. Also at higher risk are people who have been awake for 20 hours or longer, individuals who work more than one job, and those who work night shifts." Sounds like a typical emergency provider!

Points to Ponder

Seriously, however, what about the reality of a volunteer who is called out after a long day at the paying job? Or the dreadful "mandatory overtime" so common in many emergency agencies? Or 24- and 48-hour shifts in communities where you can't bank on sleeping any longer because of rising call volume? The world of emergency care notoriously ignores wellness practices among the very people who have signed on to help others.

Some ideas:

- Make getting enough rest a priority. Altering a lifestyle is a personal choice. Exercise it.
- Do whatever it takes to wring a few more hours out of each day for sleeping. Turn off the TV. Go to bed when the kids do.
- Say "no" to overtime.
- Don't drink caffeine as a habit so that it'll work for you on occasions when you really have to have something to assist you in staying awake.
- Work with the agency to eliminate destructive practices such as mandatory overtime and lousy shift structures.

Source: Syd Canan, "Sleep Deprivation and Shift Work," MERGINET. News, February 2000. *www. merginet.com.*

Health. Maintenance of consistently good health is vital for all emergency vehicle drivers. Sufficient rest and nutrition, physical fitness, and freedom from controlled substances are essential requirements for emergency vehicle drivers.

Personal Problems. A driver's personal problems can significantly affect the capabilities of an individual to function as an effective emergency vehicle driver. Problems can range from family conflicts and financial difficulties to employment problems.

To be free of any physical impairments that might inhibit the ability to drive an emergency vehicle,

> **Has the individual returned too soon from a disability or injury? Has the individual's physical fitness declined to the extent that his or her capability to recognize and react to situations is impaired?**

Age. This is the physical and mental condition of the individual as reflected by chronological age:

> **Age needs to be combined with physical fitness when evaluating an individual as a potential driver of a emergency vehicle.**

Some thoughts when considering a person's age as a factor for a potential emergency vehicle driver follow.

- At age 18 an individual usually has only a maximum of two years of driving experience.
- At age 65 or older an individual may have begun to lose certain aspects of vision or hearing.
- At age 65 or older an individual may have increasing physical limitations.

Habits. A habit is a characteristic produced by constant repetition of an action:

> **An adult has developed driving habits that can influence an individual's potential to operate an emergency vehicle safely and properly. If poor habits exist, they must be identified and corrected by constant repetition of the proper actions until the latter also become habit.**

Any of these human aspects may cause concern. It is, however, important to perform an overall evaluation of these aspects on a continuing basis. Close scrutiny of an organization's emergency vehicle drivers is a necessity. Major changes in one or more of the human aspects can occur at any time. Negative changes are usually triggered by a significant emotional event. The degree of impact and the length of time that a negative influence can persist are unique to each individual.

◆ ACQUIRED ABILITIES

DRIVING CHARACTERISTICS

The manipulative skills necessary to coordinate the steering, accelerating, and/or braking functions of maneuvering an emergency vehicle include:

> **How individuals coordinate and handle a vehicle is based on a number of driving characteristics, which they have acquired from the time they began to drive. These characteristics, good or bad, will be reflected when driving an emergency vehicle (see Figure 2.8). Characteristics that are desirable need to be reinforced, whereas a concentrated effort is needed to eliminate the bad characteristics.**

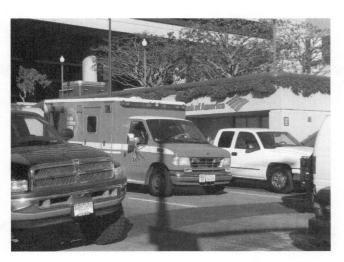

FIGURE 2.8 ◆ Emergency vehicle drivers need to be able to maneuver their vehicles safely through traffic and various adverse conditions.

MOTIVATION

A major consideration in the concept of defensive driver training is the establishment of a motivational need, including both physical and mental motivation.

Motivation provides some insight into those items that shape our actions and behavior. It appears that motivation can result from either a physical or a mental impetus, or both. Studies have also identified that motivation either can be affected by internal forces (i.e., the individual creates the impetus to undertake certain acts) or can be generated by external forces (i.e., how persons view themselves within their sphere of influence).

Everyone has a physical probability or susceptibility to experiencing a vehicle accident. If it hasn't happened, the probability exists. Just as recognizing the probability of experiencing an accident is important to an emergency driver, an understanding that individuals are, or will become, subject to behavioral traits or conditions is crucial. Recognition of this condition, which causes us to act in certain ways, is the first step to understanding mental motivation.

The concept referred to as a "psychological set" or mental rut whereby suggestion drives the brain's response is an illustration of the mental aspect of motivation. It is just as easy to get into a mental rut while driving. Because almost everyone drives on a daily basis, it becomes habit or second nature, hence, the opportunity to fall into a psychological set or mental rut (see Figure 2.9).

An individual's motive, whether driven by physical or mental considerations, results in traits being acquired over the years. These traits are the result of routine, comfort, and confidence.

Routine: "We've always done it this way," or "There was never any SOP. The way I was doing it was never questioned or corrected, so I continued to do it that way."

Comfort: "This is the easiest manner to accomplish what has to be done in the least amount of time."

Confidence: "I know the way I'm doing it may not be the safest, but I know I can get it accomplished this way. When all else fails, I will use the best-known methods that have never failed me before."

FIGURE 2.9 ◆ A driver may go through the same intersection many times during a shift; however, the traffic and conditions will change each time. Emergency vehicle drivers cannot get themselves in a rut that every emergency and non-emergency response is ever the same.

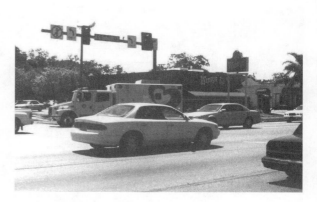

◆ DEFENSIVE DRIVING GOALS

Defensive driver training is designed to illustrate that the characteristics of routine, comfort, and confidence can be used to arrive at a safer way of doing things, especially while driving emergency vehicles. An open-minded individual with the correct attitude recognizes that there is nothing wrong with developing and implementing new methods while still retaining a sense of routine (in a safer manner), comfort (knowing one is doing something as safely as possible), and confidence (in the new methods, because they work).

What are the goals of each emergency vehicle driver? They should include the following.

1. To maintain the highest level of safety possible. Each driver is responsible for the safety of the citizens served. A driver is also fully dedicated to the safety of his or her fellow providers.
2. To be prepared for unexpected situations and conditions, which can adversely affect emergency vehicle operations. Dynamic forces are influencing emergency vehicle drivers. These include adverse weather, terrain, road conditions, and mechanical malfunction (Figure 2.10). Emergency vehicle drivers attempt, through learned responses, to limit the possible outcomes by controlling their reactions to these outside forces.

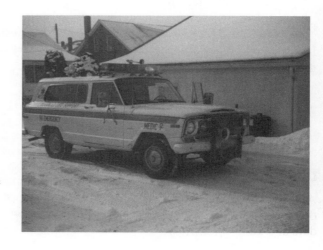

FIGURE 2.10 ◆ Adverse weather can have an effect on the driver's response and ability to maneuver the vehicle safely. Extra care and precaution need to be taken at all times.

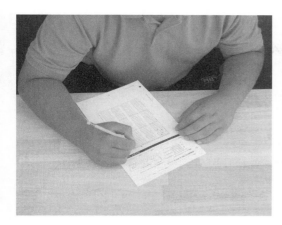

FIGURE 2.11 ◆ An emergency vehicle driver needs to demonstrate his or her competence not only behind the wheel but also by taking and passing a written exam. (*Courtesy of Prentice Hall School Division*)

3. Avoid, thorough effective training and applied practice, unnecessary legal consequences occurring as a result of emergency vehicle operations. The legal consequences of an accident may extend to individual members of the department/company, the organization, and any associated governmental unit. Consequently, legal outcomes can socially and economically ruin emergency service members as well as discredit the organization and the profession. A typical government reaction to an adverse legal outcome is to create restrictive rules and regulations affecting the type of activity involved.

Motivating, both physically and mentally, emergency drivers to adopt revised and/or new habits is a way of extending their routine, comfort zone, and confidence level. One positive approach to this motivation is to learn and apply the principles of defensive driving when operating an emergency vehicle.

DRIVING KNOWLEDGE AND PERFORMANCE

The driver should also pass a driver course written test and driving test (Figure 2.11). That should be followed by a period of on-the-job training to evaluate the driver's performance under actual job conditions. Following successful completion of the written test, the driving test, the on-the-job evaluation, and any local requirements, the supervisor should consider the driver a qualified emergency vehicle driver.

OPERATOR QUALIFICATIONS

In addition to the initial driving and medical checks drivers may have taken to qualify as an emergency vehicle driver, they should maintain the following qualifications:

- ◆ Keep their license up-to-date and valid.
- ◆ Report any violation received when driving their personal vehicle.
- ◆ Remain physically and mentally fit.
- ◆ Participate in training when available.

LICENSING

An emergency vehicle driver with an expired state driver license is of no use to the organization. Drivers need to remember to renew their license before the expiration date and keep abreast of changes in licensing requirements.

PARTICIPATION IN TRAINING

After drivers have been selected to be emergency vehicle drivers, their most important task is to improve their job performance at every opportunity. Training programs are a part of that experience. Often this is the beginning of several years of training.

DRIVER TRAINING COURSES

Driver training is an important element of selecting the right people to drive an emergency vehicle. Chapter 3 of the National Fire Protection Association's NFPA 1451 cites that a driver shall be provided with driver training and education appropriate to the driver's duties. The driver training program is not a once and done process. NFPA 1451 further delineates that driver training shall be provided for all members as often as needed, but no less than twice a year. There are a number of model driver training programs. Several fire apparatus driver training programs are discussed next.

◆ **VFIS COMPREHENSIVE DRIVER EDUCATION TRAINING PROGRAM RECOMMENDATIONS**

VFIS recommends that a formalized written statement be adopted requiring all drivers to complete a driver education and training program successfully. The program should have written objectives to address specifically the critical areas of operation for an emergency vehicle *driver*.

Organizations should reference the current applicable standards for vehicle operation (NFPA Standards, AAA Best Practices, and ASTM Standards).

The program should require all emergency vehicle drivers to meet the following minimum education and training qualifications:

1. Sixteen (16) hour driver education and training program.
   a. Eight (8) hours of classroom education. This session should cover topics that include but are not be limited to
      * Importance of driver training
      * Extent of the problem
      * Personnel selection
      * SOPs/SOGs
      * Map reading
      * Vehicle positioning
      * Legal aspects of emergency vehicle driving
      * Vehicle dynamics
      * Vehicle inspections and maintenance
      * Vehicle operations/safety
      * Written test
   b. Successful completion of a competency course (Figure 2.12). Each driver should spend sufficient time on the competency course to demonstrate proficiency in the operation of a vehicle (Figure 2.13). Drivers should demonstrate competency on each vehicle they operate. Specific tasks that should be measured are
      * Use of mirrors
      * Turning
      * Blind right side and rear positioning
      * Backing

COMPETENCY COURSE

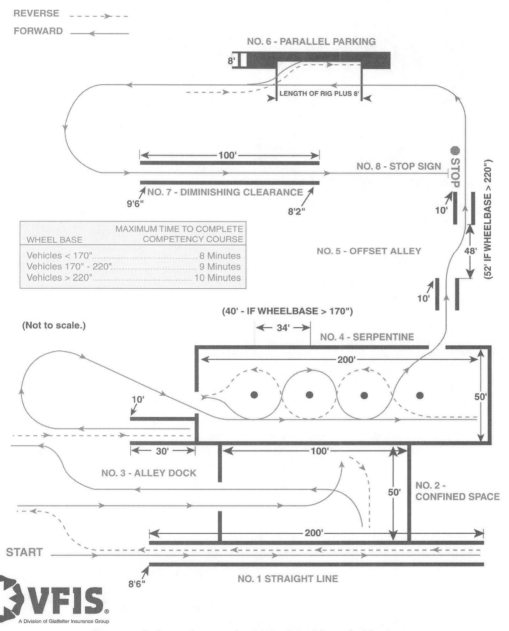

REVERSE ----→---

FORWARD ———————→

NO. 6 - PARALLEL PARKING

8'

LENGTH OF RIG PLUS 8'

100'

NO. 8 - STOP SIGN

STOP

(52' IF WHEELBASE > 220")

NO. 7 - DIMINISHING CLEARANCE

9'6"

8'2"

10'

48'

WHEEL BASE	MAXIMUM TIME TO COMPLETE COMPETENCY COURSE
Vehicles < 170"..................................	8 Minutes
Vehicles 170" - 220"..........................	9 Minutes
Vehicles > 220"..................................	10 Minutes

NO. 5 - OFFSET ALLEY

10'

(Not to scale.)

(40' - IF WHEELBASE > 170")

34'

NO. 4 - SERPENTINE

200'

10'

50'

30'

100'

NO. 3 - ALLEY DOCK

50'

NO. 2 - CONFINED SPACE

200'

START

NO. 1 STRAIGHT LINE

8'6"

VFIS.
A Division of Glatfelter Insurance Group

For more information, see instructor's guide and videotape.

© 1978, VFIS. C10:011 (Rev. 11/97)

FIGURE 2.12 ◆ This is a typical layout for the emergency vehicle driving course. (*Courtesy of VFIS*)

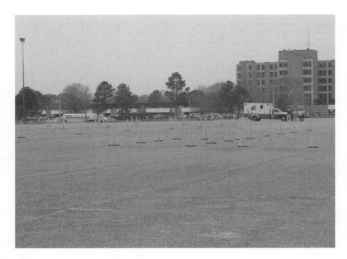

FIGURE 2.13 ◆ The competency course is an essential part of the driver training program.

- Braking and stopping
- Depth perception (front and rear)
- Height clearance
- Proper communication

2. Sufficient hands-on training (actual road driving) to demonstrate effectively the handling capabilities of emergency vehicles necessary to perform duties (Figure 2.14). Additionally, organizations providing EMS transport should conduct training with an onboard patient (simulated or actual). Eight (8) hours minimum.

3. The emergency service organization driver education and training program and procedures should be based on current recognized safety standards and departmental guidelines as well as manufacturer's suggested procedures. Additionally, the utilization of maps and practical testing with maps should be utilized.

4. Experienced drivers should minimally receive annual (actual driving) retraining and education based on their actual hands-on emergency vehicle driving activity. The type and

FIGURE 2.14 ◆ After successful completion of the competency course, drivers should then be taken on a preset route of various streets and target areas in their first response area. (*Courtesy of Ken Kerr*)

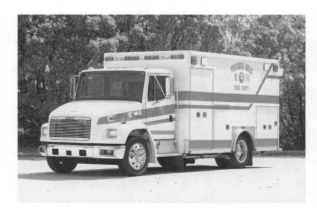

length of education and training is to be determined by the chief operating officer. Factors to review include

- Driving record
- Personnel file regarding driving-related issues
- Number of emergency calls driven
- Length of service as a driver
- Environment driven in (rural, suburban, urban)

5. Ongoing classroom education should occur at least annually and specifically address relevant safety issues (e.g., intersections, rollovers, and private vehicle use), review department SOPs/SOGs, new equipment/technology (minimum four [4] hours).

   The VFIS Emergency Vehicle Driver Education and Training program (EVDT), the Emergency Vehicle Response Safety program (EVRS), and the Dynamics of Emergency Vehicle Operations program (DEVO) can assist in complying with the above recommendations.

6. There should also be a periodic review of the hands-on skills of each driver. The frequency can vary dependent on a number of factors, which include

- Motor vehicle record checks
- Number of emergency calls driven
- Length of service as a driver
- Environment driven in (rural, suburban, urban)
- Age
- Personal auto liability coverage verification

7. Driver education and training should also be required for those individuals who are not emergency vehicle drivers (i.e., fire apparatus or ambulance drivers, etc.) but are authorized by the department or state to use red/blue lights on personal vehicles.

CALIFORNIA DEPARTMENT OF FORESTRY AND FIRE PROTECTION

The California Department of Forestry and Fire Protection (CDFFP) Academy's Basic Fire Engine Operator (BFEO) driver training program began in the 1980s as more emphasis was placed on emergency response. The BFEO driver program was replaced in 2000 with the current driving course. This change occurred as a result of several serious, avoidable apparatus crashes. Although there were no fatalities, there were some serious injuries. In all cases, the incidents were found to be driver error. Near misses also played a part in the development of the driving program. CDFFP investigators found that approximately 90 percent of vehicle crashes occurred at intersections. The current program was customized for CDFFP's needs using components of the Peace Officer Standard Training (POST) and other successful driving programs.

Full-time CDFFP drivers attend ten weeks of training at the academy. This consists of

- Orientation, one week;
- Structures and rescue, three weeks;
- Driver operations (includes pump operations), three weeks; and
- Wildland (includes apparatus placement on the line), three weeks. CDFFP also uses a large number of seasonal workers during the six-month fire season. If seasonal workers show above-average performance, the department may bring them in to complete just the driver operations module, which leads to classification as a Limited Term Engineer and allows the seasonal workers to drive the apparatus.

FIGURE 2.15 ◆ CDFFP driver operations course breakdown.

Orientation	
Orientation	3
Written Examinations	5
Performance Exams	8
Cleanup	12
Total	28
Physical Fitness	
Physical Training Sessions	8
Total	8
Pump Operations	
Pump Theory	6
Hydraulics	2
Pump Skills	17
Total	25
Vehicle Operations	
Basic Driving and Air Brakes	6
Preventative Maintenance	13
Emergency Vehicle Operations	14
Checkout Drives	8
Cross Country Driving (Field Exercise)	8
Off-Road Vehicle Operations	10
Total	59
Emergency/Fireground Operations	
Introduction to I-Zone	4
Multi-Co Drills	8
Total	12
Total	**132**

The average driver operations course consists of 30 participants with an instructor-to-student ratio of 1:4 to 6. This course is conducted entirely by the three staff instructors and two mechanics. The driver operations course consists of 132 hours, broken down as shown in Figure 2.15.

In addition to the driver operations course, the CDFFP Academy teaches the Heavy Fire Equipment Operator (HFEO) course. This six-week course covers the operation of dozers, truck/trailers, and so on. It includes the same EVOC component as the driver operations course and is taught by both staff and outside heavy equipment subject matter experts.

Drivers felt the operations course was more intense than the previous BFEO program, placed more emphasis on theory, and had more active instructor involvement. They agreed that including more theory and discussion of vehicle dynamics improved their knowledge of apparatus operation and decision-making ability by helping them learn to anticipate instead of just react. They cited the dogleg course as one example and commended the addition of the Interface Zone (I-Zone) training. An I-Zone Exercise Evaluation can be found in Figure 2.16.

Student Requirements. The driver operations course is open to driver trainees only. Driver trainees must be at least 18 years old and hold a Class B license. Because most trainees spend 6 to 7 years as firefighters first, the mean age of CDFFP drivers is the midtwenties.

I-ZONE EXERCISE EVALUATION

STUDENT _____   ENGINE NO _____

SCENARIO NO. _____ DATE _____   TIME _____

CREW OPERATIONS		POINTS	POINTS
1	Provides safety briefing to crew	2	___
2	Gives clear instructions/assignments to crew	2	___
3	Retreat signal identified with crew	2	___
4	Hoselines deployed appropriately for scenario	2	___

ENGINE OPERATIONS			
1	Doors and windows are closed	2	___
2	Code 3 and driving lights are on	2	___
3	Engine is backed in	2	___
4	Engine does not block access to other vehicles	2	___
5	Engine protection line in place and charged	2	___
6	Garden hose placed in tank	2	___
7	Ladder and roof protection lines placed in service	2	___
8	Not parked next to wood pile or debris	2	___
9	Engine positioned so propane tank not a factor	2	___
10	Not parked under powerline	2	___

STRUCTURE			
1	Windows and doors closed	2	___
2	Propane tank shut off	2	___
3	Hazardous vegetation identified and discussed	2	___
4	Hazardous wood pile or debris identified and discussed	2	___
5	Out buildings are determined and contents indentified	2	___

PUBLIC CONSIDERATIONS			
1	Number of occupants or residents are determined and contact made. Animals are identified and planned for	2	___
	TOTAL	40	___

PROCTOR _____

[Please use back for comments if necessary] Comments on back ☐

00012801.evl.doc
February 26, 2003   Page 1

FIGURE 2.16 ◆ I-Zone Exercise Evaluation.

The training chief identified a change in member demographics from an agricultural background with experience in driving tractors and bigger equipment to a college background. This shift, along with the fact that many of the trainees do not obtain the Class B license until a month or so before the class starts, contributes to a growing pool of students having little to no experience with bigger equipment.

Instructor Qualifications. All academy instructors must be California Instructor 1A and 1B trained. The instructor training program is based on the International Fire Service Training Association (IFSTA), Fire and Emergency Services Instructor manual, which in turn is based on NFPA 1041, *Standard for Fire Service Instructor Professional Qualifications.* Each component is 40 hours. California Instructor 1A covers manipulative lesson plans; 1B covers technical lesson plans. This training is offered by the state fire marshal's office. All academy instructors are also DL170 agents of the Department of Motor Vehicles (DMV) Employer Licensing Unit. The DMV audits the DL170 records for CDFFP. The testing course must be mapped out and approved by the DMV annually.

There is no standard driver training on the unit level, and these requirements do not apply to the unit driving instructors. Some units do yearly EVOC driving days, but others do not. Most of the unit training officers have received instructor training, but state certification is not required.

Recertification/Remedial Training. CDFFP currently has no requirement for recertification or repeating any portion of the driver operations course. The drivers interviewed believed that the course should be used to recertify, if it included more advanced scenarios. Although remedial training is normally handled at the unit level, unit officers can send drivers back for remedial training if they believe the drivers' skills indicate this intervention.

SACRAMENTO REGIONAL TRAINING FACILITY

In 1993, Sacramento City Fire implemented Advanced Life Support (ALS). Paramedics were recruited and trained at the fire academy, but the training did not include emergency driving. The accident frequency rate was 90 at-fault ambulance motor vehicle crashes per 1 million miles the first year of the ALS program (FEMA, 2004). This resulted in a significant increase in third-party insurance costs, in particular on the medic units.

In 1994, the Risk Management, Loss Control Safety Unit coordinated an interdepartmental EVOC between police and fire to train and certify fire EVOC instructors. After EVOC became mandatory for completion of the fire academy in 1995, a 39 percent reduction in ambulance at-fault crashes occurred.

The Sacramento Regional Training Facility provides driver training for all levels of personnel such as recruits, firefighters, drivers, captains, support staff, and law enforcement officers. The facility has an instructor-to-student ratio of 1:2. The facility develops training programs by evaluating multiple programs and customizing courses to meet the needs of the Joint Powers partners. For example, the fire instructors built a customized off-road course by adding components to the existing CDFFP and Forest Service courses.

The primary course consists of 8 hours of classroom instruction for defensive driving, 16 hours of actual course driving, and 4 hours in the simulator. The driving portion concentrates on vehicle placement and the physics of dynamics.

Fire personnel train only during daytime hours, whereas police train during both day and nighttime hours. Recruits spend approximately 90 percent of their 40-hour program behind the wheel. Vehicles used for training include police sedans, SUVs, engines, ambulances, a bus, off-road equipment, and trailer trucks. Personnel drive both their assigned apparatus and training apparatus.

Instructor Qualifications. All instructors are Fire Course Instructors IA and IB and POST certified and have completed the 40-hour National Safety Council course and an 8-hour class on law and liability issues (Figure 2.17). Although the goal is 100 percent, currently 75 percent of the instructors are certified to conduct DMV training and administer DMV examinations according to California law DL170. All instructors are cross-trained, which allows fire instructors to train police personnel and vice versa (FEMA, 2004).

RECERTIFICATION/REMEDIAL TRAINING

Fire personnel repeat the entire primary training course each year as a mandatory recertification. In addition, the Accident Review Committee can refer anyone found responsible in an at-fault incident to remedial training. Supervisors can also request remedial training for personnel. Remedial training is not a punitive action. It is used to reinforce training and is done in a positive manner.

VENTURA COUNTY (CALIFORNIA) FIRE DEPARTMENT

Ventura County Fire Training conducts seven driving courses:

- ◆ Class A Driver Training;
- ◆ Paramedic Squad Driver Training;

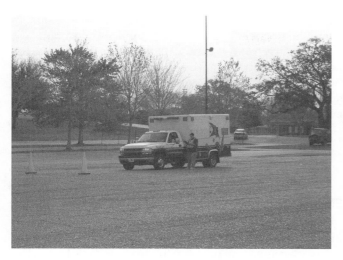

FIGURE 2.17 ◆ EVOC instructors should be cross-trained to be able to evaluate emergency vehicle operators that drive various vehicles.

- Class B Driver Training;
- Off-Road Driver Training;
- Class C Driver Training;
- Driving Simulator; and
- Tillered Truck Driver Training.

Instructor Qualifications. In addition to the instructor qualifications listed for each course, all instructors are California Fire Instructor IA and IB trained, POST certified, and certified to conduct DMV training and administer DMV examinations under the DL170 program. They have completed the Los Angeles County police simulator training and received safety officer training (FEMA, 2004).

Driving Simulator. Both Sacramento Regional Training Facility and Ventura County Fire Department have driving simulators. At the time of the site visit, Sacramento had been using the simulator for four years. Ventura County had had the simulator for two years, but the first year was fraught with technical problems, so it had been used for only one year.

The Sacramento Regional Training Facility uses the driving simulator strictly to improve drivers' decision-making processes. A simulator cannot teach the basic driving skills acquired in training exercises using actual emergency vehicles. Time has shown that errors in decision making are primarily related to intersection clearing and conflict resolution (obtaining the right-of-way). The decision-making process is reinforced as personnel complete four hours in the simulator as part of the annual re-certification process. One of Ventura County's goals for the simulator program is to educate drivers in safe driving techniques. Initially, the emphasis was on emergency driving and backing scenarios. In March 2003, it began using the scripting tool to develop scenarios that address intersection analysis, conflict management, and desired apparatus placement options at an incident (FEMA, 2004). Because the simulator was new, the Training Section was working to overcome the "video game" mentality that line personnel were exhibiting and provide the rationale to gain buy-in.

Technical Aspects: Ventura County uses a three-station mobile simulator manufactured by FAAC, Inc. At the time the unit was purchased, the simulator cost approximately $500,000, plus $20,000 for the tractor. It is housed in a 42-foot fifth-wheel RV trailer so it can be moved from location to location. Ventura County also holds a service/maintenance agreement on the simulator, which costs $10,000 annually.

It believed the additional cost to make the simulator mobile (approximately $100,000) provided a cost savings compared to stationary training by eliminating the following:

- Fuel for units to travel to training;
- Wear and tear on apparatus;
- Time saving; and
- Cost of a cover assignment from another company.

The simulator contains three stations that can be configured to represent fire engines, EMS vehicles, or other types of vehicles. This feature is useful during the scenario replay to show apparatus placement in relation to curbs and so forth. The manufacturer also programmed the graphics by incorporating pictures of actual Ventura County apparatus, so that is what is seen in the overhead view.

The Sacramento facility uses a four-station fixed Advanced Mobile Operations Simulator (AMOS) manufactured by Doron that cost approximately $750,000 at the time of purchase. This particular simulator has three flat plasma screens in each station, and each screen cost approximately $5,000. Just as the mobile simulator at Ventura County, the stationary simulator allows linking of multiple stations for interactive scenarios, programming vehicle physical responses, sounds, radio communication with other simulator "vehicles," and altering weather and day or nighttime driving through the instructor console. The stations are also equipped to interchange vehicle cab models (e.g., sedan, engine, truck, etc.). However, because vehicle dynamics are the same for a vehicle whether small or large, and only the end result differs, the only cab model used is the three-screen simulator station with sedan cab.

Training Sessions: A relatively common side effect of "driving" the simulator is simulator adaptation syndrome (SAS). SAS creates motion sickness symptoms. Ventura County experienced an incidence of 5 to 7 percent of members unable to complete the simulator exercises due to SAS. Sacramento Regional Training Facility experienced an incidence of approximately 40 percent of participants developing some motion sickness symptoms. There are a variety of methods used to reduce the incidence of SAS, with varying degrees of success. Ventura County requires all members to wear special wristbands while driving the simulator. Sacramento uses both the special wristbands and special glasses. Limiting the time the member is actually in the simulator is the most effective way to control SAS.

Each simulator session lasts 3 to 4 hours and involves a total of 20 to 30 minutes of actual simulator driving time. The session begins with an orientation process to learn to "drive" the simulator (acclimate to the cab model and graphics). The acclimation portion puts the driver through four different scenarios (Figure 2.18), each lasting approximately 2 minutes. The driver is removed from the simulator for 5 to 6 minutes following each completed scenario.

The remaining scenarios used at the Sacramento facility reflect situations requiring rapid decision making. The facility has a bank of approximately 400 usable scenarios. Most classes use 18 to 25 scenarios that focus on the most common situations with high-risk potential. These situations are usually intersection clearing and conflict resolution.

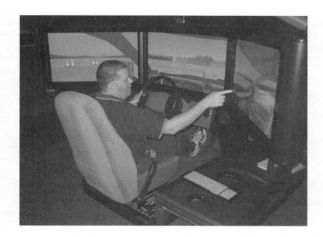

FIGURE 2.18 ◆ An instructor can use a driving simulator to illustrate certain scenarios.

If the driver makes an incorrect decision, the feedback on the screen is immediate. Both the Sacramento and the Ventura County simulators allow the instructor to play back a driver's performance through the entire scenario for review and teaching purposes.

Currently, the simulator is not used as part of a recertification program or for any type of remedial training by Ventura County. Training's short-term goal is to send all personnel through a three-hour simulator session biannually to reinforce good driving judgment. A long-term goal is to implement a nonpunitive annual driver recertification program.

The simulator is part of the driver training offered as a remedial tool through the Sacramento Regional Training Facility. The simulator's software scripting tool allows the instructor to script the scenario of the driver's actual crash. The majority of the time drivers will repeat the same actions they took in the actual crash. The instructor then reviews the "drive," discusses the appropriate response(s), and repeats simulations with new scenarios that have the same elements as the original crash.

Effects of the Training. The Sacramento Regional Training Facility was the only agency with data related to training effectiveness. From 1999 to 2003, there was a 77-percent decrease in fire department at-fault accidents. The average net savings to the city and county, after deducting the cost of operating the facility, was $2.50 to $4.00 million per year in litigation alone. This does not include savings related to such items as decreased vehicle maintenance, repair costs, workers' compensation, and downtime. In addition to hard data, the instructors receive a great deal of positive feedback from personnel, claiming the training makes them better and safer drivers both on and off duty.

Driver Requirements. All potential Ventura County Fire Department drivers must complete a task book before being eligible to take the driver's examination. The purpose of this practice is to ensure that potential drivers are familiar with all of the different models of apparatus that they may encounter and the driving course specifications. The tasks outlined in the task book are minimum requirements and are intended to provide a foundation for future learning. This practice encourages motivation and self-direction in members. They must travel to stations that house the apparatus on their own time and make arrangements with the station driver to supervise their task completion. The sections contained in the task book follow:

◆ Apparatus operator;
◆ Aerial apparatus tasks;

- Type III wildland engine tasks;
- Light and air tasks;
- Water tender/tanker tasks;
- Pumping evolution tasks;
- Specialized apparatus tasks;
- Tillered aerial apparatus tasks; and
- Aircraft crash vehicle tasks.

The completed book is submitted to the Training Section, where it is reviewed and recorded in the training database. The original book is placed in the individual's training file.

The "company" usually specifies these acquired abilities as the minimum acceptable criteria. These criteria must be either learned or demonstrated to the emergency company prior to a candidate's being sanctioned as a driver of an emergency vehicle.

The acquired abilities are typically regulatory in nature and philosophy and include the following:

Driver's License: Both knowledge and ability are prerequisites to obtaining a license. A license grants the privilege to operate a vehicle on public highways. In recent years, a number of states have added one or more criteria for obtaining the privilege of driving heavy vehicles classified as commercial with laws and statutes pertinent to emergency driving.

State and Local Laws: These laws establish the requirements for operating vehicles on public highways. A driver's license violation of one of these provisions can result in the loss of driving privileges.

Defensive Driving Techniques: An acquired ability, these techniques must be learned over time and constantly reinforced to ensure continued applicability. They include successfully completing a program that introduces and reinforces concepts such as

- Space management
- Following distance and rate of closure
- Hazard identification
- Correct braking techniques
- Evasive maneuvers

◆ VEHICLE CHARACTERISTICS

Driving any type of emergency vehicle may be a radical change for some people. It is even more complicated if the type of vehicle is drastically different from a familiar experience. For instance, an individual who has never driven a vehicle weighing over 3,500 pounds will have more to learn than just emergency vehicle driving procedures when placed in an emergency vehicle (Figure 2.19).

The ability to control and maneuver fire apparatus safely is one of the most critical aspects of an operator's responsibilities. While driving, the operator should be in control of the vehicle and take into consideration the vehicle characteristics, capabilities, and limitations (e.g., speed, road conditions, auxiliary braking systems, and weight

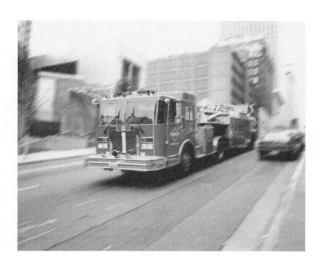

FIGURE 2.19 ◆ This photo is a good illustration of the difference in size between a fire engine and a typical passenger vehicle. (*Courtesy of Image-State/International Stock Photography Ltd.*)

transfer). Operating and controlling the vehicle at a speed from which the vehicle could be safely slowed or stopped could decrease the potential for a skid and loss of control. Based on simple physics and inertia, a top-heavy vehicle such as a tanker is inclined to tip over if the driver suddenly turns the wheel in an effort to bring the wheels back onto the road.

Some Things to Consider. The type of emergency vehicle can have a significant influence on the amount of training necessary to instill proficiency. A new emergency vehicle driver would require more time and training than a driver moving from one type of vehicle to another. It is essential that a driver receive individual training and be proficient in driving a specific emergency vehicle (Figure 2.20).

VEHICLE COMPONENTS AND FEATURES

The introductions of new technologies require a special understanding of the various vehicle components and features even for emergency vehicle drivers with years of service.

The introduction of antilock braking systems (ABS) represents a major technological advance in emergency vehicle operations. Their application to emergency vehicles requires more experienced drivers to become familiar with new and/or revised driving procedures and habits.

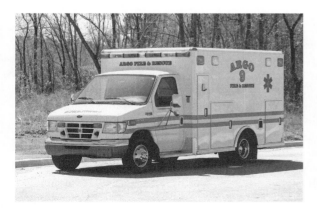

FIGURE 2.20 ◆ Emergency vehicle drivers need to learn how to drive in the vehicle they will be driving. Compare this photo to Figure 2.19, the difference between an ambulance and engine makes a difference in size and how vehicles handle. (*Courtesy of Ken Kerr*)

Certain types of vehicles require special driver training. An example would be large bus-size vehicles.

DRIVER RECERTIFICATION

Individuals may have excellent human aspects and acquired abilities at the time of selection. They may also demonstrate proficiency in all the varying components of driving emergency vehicles. But if these skills are not applied at regular intervals, competency decreases. Hence, the need for continual recertification is essential.

Driver recertification should be closely correlated to the characteristics of the organization. For example, if a driver is regularly driving an emergency vehicle under various conditions, recertification may be nothing more than a "check ride." On the other hand, if a driver has not driven a specific emergency vehicle in over 6 months or only once in 18 months, recertification may involve a complete retesting on that vehicle.

Development of a recertification program should be based on several items:

* Actual emergency vehicle driving experience
* Observed proficiency and supervisory reports compared to performance in the field
* Length of time since last recertification
* Introduction of new emergency vehicles
* Introduction of new technology on existing emergency vehicles

Although a personalized recertification program can be developed and administered, it is both difficult and time consuming to do. As a result, most emergency agencies establish one or more "thresholds" that automatically dictate recertification. Typical examples of when recertification is required include time, such as annually; amount of activity, as a driver; observed and documented competency (or lack of); and the introduction of new technology (ABS braking) or vehicles into the organization.

Driver recertification is a vital element in maintaining a valid and professional emergency vehicle driver program. Whether a personalized program or one with established thresholds is adopted, it is important that recertification of all drivers be an integral part of the program.

◆ PERSONNEL RECORDS

Not everyone can or should be an emergency vehicle driver. The selection process for an emergency vehicle driver candidate is a critical part of the emergency vehicle driver training program.

It should be recognized that age, maturity, and experience, as well as other human aspect factors identified, are all different and not necessarily related.

A record of each individual's human aspects and acquired abilities should be compiled and stored in a central location that is convenient and secure for the organization. The personnel file should contain the qualifications of each individual. The information in the file can then be used as a means to select an emergency vehicle driver, identify an individual requiring additional training, and alert the organization to one who is in need of recertification.

TRAINING RECORDS

A key component of the personnel file is the training record for each individual. Most companies not only keep track of classes attended but also have some type of evaluative system so that competency and proficiency can be monitored.

Typically the training records include the following:

- ✦ Classes attended (proficiency not verifiable)
- ✦ Classes successfully completed (proficiency at time measured via testing or simulation)
- ✦ Certification (proficiency measured and certified by the organization)
- ✦ Licensing (proficiency measured and licensed by the agency)

Each individual's personnel file, including those of drivers and vehicle technicians, becomes a legal document. It can be utilized either on behalf of the emergency company or against the company. It should be emphasized that the absence of any documentation presents the potential for a high degree of liability and, in the opinion of some legal minds, a greater liability.

The information in the personnel files of emergency workers should relate to their qualities and capabilities as emergency vehicle drivers. This information should address several issues.

Physical Capability

Is the driver physically able to perform the function of an emergency vehicle driver?

Driving Record

Does the individual have a good driving record?

This is important for several reasons. First, one's driving record is an indication of whether or not a person has demonstrated respect for motor vehicle operations and laws. Second, the action of researching a driving record serves as a protection for the person who is authorizing the candidate to be an emergency vehicle driver for the ESO.

Some control measures that should be undertaken to determine the driving record for each potential and existing emergency vehicle driver include:

- ✦ Checking motor vehicle records (MVRs) even before a person can begin training
- ✦ Checking MVRs on an ongoing basis, at least annually
- ✦ Making a photocopy of each emergency vehicle driver's operator's license and placing it in the driver's personnel file on a yearly basis

The organization needs to establish SOP/SOGs to determine whether individuals' previous offenses prevent them from driving a company emergency vehicle.

SUSPECTED DRUG AND/OR ALCOHOL ABUSE

These issues involve ESO just as they do society in general. However, they are particularly important to organizations entrusted with the care and transportation of the public. An ESO should have a substance abuse policy that includes the conditions under which an individual can be tested and disciplined if necessary.

One excellent criterion routine for testing in emergency operations is this: In the event a vehicular accident occurs, the driver is tested. The reasoning is that the existence of the accident constitutes "reasonable cause" for the company to require testing. In addition, it provides both the emergency vehicle driver and the company with a "defense" of no such substance abuse should a plaintiff allege the possibility of drug or intoxicant use by the emergency vehicle driver.

◆ **CASE STUDY RECAP**

Seeing the headline "Emergency Vehicle Operator Is Arrested for DUI" is never something a chief wants to read in the local newspaper. It is important to have a designated individual on staff to handle all media calls. A prepared statement prior to the first call is always more appropriate than trying to improvise when the first reporter calls. It is always best to identify and recognize the situation, and in most instances the best thing to do is to follow policy regarding an internal investigation into the incident. Never be judgmental or conclude immediately the person is innocent or guilty but state that you are conducting an investigation. This type of press is never good for an organization, but how you handle it will make the difference. Prepare ahead of time what to do in these situations. It is difficult to prevent personnel from doing inappropriate things off duty; however, the leadership of the organization should have appropriate standard operating guidelines in place, and personnel must be educated that what they do off duty can have a detrimental effect on the organization.

◆ **SUMMARY**

Emergency vehicle drivers are selected based on their qualifications to perform the duties required of them. A driving record check and a license check are preconditions to hiring. A medical evaluation should be required to determine physical ability to perform the job under all conditions.

The driver should pass an emergency vehicle driver course written test and driving test, and then pass the on-the-job driving evaluation. The driver is expected to be mentally and physically fit for every response. Personal appearance and hygiene have a lot to do with how well drivers perform their job. The emergency vehicle driver has an important job to do, driving an emergency vehicle, and taking a training course will offer the emergency vehicle driver the training designed for all aspects of that job. The training should be presented in the classroom, behind the wheel, and on the job. When a driver has successfully completed all three modules, met all local and state requirements, and been recommended by the supervisor, the driver should be considered a qualified emergency vehicle driver.

Review Questions

1. What is the most important aspect of emergency driving?
2. What are the major components of an emergency driving program?
3. What are the four categories of human characteristics that contribute to vehicle crashes?
4. When should motor vehicle record checks be conducted on drivers?
5. What are some of the types of unwanted attitudes for emergency vehicle drivers?
6. Describe what traffic psychology is.
7. What are some of the factors that detract from driver readiness?

8. List the eight ways to maximize sleep during the day.
9. What three traits result over the years from driving as it relates to motivation?
10. What qualifications should emergency vehicle drivers possess?
11. List the eleven components of a driver training program.
12. What eight tasks should be measured in the competency course?
13. Describe at least three areas a recertification program should be based on.
14. Describe four things a training record should include.

References

Canan, Syd. February 2000. "Sleep deprivation and shift work." MERGINET. News.

Cyan, S. 2000. *Sleep deprivation, shift work, and sweet dreams.* Retrieved October 6, 2004, from http://www.merginet.com/tgp/2000/0002/feature-sleep.shtml

Dernocoeur, Kate. 2005. "Shift workers" Retrieved October 13, 2005, from http://www.merginet.com/emsnewsfiles/174_Kate_Dernocoeur_20020704.shtml

FEMA. 2004. *Emergency Vehicle Safety Initiative FA-272.*

James, L. 2004. *Traffic psychology.* Retrieved November 12, 2005, from http://www.soc.hawaii.edu/LEONj/leonj/leonpsy/traffic/tpintro.html

Land Transport Safety Authority. November 2003. *Fatigue and driving.* Retrieved November 5, 2004, from http://www.ltsa.govt.nz/factsheets/24.html

National Sleep Foundation. Spring 2000. *Sleep matters.* Retrieved December 15, 2004, from http://www.sleepfoundation.org

NFPA. 2002. *NFPA 1451, Standard for a fire service vehicle operations training program.* Quincy, MA: National Fire Protection Association.

NHTSA Expert Panel. April 1998. *Drowsy driving and automobile crashes.* Retrieved November 5, 2004, from http://www.nhtsa.dot.gov/people/injury/drowsy_driving1/Drowsy.html

North Carolina NIOSH. 2001. "Career fire fighter dies in tanker rollover." Retrieved December 10, 2004, from http://www.cdc.gov/niosh/face200241.html

Rules, Regulations, and the Law

CHAPTER 3

Objectives

After completing this chapter, you should be able to:

- Identify types of laws that apply to emergency vehicle operations.
- Identify how specific laws apply to emergency vehicle operations.
- Identify the changing legal climate that exists and its impact on emergency vehicle drivers and their organization.
- Identify the primary legal principles that affect drivers and recognize their implications on emergency vehicle operations.
- Identify the specific state driving laws that affect the emergency and related vehicle driver.
- Identify the individual state laws, local ordinances, standards, and requirements that impact emergency vehicle driver training and operations.

Case Study

Junior Volunteer Fire Fighter Is Killed While Responding to a Brush Fire with an Intoxicated Driver—Wyoming

On May 22, 2003, a 16-year-old female junior firefighter died after the tanker truck she was riding in overturned while responding to a brush fire. The tanker truck drifted off the roadway, causing the driver to lose control of the truck and to overturn. The driver crawled out a window. The victim was ejected and trapped beneath the front passenger door. She was extricated by emergency personnel and transported to a county hospital where she was pronounced dead on arrival.

◆ INTRODUCTION

As an emergency vehicle operator, you are responsible for the safe and efficient preparation for and response to the incident and the transportation of your crew and patients. At the same time, emergency responders must look out for the safety of the public. The very nature of this profession requires emergency responders to work with others during a time of crisis. With this responsibility come certain risks. Emergency responders need to be aware that they are being held "legally accountable" for their actions at all times while performing their job.

One does not have to go far to realize the extent of the problem. In just a two-month period alone at least four EMS and fire service personnel died in emergency vehicle collisions and related vehicular incidents. Stemming from unsafe driving practices to the lack of seat belt use, these and most emergency-related vehicle incidents may have been avoided.

Too often the subject of driving is taken for granted. According to a leading insurance company, many emergency vehicle drivers feel the sole source of the emergency response problem is the general public's failure to yield properly to emergency vehicles. Emergency vehicle drivers tend to see this as the cause of motor vehicle accidents with emergency vehicles. Although the public is under a certain amount of obligation to both understand and execute compliance with motor vehicle laws, it is not realistic or practical to expect the general public to react properly every time it encounters an emergency vehicle (VFIS, 1997). Many drivers from the general public are rarely overtaken by vehicles making a light and siren response, so they have little experience in how to react. Regardless of the public responsibility to yield the right-of-way, every emergency response requires the emergency vehicle operator to assure that he or she has been granted the right-of-way prior to exercising any privileges afforded in the law.

Virtually every national organization representing the emergency services industry has addressed the operation of emergency vehicles and even nonemergency vehicles used for emergency organization and response operations. So why is it that the issue of emergency vehicle operations continues to be at the forefront of all emergency-related risk concerns?

When someone is granted rights and privileges not given to everyone, that person is expected and required to perform at a higher standard of care while exercising these privileges. This particularly applies to any emergency vehicle operation. Under state motor vehicle statutes, emergency vehicle drivers are usually granted privileges that permit them to be exempt, with qualifications, from certain laws. Some special privileges are

- Permission to proceed through a red traffic signal or stop sign
- Ability to exceed the posted speed limit
- Right to travel against the normal flow of traffic
- Park on roadways regardless of traffic flow

Training emergency vehicle drivers in their legal responsibilities is absolutely imperative. The number of lawsuits and criminal allegations surrounding emergency-related vehicle operations continues to rise.

There is a variety of local, state, and national rules, regulations, and laws that impact emergency vehicle driver training and operation. These are generally classified into five categories:

1. State motor vehicle and traffic laws
2. Nationally recognized standards
3. State and federal occupational safety and health regulations
4. Local ordinances
5. Organizational policies, procedures, and guidelines

◆ CHANGING LEGAL CLIMATE

For decades, many aspects of American society depended on the concept of public kindness—if a person or organization undertook an action on behalf of someone else in its community, it was not, in most cases, sued when something went wrong. Unfortunately, the basic concept of public kindness no longer exists.

When something goes wrong, no matter what is being attempted, the aggrieved party wants restitution and goes to the court system to obtain satisfaction. Lawsuits impacting emergency response are increasing and tend to include any and all parties involved:

- Organization as a whole
- Emergency vehicle operator
- Officer of the vehicle
- Vehicle crew members
- Chief executive of the organization
- Board of directors, commissioners

Another legal concept being challenged successfully in many areas of the country is sovereign immunity, which is reflected in the old adage of "the king can do no wrong."

In our society, the king is represented as the government and state laws that essentially exempt, from suit, most government actions under sovereign immunity statutes. As the years have passed and with the disappearance of the public kindness concept, exceptions to immunity have developed. In some states, the entire sovereign immunity principle has been voided, whereas in others, if the government entity has incurrence, immunity is, by definition, waived.

The original concept of the king can do no wrong has now been changed in many areas to mean "the king shall do no wrong." Lawsuits against emergency service organizations have increased significantly in recent years. These suits often include all parties: the emergency service organization, the emergency vehicle operator, any officer or supervisor, and the chief executive of the emergency service organization (Figure 3.1). This is not to imply that the general public has no responsibility when involved in a collision with an emergency response vehicle.

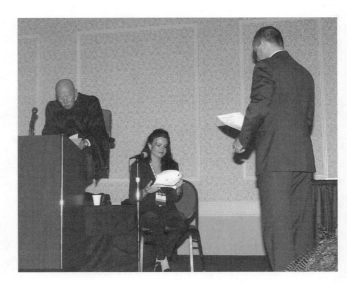

Figure 3.1 ◆ Courtroom scene with emergency vehicle driver on the stand.

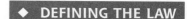

The NHTSA National Standard Curriculum for Emergency Vehicle Operators Course references some of the types of regulations covering emergency vehicle operation and how the regulations guide the decisions emergency responders make while performing their jobs.

TYPES OF REGULATIONS

Several types of regulations tell how to conduct emergency vehicle operations. These regulations are for all types of emergency vehicles.

- ◆ Constitutional laws come from the U.S. Constitution. The Constitution guarantees the rights of the individual. These laws explain patients' rights before, during, and after transport.
- ◆ Statutory laws come from legislative acts. Each state has laws or statutes that tell how to operate emergency vehicles. The laws vary from state to state. For example, each state's Motor Vehicle Code contains laws about traffic regulations. The code may dictate exceptions to these laws for operators, such as special procedures for proceeding through red traffic lights or parking in a no parking zone.
- ◆ Ordinances are enacted by a governing municipal body or its agent. These ordinances usually include city or county codes. For example, in some cities, the use of "Jake brakes" is not permitted.
- ◆ Rules and regulations that have the force of law are enacted by an agency. The rules and regulations are intended to provide more information about statutory laws, the do's and don'ts, and parameters. These are often referred to as the organizational policies, procedures, and guidelines or standard operating procedures (SOP) or standard operating guidelines (SOG). For example, an organization may have specific guidelines about when to use sirens. SOP/SOGs are discussed further in Chapter 4.

UNDERSTANDING THE REGULATIONS

There are things about emergency vehicle operation laws that every emergency responder needs to know, such as how the laws work and when they are exempt from doing what the law says to do. With so many regulations dictating how to operate emergency vehicles, emergency responders must know which law applies in a given situation. It may seem to emergency responders that there is a conflict of policy about how to do the job. Some suggested guidelines for emergency and related vehicle operators follow.

All organizational policy should incorporate the principles of state laws, local ordinances, rules, and regulations into guidelines for the emergency vehicle operator.

This means that all organizational policies and procedures should include and must not contradict federal, state, and local laws concerning the vehicle operation under all conditions. ESO policies may be formal or informal, but all policies should be in writing to provide protection from liability issues. As an emergency or related vehicle operator, you must know your organization's policies.

Let's see what some of the local policies are concerning vehicle operation. Chapter 4 discusses what makes up these policies in more detail.

Here are some local organization SOP/SOGs to consider:

- ◆ Policy on emergency vehicle driver training
- ◆ Emergency and nonemergency response protocols
- ◆ Navigating intersections

- ◆ Use of privately owned vehicles
- ◆ Speed and space management
- ◆ Seat belt use
- ◆ Parking and placement of vehicles
- ◆ What to do if involved in an collision

There are times when the emergency responder will be exempt from certain components listed in the regulations. As part of the job, emergency responders are required to make decisions concerning the operation of the vehicle. Good training provides the knowledge and ability to make appropriate decisions when faced with an emergency situation. Knowing ahead of time that what the law says does not apply in a given situation is important. Keep the following three principles in mind when approaching the idea of exemptions:

1. Emergency and related vehicle drivers are subject to all traffic regulations unless a specific exemption is made in the state or local statutes.
2. Exemptions are legal only in the emergency mode.
3. Even with an exemption, emergency and related vehicle drivers can be found criminally or civilly liable if involved in a crash.

Some examples of emergency vehicle exemptions to laws include proceeding through red lights/stop signs at controlled intersections, exceeding a posted speed limit, parking in a no parking zone, and violating traffic flow and turning procedures. These do not negate the rules of "due regard."

Point to Ponder

What is meant by *specific exemption*?

Answer: A specific exemption is a statement that appears in the statutes and specifies an exception to the rule such as "The operator of an authorized emergency vehicle may park in a no parking zone as long as the operator does not endanger life or property" (NHTSA, 1994).

◆ INTERPRETING THE LAW

Specific laws and how they are interpreted by emergency and related vehicle operators are important to overall compliance. Understanding how the emergency responder can be held legally liable and what patients' rights are during an ambulance transport are essential.

The three principles of law specifically affecting emergency vehicle drivers that apply in almost every state and instance follow.

- ◆ Emergency vehicle drivers are subject to all traffic laws unless a specific exemption is provided.
- ◆ Exemptions for emergency vehicle drivers apply only when the emergency vehicle is responding to a true emergency.
- ◆ Emergency vehicle drivers can be found criminally or civilly liable if involved in an accident, even if they are operating under the provisions of an exemption.

In addition to these principles, a number of legal terms have significant impact on emergency vehicle operations. Knowledge and understanding of these terms and concepts affecting emergency vehicle operators are very important. According to the NHTSA, the following specific terms should be understood:

- True emergency
- Due regard
- Negligence
- Gross negligence
- Willful and wanton
- Vicarious liability

TRUE EMERGENCY SITUATION

According to the **NHTSA, true emergency** is defined as a situation in which there is a high probability of death or serious injury to an individual or significant property loss.

In some situations, others—not the emergency responder—decide whether a true emergency exists. However, even in emergency situations, the emergency responder is still responsible for operating the vehicle in a prudent and safe manner.

Situations in which others determine the "nature of the emergency" include

- Emergency dispatch protocols (hot, cold) for fire and EMS
- Information from a dispatcher (e.g., While en route to an emergency, the status of the emergency may change—from emergency to nonemergency—and this information is relayed to you by the dispatcher.)
- Affiliated emergency service operator requests (e.g., Another emergency service may ask for your assistance because its service cannot handle the emergency.)
- Medical facility physician's decision

Situations in which the emergency responder must decide what is a true emergency are the exception rather than the rule. However, if faced with these situations, keep these points in mind.

Ask yourself these questions:

- Is there a high probability of death or serious injury to the patient?
- Will my actions reduce the seriousness of the incident?

Examples

- *True emergency*. Residential fire with reported persons trapped.
- *True emergency*. Dispatcher reports individual who is highly allergic to bees is stung by a bee
- *Nonemergency*. Automatic fire alarm sounding.
- *Nonemergency*. A person falls and breaks an ankle.

LAW OF DUE REGARD

All crew members and patients have the right to know that, while being entrusted in the care of the emergency responder, that responder is exercising **due regard** for their safety. If ever a crash should occur while operating an emergency vehicle, the courts will judge the actions of the emergency vehicle crew according to this principle (Figure 3.2). Essentially, due regard means that no one gets hurt, no damage is caused, and safe passage is assured. This concept applies when responding to an incident, transporting patients, and returning from the incident.

FIGURE 3.2 ◆ Judge overseeing the case.

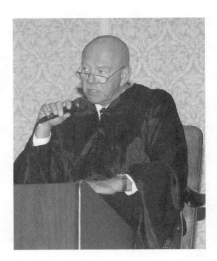

Deciding whether an emergency vehicle operator has exercised due regard for the safety of others is always based on the specific set of circumstances. Certain rules, however, should act as guidelines for all emergency responders' actions regardless of vehicle type. Always keep these points in mind when thinking about the law of due regard and the safety of others.

Ask yourself these questions:

- Am I responding like others will in the same situation?
- Am I giving enough notice of my vehicle's approach to allow other motorists and pedestrians to clear a path and protect themselves? *(Notice is given by using appropriate signaling equipment [i.e., audible and visual warning devices] in accordance with statutes. Enough is difficult to define. If motorists have the windows up; have the heater, air conditioner, or radio on; are using cell phones; or other distractions exist; it may take them a long time to acknowledge your presence and respond.)*
- Am I using the signaling equipment appropriately?
- Is it necessary to use it?
- Can motorists and pedestrians hear and see my signals?
- Am I using extreme caution?

The emergency and related vehicle operator must never travel at a speed that does not permit complete control of my vehicle.

Examples

- *No regard for safety.* When returning to the station at the end of a run, an ambulance proceeds through a red light after slowing to 10 mph. This situation indicates the operator had no regard for safety of others. No true emergency exists and the operator is violating a traffic law.
- *Due regard for safety.* While en route to an emergency, the fire engine lights are flashing, the siren is on, and the fire engine is traveling within posted speed limits. The fire engine approaches an intersection with a red light, stops, checks for other motorists and pedestrians, and proceeds through the intersection with extreme caution. In this case an emergency exists, and the correct procedures were followed to ensure the safety of others.

NEGLIGENCE

Emergency responders may also be held liable in a court of law if they were in some way careless while performing their duties as emergency vehicle operators. **Negligence** is defined as the legal deficiency or wrong that results whenever a person fails to exercise that degree of care that a prudent person would use under similar circumstances. The negligence may be viewed as slight, ordinary, or gross, to be determined by the courts.

This means that something that should have been done was not done or was done incorrectly by the emergency or related vehicle operator. As a direct result, a person was injured or killed or property was damaged. No court can replace lives, but it can attempt to compensate the injured or their families with money.

In a lawsuit involving negligence, proving operator negligence is difficult. Certain facts must be established in the case to prove that the negligence was willfully done. To avoid being caught in a negligence issue, keep the following in mind.

Ask yourself these questions:

- Do I have a "duty to act" toward the other person?
- What must I do to avoid a "breach of duty"? *(For example, you must not fail to respond.)*
- How can I avoid the other person suffering injury or loss because of my duty? *(The actual cause of the other person's injury or loss must be a direct result of breach of duty, such as a violation of a traffic regulation.)*

Case Examples

- *Example 1.* An ambulance was transporting a young girl with an injured arm to the hospital when it crashed with another vehicle. The operator of the ambulance was at fault. The crash caused an additional injury to the child. The operator could be found negligent.
- *Example 2.* An aerial truck inspection was done and the operator noted in writing that the tire had a problem. A run was called in and the operator drove the vehicle knowing the tire was bad. During the run, the operator was involved in a crash as a result of the bad tire. The operator could be found negligent.

There are varying degrees of negligence. **Gross negligence** is reckless disregard of the consequences of an act to another person. It occurs when a person's actions (or lack of action) result in the failure to exercise even a slight degree of care. **Willful and wanton** means intentional or with careless indifference (considered the most serious form of negligence). **Vicarious liability** is legal liability placed on one person for the acts committed by another person.

Usually a court judges the actions of an emergency vehicle driver based on two primary considerations:

1. Was the emergency vehicle responding to a true emergency?
2. Did the emergency vehicle driver exercise due regard for the safety of others?

If the answer to both of these questions is yes, the emergency vehicle driver has demonstrated a responsible and professional attitude through subsequent action(s).

◆ OTHER LEGAL LIABILITY ISSUES

As part of the team, the emergency responder has other responsibilities during the incident that may carry legal implications if carried out in an inappropriate manner.

Every ESO must consider other factors, which include

- Failure to report crashes or using improper reporting procedures (must follow state guidelines)
- Exceeding load capacity of the vehicle (must follow vehicle weight restrictions)
- Failure to conduct/record vehicle inspections
- Failure to provide training (must not operate any vehicle when the emergency responder has not completed operator training)
- Responsibility for passenger possessions
- Failure to maintain training records

◆ CERTIFIED DRIVER'S LICENSE (CDL)

A certified driver's license (**CDL**) is typically required for anyone who operates a vehicle in excess of 26,001 pounds. Obtaining a CDL has long been considered cumbersome and unrealistic to the majority of ESOs. In some instances, the ESO has the attitude that is geared at a false sense of losing volunteers, because it enforces having highly skilled and trained emergency vehicle operators.

Many states provide exemptions to emergency service personnel from the CDL requirement. As an example, Pennsylvania's Department of Transportation regulation states that firefighters who have a certificate of authorization from their fire chief while operating fire or emergency vehicles registered to the fire department are exempt from the CDL requirements. Persons can obtain specific state-, territory-, or country-specific information from the respective emergency service governing body or vehicle transportation agency. Much of this information is also readily available on the Internet.

◆ SPECIFIC MOTOR VEHICLE OPERATION LAW

All states have statutes governing the operation of motor vehicles. It is important for emergency responders to understand the statutes dealing with operating an emergency vehicle in their specific jurisdiction (Figure 3.3).

Know Your Motor Vehicle Laws

As the operator of an Emergency Vehicle, you may (in most states and territories):

- Exceed the maximum posted speed limits,
- Proceed past a red light or stop sign,
- Travel against the flow of traffic,
- Park or stand irrespective of the law,

As long as you do it with "*Due Regard*" for the safety of everyone.

FIGURE 3.3 ◆ Privileges granted to emergency responders by motor vehicle laws vary from state to state. The chart references a common theme held in most states, territories, and other countries. Drivers must be trained on specific state laws, local ordinances, and/or governing rules and regulations.

Legal issues surrounding emergency and related vehicle operation is a serious subject. The emergency responder and other responding parties can be sued. However, knowing the laws makes a difference and helps you to act "legally smart."

◆ **STANDARDS AND POSITION STATEMENTS**

Several national standards and national trade organization position papers govern emergency and related vehicle driving procedures. This section takes a cursory view of some of the top standards and position statements.

The NHTSA National Standard Curriculum for Emergency Vehicle Operators Course (EVOC) is referenced throughout this book. This EVOC program is considered to be the main national EMS-related document to benchmark EMS driver training requirements.

The National Fire Protection Association (NFPA) standards NFPA1002, *Standard on Apparatus Driver/Operator Professional Qualifications,* and NFPA 1451, *Standard for a Fire Service Vehicle Operations Training Program*, provide the primary foundation for fire service driving–related subjects.

NFPA 1002 identifies the minimum job performance requirements for driver operators of fire department vehicles. The purpose of this standard is to specify the minimum job performance requirements for service as a fire department vehicle driver, pump operator, aerial operator, tiller operator, wild land apparatus operator, and aircraft rescue and firefighting apparatus operator.

The National Association of EMS Physicians and the National Association of State EMS Directors have a standing position statement titled, "Use of Warning Lights and Sirens in Emergency Medical Vehicles." This document provides an official position and rationale for the responsible use of warning lights and sirens. The position paper contains 11 specific positions with supporting rationale.

In 2004, the International Association of Fire Chiefs issued a zero-tolerance policy for the consumption of alcohol in the fire and emergency medical services. The policy needs no explanation—zero tolerance. The consumption of alcohol and subsequent operation of emergency and related vehicles is believed to be a major problem in the emergency services arena. In Pennsylvania, when an individual's driver's license has been suspended for a conviction of driving under the influence of alcohol or drugs, the person is prohibited from driving an ambulance for a period of four years and must successfully repeat an emergency vehicle operator's course of instruction approved by the Department of Health EMS Office.

The American Ambulance Association (AAA) has a position statement on EMS driving (Figure 3.4). According to the **AAA,** it is positioning itself to educate its members regarding the high incidence of collisions and provide them with information, technical assistance, and industry "best practices" to substantially reduce or eliminate the risk of ambulance collisions.

The AAA recognizes that there may be many causes of ambulance collisions. The AAA also recognizes that a systems approach to safe EMS driving (for which there is scientific evidence) can significantly reduce the risk of collisions and the resultant death or injuries.

American Ambulance Association Position Statement on EMS Driving

Issue:

In the 21st century health care environment in the United States, health care providers are attempting to find solutions and systems to reduce the unintended deaths and injuries to hospitalized patients described by the 1999 Institute of Medicine study. Likewise, ambulance providers are challenged to look carefully at themselves to reduce the incidence of death and injury to patients, ambulance service employees and the public due to collisions between ambulances and other vehicles and/or stationary objects.

AAA Position:

The American Ambulance Association is positioning itself to educate its members regarding the high incidence of collisions and provide them with information, technical assistance, and industry "best practices" to substantially reduce or eliminate the risk of ambulance collisions.

The AAA recognizes that there may be many causes of ambulance collisions. The AAA also recognizes that a systems approach to safe driving can significantly reduce the risk of collisions and the resultant death or injuries. The AAA also acknowledges that there is scientific evidence that supports a systems approach to safe EMS driving.

Background:

Leaders in the ambulance industry and those who insure the industry are acutely aware of the significant risks associated with driving ambulances, especially under emergency conditions. According to leading insurers of ambulance services, annually, over 10,000 ambulance related collisions occur that result in injury or death. The rate of ambulance collisions per miles driven is believed to be several times that of civilian drivers.

Current studies focus on how to make ambulances structurally more crash worthy and how to make a safer patient compartment. This increases survival rates for crew and patients after a crash has occurred; however, this does little to address the issue of accident prevention. Enough scientific evidence currently exists to easily understand the multiple risk factors involved in EMS driving and how they can be mitigated.

The benefits of a systems approach to safe ambulance driving practices are significant. First and most importantly, safe driving systems reward EMS staff and management in upholding the first tenet of medicine, "do no harm to your patient"; second, the safe ambulance driver reduces the risk to himself or herself and his or her partner and passengers; third, it creates a safer more stable work platform for treating patients while the vehicle is in motion; and finally, it reduces the risk to the driving public at large.

The American Ambulance Association recognizes the serious issue of vehicle collisions in EMS and is committed to helping ambulance providers significantly reduce collisions. The AAA will provide educational sessions, publicize best practices, publish articles, provide website links and a bibliography, and work with other agencies and associations to address this issue.

The AAA Professional Standards and Research Committee is authorized to develop the above concepts to assist the AAA membership in reducing ambulance vehicle collisions.

Conclusion:

The AAA recognizes the hazards of driving an ambulance under emergency and non-emergency conditions and that many of the thousands of collisions occurring annually may be preventable. The AAA also recognizes that there is science and/or a body of knowledge that supports the implementation of a safe EMS driving system. The AAA will strive to provide the educational focus to significantly change the incidence of ambulance crashes across the nation by being a leading advocate of vehicle and crew safety systems available today.

Board Action: Approved by the AAA Board of Directors on May 6, 2002.

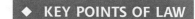
◆ **KEY POINTS OF LAW**

Several key areas play integral roles in the operations of emergency and related vehicle response. Every ESO and emergency responder should keep the following in mind:

* Federal, state, provincial, and local laws dictate emergency vehicle operation.
* ESO requirements must incorporate and not contradict federal, state, or local requirements.
* There are certain situations in which the emergency vehicle operator may be exempt from the regulations. Know the exemptions for your state.

When interpreting rules, regulations, and the law, emergency and related vehicle operators

* Must exercise due regard for the safety of the crew, patients, passengers, and general public.
* Should not operate under emergency response conditions unless a true emergency exists.
* Need to "think safety" to avoid negligence charges.

By knowing and adhering to specific federal, state, and local laws, emergency responders can protect themselves against potential liability situations.

◆ **INTERNATIONAL PERSPECTIVE AND APPLICABLE GUIDELINES**

The issues addressed in this text are echoed around the globe. From Canada and Europe to Asia, Iceland, and the Orient, safe driving practices are stressed. Many international ESOs and emergency service colleagues reference these same issues and best practices.

◆ **NIOSH RECOMMENDATIONS/DISCUSSIONS**

These recommendations and discussions are the NIOSH findings as a result of the opening case study.

RECOMMENDATION #1

Fire departments should adopt the International Association of Fire Chiefs' Zero-Tolerance Policy for Alcohol and Drinking to prohibit the use of alcohol by members of any fire or emergency services agency/organization at any time when they may be called upon to act or respond as a member of those departments. Departments should develop written policies and have procedures in place to enforce this policy.[1-4]

Discussion. Fire departments should strictly prohibit any members of the fire department from responding to a call if they have been drinking. According to the International Association of Fire Chiefs' (IAFC) policy statement (#03.04), Zero-Tolerance for Alcohol & Drinking in the Fire and Emergency Service (2004), "if someone has consumed alcohol within the previous eight (8) hours, or is still noticeably impaired by alcohol consumed previous to the eight (8) hours, they must voluntarily remove themselves from the activities and function of the fire or emergency services agency/organization, including all emergency operations and training."

In addition, the IAFC policy states, "No member of a fire & emergency services agency/organization shall participate in *any aspect of the organization and operation of the fire or emergency agency/organization* under the influence of alcohol, including but not limited to any fire and emergency operations, fire–police, training, etc."

IAFC further recommends that fire and emergency service agencies/organizations develop written policies and have procedures in place to enforce such policies. These policies should include provisions for testing blood alcohol on individuals involved in an incident that results in "measurable damage to apparatus or property or injury/death of agency/organization personnel or civilians."

RECOMMENDATION #2

Fire departments should develop and enforce standard operating procedures (SOPs) that require mandatory use of seat belts in all vehicles.[5-9]

Discussion. Fire departments should develop and enforce SOPs on the use of seat belts. The SOPs must apply to all persons riding in emergency vehicles and should state that all persons must be seated and secured in an approved riding position whenever the vehicle is in motion. An operator who is properly secured by a seat belt has a better chance of maintaining control of the vehicle in an emergency situation and of surviving a crash. In its publication *Safe Operation of Fire Tankers,* the USFA cites a Department of Transportation (**DOT**) study of seat belt use that revealed the following statistics: (1) Seventy-five percent of the people ejected from vehicles suffer fatal injuries; (2) 80 percent of fatalities in rollover incidents involve occupants being ejected from the vehicle; and (3) in a rollover incident, occupants are 22 times more likely to be thrown from the vehicle if they are not wearing their seat belts. The victim and the driver in this incident were not wearing seat belts and the victim was ejected from the tanker. Wyoming has a mandatory seat belt law, and the Learning-for-Life Program, the parent organization for the Explorers, requires that members wear seat belts when riding in fire vehicles.

RECOMMENDATION #3

Fire departments should develop or revise existing SOPs to specify permissible and nonpermissible tasks and activities for youth members participating in junior fire service programs.[2,4,8,10,11]

Discussion. Junior fire/emergency service programs such as Learning-for-Life's Explorers provide young people with work-based learning experiences to help them become responsible and caring adults. The Fire Explorer Program in particular gives participants the opportunity to experience the fire service firsthand and often provides future firefighter recruits. Each Explorer post (a sponsor such as a fire department) must follow the guidelines set forth by the parent organization (i.e., Learning-for-Life) as well as the policies and procedures of the specific fire department. Programs involving junior firefighters must be cognizant of the local and state laws for protection of youth from hazardous conditions and should specify the permissible and nonpermissible tasks and functions for youth. Guidelines and procedures should be in writing, readily available to members of the fire department, and incorporated into departmental SOPs. In *Junior Fire and Emergency Services*, VFIS[a] (p. 23) states, "Sound safety policies must be in place to stipulate what youth members are permitted to do and prohibited from doing in and around the fire station, en route to and from emergencies, and on the emergency scene. These policies must be consistent with fire department regulations, and State laws, and in the case of organizations which are Explorer Posts, must be consistent with guidelines from the Boy Scouts of America. These policies should be established through a comprehensive set of laws before group activities are initiated."

The volunteer department did not have written SOPs; however, it did have a copy of the written policies (i.e., activities and function, bylaws, and training requirements) for Explorers working at this post. The written guidelines for Explorer members state that Explorers with appropriate training are permitted to respond to various emergency calls including structural and wild land fires, although they are prohibited from participating in fighting uncontrolled fires. Explorers are permitted to respond to wild land fire scenes if they have received training in Standards for Survival or the equivalent, and Truck & Equipment Orientation. The victim had taken Standards for Survival but not Truck & Equipment Orientation. These guidelines also included a provision that at least two adults must be present for all activities involving Explorers.

Fire department personnel should be made aware of the requirements, responsibilities, and permitted activities of junior firefighters (e.g., Fire Explorers) to help ensure that they are assigned appropriate tasks and are appropriately supervised. Adequate supervision of the victim was not provided at the fire station or during the response in the tanker.

RECOMMENDATION #4

Fire departments should provide training to driver/operators as often as necessary to meet the requirements of NFPA 1451, and incorporate specifics on rollover prevention in standard operating procedures (SOPs).[5,12,13,14]

Discussion. NFPA 1451 § 5.3 states that fire department personnel must be trained in and exercise applicable principles of defensive driving techniques under both emergency and nonemergency conditions. SOPs for driving fire department vehicles during nonemergency travel and emergency response should include, but not be limited to, the principles of skid avoidance and the effects of liquid surge, load factors, general steering reactions, and speed on vehicle control. Common causes for loss of control are driving too fast for road conditions, failing to appreciate weight shifts of heavy emergency vehicles/apparatus properly, driver distraction, and failing to anticipate obstacles.

Driver training should incorporate vehicle characteristics, capabilities, and limitations. Tankers, for example, tend to be heavier and to have a higher center of gravity than other fire vehicles. Both of these factors affect the driver's ability to control a tanker. Based on simple physics and inertia, a top-heavy vehicle such as a tanker is inclined to tip over if driven through a curve at an unsafe speed or if the driver suddenly turns the wheel in an effort to bring the wheels back onto the road. VFIS lists some vehicle rollover prevention points to increase drivers' ability to maintain control of a vehicle should they run off the road onto the shoulder. VFIS cautions that the vehicle should be slowed gradually by taking the foot off the accelerator, feathering the brakes, and downshifting. Only after the vehicle has been brought down to a safe speed[b], should it be gently steered back onto the road.

Frequency of Training. Driver training should be documented and given in accordance with NFPA 1451, *Standard for a Fire Service Vehicle Operations Training Program*, and NFPA 1002, *Standard on Apparatus Driver/Operator Professional Qualifications*. These standards state that departments should establish and maintain a driver training education program, and each member should be provided driver training not less than twice a year. During this training, each driver needs to operate the vehicle and perform tasks that the driver/operator is expected to encounter during normal operations to ensure the vehicle is safely operated in compliance with all applicable state and local laws.

RECOMMENDATION #5

Fire departments should select and utilize only the safest drivers to operate emergency vehicles.[5,15]

Discussion. Emergency vehicles are one of the most important assets to a fire organization. According to **USFA** statistics, 25 percent of all firefighter fatalities occur in emergency or privately owned vehicles. The safe operation of these vehicles, particularly during emergency response, depends greatly on the ability and skills of the driver. According to the VFIS communiqué, *Emergency Vehicle Driver Selection Criteria* (2000), "Knowing drivers' on and off duty driving habits and records is an important tool in both selecting and maintaining the safest drivers for your emergency vehicles. Routine administrative reviews of all drivers' MVRs[c] is the most effective way to know specific driving habits of individual drivers." VFIS recommends reviewing MVRs annually (minimally every three years) and that copies be retained in each member's personnel file. VFIS further recommends that those convicted of a Class A[d] violation have their (fire vehicle) driving privileges suspended for 18 months.

RECOMMENDATION #6

Fire departments should use caution when retrofitting non–fire service apparatus to serve as tankers and, when this a necessity, ensure that the vehicle does not exceed its load-carrying capacity and meets the requirements of NFPA 1901, Standard for Automotive Fire Apparatus.[5,16,17]

Discussion. Retrofitting non–fire service vehicles such as fuel oil or gasoline tankers is a common practice among fire departments with limited financial resources. The USFA cautions the fire service that converting surplus vehicles designed for another purpose to water tankers may create serious maintenance issues. If, for example, the vehicle has been donated because it is worn out and the donor did not want to deal with maintenance issues, the department that acquires it may be starting with a vehicle in "questionable mechanical and safety condition." Even if the donated vehicle is in excellent condition when acquired by the fire department, the chassis may not be designed to safely carry water. Water weighs 8.3 lb/gal—more than fuel oil (7.12 lb/gal) or gasoline (5.6 lb/gal). This extra weight can create substantial safety issues for the vehicle. To determine whether the chassis can safely carry a load, subtract the unloaded weight of the vehicle from the maximum weight it is rated to carry (**GVWR**, or gross vehicle weight rating). Load-carrying (payload) capacity (amount left to carry passengers, water, equipment and so forth) = GVWR − unloaded weight of vehicle. The vehicle involved in this incident had a GVWR of 50,000 pounds. If we assume an unloaded weight[e] of 16,800 pounds for this chassis, the load-carrying capacity is 50,000 pounds − 16,800 pounds or 33,200 pounds. The weight of the water in a full 4500-gallon tank is 37,350 pounds. In this incident, therefore, the load-carrying capacity of the chassis was exceeded. Although it is unknown whether exceeding the load-carrying capacity contributed to this incident (it was not identified in the state highway patrol report), some cautionary comments are in order. According to the National Highway Traffic Safety Administration (NHTSA), "It is very dangerous to drive *any* vehicle whose load carrying capacity has been exceeded. Too much weight in a vehicle can cause difficulty steering and braking. It can also compromise a vehicle's safety by causing the tires to wear more quickly and unevenly and suspension parts and axles to wear more quickly. In extreme cases, overloading may cause catastrophic failure of any of these components."

Niosh references

[a]Volunteer Fireman Insurance Services.

[b]According to USFA/FEMA (p. 113), the appropriate speed at which to remount the paved surface is estimated to be 20 mph or less.

[c]Motor vehicle report.

[d]According to VFIS, examples of Type A violations include driving while intoxicated, driving under the influence of drugs, and negligent homicide arising out of the use of a motor vehicle (gross negligence).

[e]The unloaded weight estimate is based on a conversation with a representative of the company that sold this particular vehicle to its original owner.

◆ **CASE STUDY RECAP**

There are many circumstances surrounding this case study ranging from safe driving practices and seat belt use to alcohol-related activities. Driving rules, regulations, and laws exist to provide recognized safe practices and behaviors for all users of the roadway. As depicted in the beginning of this chapter, NIOSH investigators concluded that, in order to minimize the risk of similar occurrences, fire departments (all ESQs) should do the following.

- Adopt the International Association of Fire Chiefs' Zero-Tolerance Policy for Alcohol and Drinking to prohibit the use of alcohol by members of any fire or emergency services agency/organization at any time when they may be called on to act or respond as a member of those departments. Departments should develop written policies and have procedures in place to enforce this policy.
- Develop and enforce standard operating procedures (SOPs) that require mandatory use of seat belts in all vehicles.
- Develop or revise existing SOPs to specify permissible and nonpermissible tasks and activities for youth members participating in junior fire service programs.
- Provide training to driver/operators as often as necessary to meet the requirements of NFPA 1451, and incorporate specifies on rollover prevention in standard operating procedures.
- Select and utilize only the safest drivers to operate emergency vehicles.
- Use caution when retrofitting non–fire service apparatus to serve as tankers and, when this is a necessity, ensure that the vehicle does not exceed its load-carrying capacity and meets the requirements of NFPA 1901, *Standard for Automotive Fire Apparatus.*

◆ **SUMMARY**

Driving is a privilege, thus any special provision granted to an emergency or related vehicle operator should be viewed as a supreme privilege. Exercising these supreme privileges allows the emergency or related vehicle operator to do things that the average driver on the roadway cannot do and seldom knows what to do when approached by a vehicle under emergency response conditions. As an emergency vehicle operator, you are responsible for the safe and efficient preparation of and response to the incident.

The responsibility goes well beyond response. The transportation of your crew, patients, family members, and the general public along the way remain critical components of the driving process.

Emergency responders need to be aware that they are being held "legally accountable" for their actions at all times while performing their job. One does not have to go far to realize the extent of the problem. Virtually every national organization representing the emergency services industry has addressed the operation of emergency vehicles and even nonemergency vehicles used for emergency organization and response operations.

Rules, regulations, laws, and ordinances exist to maintain order and keep everyone as safe as possible. Prudent driving habits reflect adherence to these laws and standards and will permit a friendly driving and legal environment. The education and training of emergency and related vehicle drivers in their legal responsibilities is absolutely imperative.

Review Questions

1. What are four primary exemptions granted by law (in many states) to emergency vehicles under emergency response conditions?
2. What is the difference between rules, regulations, and law?
3. Define a true emergency.
4. What is due regard?
5. How does vicarious liability affect the emergency vehicle driver?

References

International Association of Fire Chiefs. 2004. *Policy statement #03.04: Zerotolerance for alcohol & drinking in the fire and emergency service*. Retrieved December 3, 2005, from http://www.iafc.org

New York State Motor Vehicle Code. April 10, 2005.

NFPA. 2002. *NFPA 1451, Standard for a fire service vehicle operations training program*. Quincy, MA: National Fire Protection Association.

NFPA. 2003. *NFPA 1002, Standard on apparatus driver/operator professional qualifications*. Quincy, MA: National Fire Protection Association.

NHTSA. 1994. *NHTSA ambulance operator driver training program, national standard curriculum*. Washington, DC.

NIOSH. 2001. *NIOSH Hazard ID: Fire fighter deaths from tanker truck rollovers*. Cincinnati, OH: U.S. Department of Health and Human Services, Public Health Service, Centers for Disease Control and Prevention, National Institute for Occupational Safety and Health, DHHS (NIOSH) Publication No. 2002-111.

North Carolina Motor Vehicle Code. April 10, 2005.

Pennsylvania Department of Health EMS Office. March 24, 2004, *EMS Information Bulletin #12*.

Pennsylvania Motor Vehicle Code. April 10, 2005.

USFA/FEMA. 2003. *Alive on arrival: Tips for safe emergency vehicle operations*. Emmitsburg, MD: U.S. Fire Administration.

VFIS. 1997. *Emergency Vehicle Driver Training Program*. York, PA.

VFIS. 2000. *Technical reference communiqué—Emergency vehicle driver selection criteria*. Retrieved April 10, 2004, from http://www.vfis.com.

Wilbur, M. 2004. *Driving with due regard—How does it affect you, the emergency vehicle operator?* Retrieved December 3, 2005, from http://www.firehouse.com

Policy,
Procedures,
and Guidelines

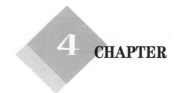

Objectives

After completing this chapter, you should be able to:

- List the difference between policy, procedure, and guideline.
- Identify the reasons that written SOP/SOGs are important to operating an effective driver training program.
- Identify the subject areas for written SOP/SOGs that impact the certification, operations, and recertification of emergency vehicle drivers.
- Identify written SOP/SOGs that impact emergency and related vehicle response procedures.

Case Study

During their daily vehicle check, the crew started the ambulance and thought it made an unusual sound. With no policy as to what to do, crew members wrote off the sound as a fluke and continued their check without a second thought to the unusual sound. Later that morning the crew was dispatched to an emergency. While en route the ambulance started making the same sound and then suddenly lost power. The driver managed to get off the roadway and notified dispatch to send another ambulance to the original emergency incident.

In today's society it is essential that all emergency service organizations develop, adopt, and implement policy with supporting standard operating procedures and guidelines. The principle of public kindness is no longer an acceptable practice, and concepts such as sovereign immunity (individual versus government) have been significantly limited and narrowed by the courts.

Many of the federal, state, and provincial laws allow for suits against individual leaders of emergency service organizations. Terms such as *duty of care, breach of omission or commission,* and *joint and several liability* are entering the vocabulary of emergency service personnel.

Policy with supporting procedures should be addressed first and foremost. Sound, practical policy is essential. Organizational leadership must understand the importance of this critical risk area, develop policy for compliance, educate personnel on policy and safe, defensive low-force driving, hold staff accountable, reward good behavior, and remediate as warranted.

One important way to prepare for this challenge is to develop, adopt, and implement a comprehensive set of standard operating procedures/standard operating guidelines (SOP/SOGs) that support the ESO policy (Figure 4.1).

During the process of compiling SOP/SOGs, the difference between these varied documents may become blurred. For instance, often the distinction between policy and procedure does not seem so clear. Policy is different from SOP/SOG. All procedures and guidelines come with policy. Policy can be viewed as the attitude, philosophy toward the organization's personnel, and intent of top management. It provides a framework and guidance to organization personnel in making decisions. In the evaluation of policy, it is essential to obtain input from the organization's members. This basic principle sets the stage for buy-in by the emergency responders.

Anywhere ESO Any Town Administrative Procedures & Guidelines	Subject	Policy and SOP/SOG Development
	Guideline Number	
	Adopted	
	Effective Date	
	Revised	
	Due for Revision	
	Pages	1 of 1

Purpose: To assure sound policy with supporting procedures and/or guidelines are developed, implemented, and enforced for the protection of the <**ESO NAME**> and its personnel.

Scope: All <**ESO NAME**> personnel.

Responsibility: The fire company administration is responsible for authorizing and ensuring that these provisions are followed.

Functions:
1. All administrative policy is developed by the <**ESO NAME**> BOD.
2. Questions and suggestions pertaining to administrative policy shall be directed to the <**ESO NAME or DEPARTMENT**>.
3. All operational policy is developed and approved by the Fire Chief and ratified by the <**NAME**>.
4. Questions and suggestions pertaining to operational policy shall be directed to the Fire Chief.
5. All <**ESO NAME**> members are responsible to adhere to established policy and play a vital role in policy compliance.
6. All officers, elected and appointed, are responsible to educate members on all policy.
7. All officers, elected and appointed, are responsible to enforce all policy.
8. Policy that is no longer effective or in effect should be removed from the policy manual and all members notified in writing.
9. Policy revisions follow the same format and process as defined in #1 and #3 above and adhere to the <**ESO NAME**> SOP Refinement Policy (#____).

FIGURE 4.1 ◆ Imprint of sample SOP.

RECOMMENDATION #1

According to NIOSH, fire departments should develop standard operating procedures as they relate to responding to or returning from an alarm and monitor to ensure their use.

Discussion. Driver/operators of emergency vehicles are regulated by state laws, city ordinances, and departmental policies. All members of the department should study and be familiar with departmental policies and procedures as they relate to fire emergency vehicles. Department policies state that when responding to emergencies, all traffic laws must be observed. All drivers should also have a thorough knowledge of the rules governing speed for emergency vehicles in their own jurisdictions and the jurisdictions of their mutual-aid partners. Unless specifically exempt, emergency vehicle driver/operators are subject to any statute or ordinance that governs any vehicle operator. Statutes usually describe those vehicles that are in the emergency category; this classification then covers all fire department vehicles when responding to an emergency.

◆ **TERMS**

To aid in the development of SOP/SOGs, understanding specific definitions of terms is essential.

Policy: A guiding principle or course of action adopted toward an objective or objectives. Describes the general principle that will guide behavior (management's intent). A definite course or method of action to guide and determine present and future decisions.

Procedure: Prescribes specific ways of doing specific activities. That which regulates the formal steps in an action. A series of steps followed in a particular order.

Guideline: A statement, indication, or outline of policy by which to determine a course of action. Any guide or indication of a future course of action. Guidelines can often be tailored to specific circumstances.

Rule: A principle set up by authority, prescribing or directing action or forbearance (do's and don'ts).

Regulation: A rule or order prescribed by authority to regulate conduct.

The following are questions to be asked regarding policy:

- Is it founded on sound judgment?
- Is it reasonably attainable?
- Is it within legal and/or regulatory boundaries?
- Is it definite, positive, and clear?
- Does it need further definition or explanation to those affected?
- Is it applicable to all organizational units?
- Is it flexible?
- Should it be flexible?
- Does it reflect the general thinking and enforcement philosophy of all levels of personnel?
- Will or must it be supported by procedures, guidelines, rules, and regulations?
- Can it be enforced?
- Will it be enforced?

The following is a visual reference for the difference in terms (Figure 4.2).

FIGURE 4.2 ◆ Schematic depicting ability to get from Point *A* to Point *B*.

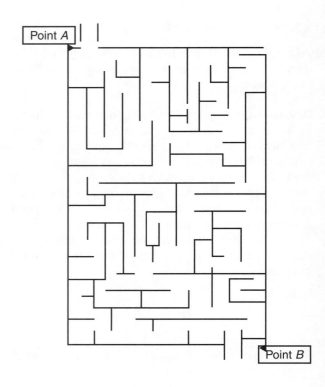

EXAMPLE

Policy: Go from Point *A* to Point *B*.
Procedure: Begin at Point *A*, go to Point *B* by following the prescribed directions.
Guideline: Begin at Point *A,* go to Point *B* but does not give explicit directions as a procedure.
Rules and regulations: Do not cross any line, do not backtrack.

◆ CONDUCTING A NEEDS ASSESSMENT

Whether it is the starting point or part of the process, policy development and the SOP/SOG process should include a *needs assessment*. The need exists in every ESO; the real question is what SOP/SOGs most apply to the ESO. Every emergency service organization should periodically conduct a formal review of policy and SOP/SOGs. These assessments should be handled by top management for policy and a task group/committee of organizational members representing all ranks and possibly other applicable agencies (e.g., an attorney or policy analyst from the local government). The product of this formal review results in a document that can be used as a "road map" for enhancing or developing new policy and SOP/SOGs.

The needs assessment process must be consistent and systematic. The product should include a written analysis of current policy and SOP/SOGs, recommendations, and the rationale for changes (if any); priorities; and a plan for action. Although major changes in legal and/or operational requirements will prompt a formal needs assessment, the process should be performed annually to help keep SOP/SOGs current and valid.

While prioritizing, it is important to remember that SOP/SOGs must reflect reality. Creating SOP/SOGs that cannot be implemented with existing resources serves little purpose and may create a safety hazard. Revisions to critical safety SOP/SOGs should receive a high priority in the action plan because they influence the safety of responders and the effectiveness of overall operations.

◆ FORMULATION PROCEDURE

Decrees issued from those in charge often do not receive widespread support. To expect the members of an emergency service organization to support SOP/SOGs enthusiastically when they are formulated and issued without member support and involvement is not realistic. However, the formulation procedure can be an integral component in having effective and realistic SOP/SOGs that are supported.

Although the exact methods used to develop SOP/SOGs will vary, certain strategies will help define a successful process. The needs assessment process establishes the foundation for the SOP/SOG development effort. Various organizations have found the following recommendations very effective in developing and implementing effective SOP/SOGs.

- Inform the membership as to the need to develop, adopt, and implement SOP/SOGs and how the process is undertaken.
- Build the development team. Commit to utilizing task forces, committees, or guideline groups involving the members of the organization.

SOP/SOGs are most effective when members of the organization are included in the development process. As a general rule, organizations should get input from all groups potentially affected by the SOP/SOG.

A key variable in determining success or failure during implementation is keeping the product *user friendly*. The following are some suggestions to help attain this goal:

- *Level of detail:* SOP/SOGs should provide only broad procedural guidelines, not specific details of task performance.
- *Clarity and conciseness:* SOP/SOGs must be clear, concise, and written in plain English language. Clear and simple statements are the best way to describe actions in SOP/SOGs using language that members can easily understand.
- *Target audience:* Generally, SOP/SOGs should be written to address the needs and educational level of the majority of the organization members.
- *Flexibility and ambiguity:* To be effective, organizational guidelines (SOGs) must be clear and concise. An organization's SOGs should be precise but inherently flexible, permitting an acceptable level of discretion that reflects the nature of the situation and the judgment of the incident commander.

A related issue involves the use of the terms *shall* and *may* when writing SOP/SOGs. An action preceded by the word *shall* is generally considered to be an inviolate rule (SOP), whereas using the term *may* implies greater flexibility and discretion by personnel (SOG).

A "cardinal rule" of SOP/SOGs is that they must be **doable**!

Simply put, SOP/SOGs must be written in a specific format so that those individuals expected to comply can do so in an easy, practical way.

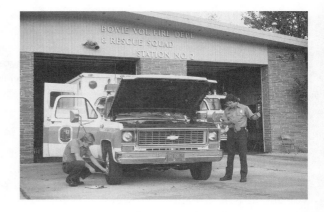

FIGURE 4.3 ◆ EMS crew conducting a routine vehicle inspection. (*Courtesy of Pearson Education/PH College*)

A standard header format for SOP/SOGs helps streamline the writing process. Different formats may be used for SOP/SOGs depending on the intended audience and purpose. Several items are usually included in an SOP/SOG:

- Numbering system
- Page numbers
- Effective date
- Expiration/review date
- Title
- Description of purpose or rationale statement (ESO policy)
- Authority signature(s)
- Scope
- General procedures or guidelines
- Specific procedures or guidelines
- References (A sample format can be found in Figure 4.5 at the end of the chapter.)

◆ PERIODIC REVIEW

Standard operating procedures and guidelines are not static documents. All SOP/SOGs need to be regularly reviewed and updated. This is not to suggest that every SOP/SOG should be changed annually; but each one should be checked for updating, correcting, fine-tuning, or otherwise changing if necessary. The process of having the SOP/SOGs reviewed and revised is more important than how many SOP/SOGs are changed. Change just for the sake of change is not recommended. Personnel become familiar and comfortable operating under established procedures/guidelines. If these are valid, they should be left in place.

Evaluation is not the same as performance monitoring. The purpose of performance monitoring is to make sure that personnel comply with the SOP/SOG and perform it correctly, in effect asking, "Are we doing things right?" Evaluation on the other hand, looks at the same employee action but asks, "Are we doing the right thing?" The goal in this case is to assess and redesign the SOP/SOG.

Most organizations strive to review SOP/SOGs annually. If the resources are available, this is desirable. Many smaller organizations conduct an annual review but

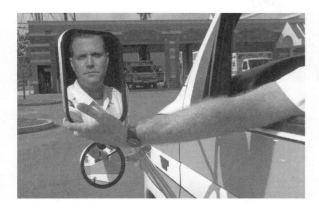

FIGURE 4.4 ◆   The driver sets the mirror to enhance safe operations based on ESO driving policy. (*Courtesy of Pearson Education/PH College*)

only cover one-half of the SOP/SOG manual. This provides a biannual review, and if individual SOP/SOGs are changed when it becomes necessary, the members will be able to digest the changes better.

Employees expect a safe working environment. According to the National Highway Traffic Safety Administration (NHTSA), ambulance operators need to be trained with the knowledge and skills to operate their vehicles so that their vehicle, equipment, crew, and patients will be delivered safely and efficiently (1994). **NHTSA** also emphasizes the importance of safety of the public and that it be assured during all phases of the delivery of the emergency medical services (EMS) involving the ambulance. This same categorization can be applied to all ESOs and response scenarios.

The Firefighter Life Safety Summit held in Tampa, Florida, in March 2004, produced 16 major initiatives to give the fire service a blueprint for making changes. Many of the initiatives can be applied to policy and SOP/SOG needs, but initiative 11 specifically identifies the need for driving-related policy: Develop and champion national standards for emergency response policies and procedures. The National Association of Emergency Medical Technicians (**NAEMT**) also lists on its Web site a number of policy recommendations related to safe driving practices.

The ESO can provide that environment by sincerely believing and promoting that nothing supercedes safety, *absolutely nothing!* Establishing policy sets the stage for the safe work environment (Figure 4.4). The supporting procedures should be clear and attainable by the majority of personnel. Leaders must lead by example. Be sure you lead in the right direction, because personnel will follow your lead.

◆ COMPLIANCE/ENFORCEMENT

Compliance to and enforcement of policy and applicable SOP/SOGs are based on management's leadership abilities. Setting the example is critical to compliance and will decrease the likelihood of additional enforcement. Every person in the ESO should be educated on policy and expected actions. Supervisors and line officers as middle management must lead by example and account for the actions of every responder. Emergency responders want a safe work environment and thus have expectations as to what is expected of them. Safety is considered personal, but leaving compliance solely to the driver and crew could be disastrous for every facet of the ESO.

◆ ADOPTION OF SOP/SOGS

The need to adopt SOP/SOGs is not always obvious to everyone. Consider the following basic reasons for adoption:

- All personnel understand what is expected or required.
  - Eligibility qualifications and certification requirements to become an emergency vehicle driver.
  - Training schedule, expectations, and requirements for emergency vehicle drivers.
  - Annual requirements for maintaining certification.
  - General conduct and obligations of drivers.
- Intended compliance with all necessary requirements is identified.
  - Not a guarantee of compliance.
  - Indication of organization's intent to follow applicable laws.
  - SOP/SOG examples.
    - Compliance with organizational rules and requirements.
    - Compliance with legal jurisdictions.
    - Compliance with other professional standards.
- Written and maintained.
- Preplanned and agreed-upon actions.
  - Personnel and vehicles are variable at any incident.
  - Drivers should have standardized procedures for response and arrival operations.
  - Incident commanders should not have to worry about the actions of drivers.
- Resource documents on which to base training.
  - Predetermined procedures and responsibilities allow the driver to train and practice in accordance with SOP/SOG.
    - Prospective drivers can identify the training requirements necessary to qualify as an emergency vehicle driver.
    - All drivers can be informed and trained to identify which vehicle responds to various types of incidents.
    - Existing emergency vehicle drivers can identify the requirements for retraining and certification to additional vehicles within the organization.
- Required anticipated actions.
  - It is easier and less stressful to brainstorm certain situations and their solutions in a quiet setting.
  - Critical tasks of inspection and maintenance can be scheduled.
  - Pretrip, response, and posttrip responsibilities can be identified and detailed.
  - Inappropriate driving actions and/or conflicting actions that might lead to emergency vehicle collisions can be eliminated or at least minimized.

◆ SOP/SOG SUBJECT AREAS

The following are suggested subject areas to develop policy and support SOP/SOGs.

- Eligibility requirements for drivers
  - Age, experience, and performance standards for new applicants
  - Motor vehicle record checks
  - Personal auto insurance verification
  - Necessary steps to maintain emergency vehicle certification

- Procedure to expanding an existing certification to other vehicles
- Recertification procedures for existing drivers
- Testing and proficiency requirements for drivers
  - Classroom training and written examination
  - Simulation training
  - Competency course training and testing
  - On-the-road training and testing (nonemergent, emergent, without patient onboard, patient onboard)
  - Annual training and/or driving for certification maintenance
- Emergency response procedures
  - Emergency vehicle response per type of incident
  - Application of state traffic laws to emergency incident response
  - Emergency incident scene operations
  - Off-road emergency vehicle operations
  - Private and administrative vehicle response
- Customary and/or ordinary procedures
  - Vehicle inspection and maintenance procedures
  - Nonemergency travel
  - High-hazard operational procedures
- Special situations
  - Inclement weather operations
  - Night operations
  - Special location considerations
  - Accident reaction and reporting procedures
  - Vehicle malfunction procedures

The following are key topics to be considered when developing SOP/SOGs.

1. Recommend local authority having jurisdiction should review any pertinent written SOP/SOGs for compliance.
2. Have legal counsel and local governing body should review policies prior to adoption.
3. The authority having jurisdiction should have written policies governing speed and the limitations to be observed during all facets of the response including inclement weather and various road and traffic conditions.
4. At no time should driving regulations be less restrictive than state motor vehicle laws.
5. Drivers of ESO vehicles should bring the vehicle to a complete stop and shall not proceed until it is confirmed that it is safe to do so for any of the following situations:
   - Any "stop" signal (i.e., sign, light, or traffic officer)
   - Blind intersections
   - Intersections where the operator cannot account for all lanes of traffic (vehicle and pedestrian)
   - A stopped school bus with flashing warning lights
6. Responding emergency vehicles should stop at all railroad crossings to ensure that a safe crossing can be made.
   - The driver should obey all railroad crossing signals even when responding to emergencies.
   - Vehicles should not be driven around railroad crossing gates.
7. The driver should maintain a distance in front of the vehicle that is at least equal to the minimum travel distance necessary to stop the vehicle without contacting another object.
8. ESO vehicles following each other should maintain an adequate distance to avoid rear-end collisions.
9. Overtaking and passing other vehicles during emergency response should be accomplished with extreme caution (due regard).

Anywhere ESO Any Town Administrative Procedures & Guidelines	Subject	Driver Training
	Guideline Number	
	Adopted	
	Effective Date	
	Revised	
	Due for Revision	
	Pages	1

Purpose: To assure that every volunteer or employee acknowledges the seriousness of the use and safe operation of all privately owned vehicles during <**ESO NAME**> functions.

Scope: All <**ESO NAME**> personnel.

Responsibility: It is the responsibility of all <**ESO NAME**> personnel who own and operate their own respective vehicles to adhere to this policy for response to and returning from <**ESO NAME**> events and acknowledge such in writing.

Policy:

A. Valid Driver's License and Insurance Coverage

No volunteer or employee of <**ESO NAME**> shall operate a <**ESO NAME**> vehicle or mobile unit of any kind without the appropriate, valid <**STATE**> Driver's License, and appropriate personal vehicle insurance coverage.

<**ESO NAME**> will conduct annual Motor Vehicle Record checks and personal insurance verification on all <**ESO NAME**> personnel.

B. Driver Training Requirements
1. Driver candidates must comply with Section A. above.
2. Driver candidates for <**ESO NAME**> vehicles must have at least five years' driving experience prior to entering the department's training program.
3. Candidates must successfully complete an approved Emergency Vehicle Driver Training program approved by <**ESO NAME**> and demonstrate satisfactory handling of each qualified vehicle prior to approval.
   a. Initial education and training should consist of not less than 16 hours.
4. Annual refresher training is required.
   a. Annual updates may occur in any of the following approved formats.
      i. Classroom
      ii. Video
      iii. CD
      iv. Tailboard Safety Talks
5. Only the lead driving instructor of the <**ESO NAME**> can authorize driver candidate approvals and certify compliance with education and training requirements.

Record Keeping

All driving records will be maintained in the volunteer or employee's respective training files.

Monitoring and Remediation
1. All drivers will be monitored for policy compliance. <**ESO NAME**> encourages drivers and other personnel to communicate incidents, both real and near misses, to a company officer.
2. <**ESO NAME**>'s position is to positively address any incident to avoid more serious incidents in the future.
3. Remedial training may occur by any of the previously mentioned training methods and/or one-on-one to facilitate appropriate response to the incident.

FIGURE 4.5 ◆ This sample SOP depicts the ESO's intent for a safe driving policy.

10. While en route to transfers, vehicles, should be operated in a nonemergency mode, and the driver shall obey all traffic laws.
11. Every ESO should identify the types of responses that will be made in a nonemergency mode.

◆ SAMPLE SOP/SOG

Figure 4.5 depicts an example of an SOP/SOG for various aspects of emergency and related vehicle operations. It is by no means inclusive of all driving-related needs. Use the example to hone or develop your department-wide policy and SOP/SOGs.

◆ CASE STUDY RECAP

When left unaddressed, issues that affect safe operations may be left to the decision of inexperienced personnel. The case study depicted a crew who recognized an unusual sound with the vehicle while conducting a routine inspection. Not knowing how to broach the issue of the unusual sound, the crew "wrote off" the sound as a fluke and no action was taken, resulting in the vehicle breaking down during a response. Policy, procedures, and guidelines that address vehicle inspections and routine checks should provide crews with action steps to correct any noted deficiency.

◆ SUMMARY

Personnel not only need to know but also want to know what is expected of them in everyday functions of the ESO. Organizational leadership must understand the importance of this critical risk area, develop policy for compliance, educate personnel on policy and safe, defensive low-force driving, hold staff accountable, reward good behavior, and remediate as warranted. Sound administrative policy supported by clear, concise, doable SOP/SOGs that are followed and enforced will set the stage for safe, effective, and efficient operations.

Review Questions

1. What is the definition of policy?
2. What is the difference between standard operating procedures and standard operating guidelines?
3. How can an ESO best obtain buy-in from the personnel expected to adhere to the SOP/SOGs?
4. When should a policy, SOP, or SOG be taken out of circulation?
5. How long should it normally take to develop and implement an SOP/SOG?
6. What is the purpose of having a policy statement?
7. What is the main principle behind how a standard operating procedure works?
8. What is the main principle behind how a standard operating guideline works?
9. What are five key components recommended for use in the header format?
10. Why is it important for all personnel to follow safe driving SOP/SOGs?
11. Who has the primary responsibility for SOP/SOG development?

■ ■

References

FEMA and National Fallen Firefighters Foundation. April 14, 2004. Firefighter Life Safety Summit Initial Report. Tampa, FL.

FEMA/USFA. *Developing SOP/SOG manual.* Retrieved December 3, 2004, from http://www.usfa.fema.gov/downloads/pdf/publications/fa-197.pdf

Jenaway, B. Ph.D. November 2005. "Best practices in vehicle safety." *NVFC.*

National Association of EMTs Web site. December 2004. http://www.naemt.org.

NHTSA. 1994. *Emergency vehicle operators course (ambulance)—National standard curriculum.*

Patrick, R.W. Spring 2003. "Principles of standard operating procedures." *VFIS News.*

Patrick, R. W., October 2003. "General safety." *EMS Magazine.*

VFIS. 2002. *Developing and implementing SOPs and SOGs.* York, PA.

Emergency Vehicle Characteristics and Driving

5 **CHAPTER**

Objectives

After completing this chapter, you should be able to:

+ Define the different types of emergency vehicles.
+ Describe the operations of an emergency vehicle.
+ Discuss the characteristics of an emergency vehicle.
+ Describe how to avoid vehicle crashes.
+ Discuss the different types of road surfaces.
+ Describe how to correct various types of situations you may encounter while driving an emergency vehicle.

Case Study

On August 19, 2001, a 52-year-old male volunteer firefighter (the victim) died after he lost control of the tanker truck he was driving when the right front tire ruptured, resulting in a blowout. The road on which the truck was traveling was an interstate highway comprised of two eastbound and two westbound lanes. The surface of the highway is constructed of a large, coarse, bituminous material. The highway had fog edge lines, rumble strips, and paved shoulders, and it was straight and level in the area of the collision. The road had a posted speed limit of 65 mph for cars and 55 mph for trucks. Weather conditions on the day of the incident were clear and the highway was dry. The truck struck a large boulder and tree, entrapping the victim in the cab. He was extricated from the truck, and the medical examiner pronounced him dead at the scene.

◆ **INTRODUCTION**

Based on simple **physics** and **inertia**, a top-heavy vehicle such as a tanker is inclined to tip over if the driver suddenly turns the wheel in effort to bring the wheels back onto the road. According to VFIS of York, Pennsylvania, only after the vehicle has been slowed to a safe speed, should it be gently steered back onto the road. The most common causes for skids are driving too fast for road conditions, oversteering, failing to properly appreciate weight shifts of heavy emergency vehicles/apparatus, overbraking, and failing to anticipate obstacles. This chapter discusses the physical dynamics of operating an emergency vehicle.

◆ EMERGENCY MEDICAL, FIRE, AND SPECIALTY APPARATUS

AMBULANCE TYPES

The KKK-A-1822C Federal Specification standards, published by the General Services Administration (GSA), recognize three types of ambulances—Type I, Type II, and Type III. A Type I ambulance has a conventional truck, cab chassis with a modular body (Figure 5.1). A Type II ambulance is a standard van with an integral cab body (Figure 5.2). A Type III ambulance has a cutaway van with a cab chassis with an integral or containerized modular body ambulance (Figure 5.3).

The Star of Life emblem may be displayed on the ambulance when the manufacturer certifies to the purchaser that the ambulance, its components, and its equipment meet or exceed the tests in the KKK specification. This emblem certifies that the ambulance meets minimum specifications and has passed certain tests, as well as design, performance, equipment, and appearance requirements.

If drivers usually operate the same type of ambulance, they will get to know all of the operating equipment and how to use it in a variety of situations. If drivers are assigned to drive a type of ambulance they have never driven before, the supervisor (or another qualified operator) should give drivers an orientation to the new ambulance. Drivers should have an opportunity to PRACTICE driving the new ambulance type and pass a written and performance test before they operate the ambulance.

FIRE APPARATUS

Fire apparatus come in a wide variety of styles and types. The Fire Apparatus Manufacturers' Association uses the following definitions for fire apparatus.

Tanker (Elliptical or Rectangular). A vehicle designed primarily for transporting (pick up, transporting, and delivering) water to fire emergency scenes to be applied to other vehicles or pumping equipment (NFPA 1901 3.3.109) (Figure 5.4).

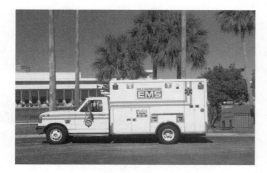

FIGURE 5.1 ◆ Type I ambulance. (*Courtesy of Pearson Education/PH College*)

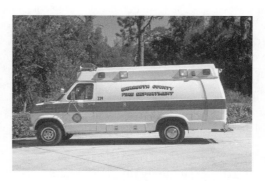

FIGURE 5.2 ◆ Type II ambulance. (*Courtesy of Pearson Education/PH College*)

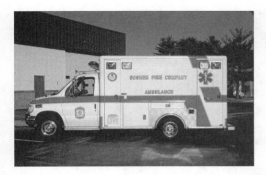

FIGURE 5.3 ◆ Type III ambulance. (*Courtesy of Pearson Education/PH College*)

Pumper. Fire apparatus with a permanently mounted fire pump of at least 750 gallons per minute (gpm) capacity, water tank, and hose body whose primary purpose is to combat structural and associated fires (NFPA 1901 3.3.136) (Figure 5.5).

Rescue Pumper. Fire apparatus with a permanently mounted fire pump of at least 750 gpm capacity, water tank, and hose body whose primary purpose is to combat structural and associated fires (NFPA 1901 3.3.136).

Mini Pumper Initial Attack. Fire apparatus with a permanently mounted fire pump of at least 250 gpm capacity, water tank, and hose body whose primary purpose is to initiate a fire suppression attack on structural, vehicular, or vegetation fires, and to support associated fire department operations (NFPA 1901 3.3.88).

Brush Trucks. Fire apparatus designed for fighting wildland fires off-road that is equipped with a pump having a capacity normally between 10 gpm and 500 gpm, a water tank, limited hose and equipment, and that has pump and roll capability (NFPA 1906 1.7.93) (Figure 5.6).

Rescue, Walk-in. Special services fire apparatus is a multipurpose vehicle that primarily provides support services at emergency scenes (NFPA 1901 3.3.153). These services could be rescue, command, hazardous material containment, air supply, electrical generation and floodlighting, or transportation of support equipment *and personnel* (NFPA 1901 A.3.3.153).

Rescue, Non Walk-in. Special services fire apparatus is a multipurpose vehicle that primarily provides support services at emergency scenes (NFPA 1901 3.3.153). These serv-

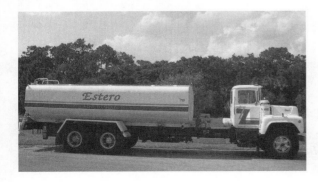

FIGURE 5.4 ◆ In the eastern part of the United States this is referred to as a tanker; in the western part a water tender.

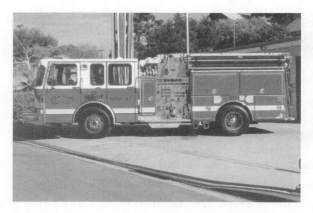

FIGURE 5.5 ◆ Many agencies refer to this piece of apparatus as a pumper or engine; some areas call it a wagon depending on the function of the vehicle and the agency. Nonetheless the vehicle typically handles in the same manner. (*Courtesy of Dorling Kindersley Media Library*)

ices could be rescue, command, hazardous material containment, air supply, electrical generation and floodlighting, or transportation of support equipment (NFPA 1901 A.3.3.153).

Snorkel. Sometimes people refer to any water tower, aerial ladder, or elevated platform as a Snorkel. This is inaccurate. A Snorkel is a brand name of articulating boom with a platform (Figure 5.7). It usually has the ability to spray water from the platform permanently plumbed into the system. There are several types of aerial devices. Some are just large extension ladders; others are ladders with a platform on the end. The articulating boom has the most versatile reach, but rescue efforts are slowed because the platform must be raised and lowered to bring people to the ground. A ladder or a platform on a ladder has the ability to allow a steady stream of people to exit the upper floors of a building without the need to go up and down itself. Just about any aerial device can be configured to be an elevated nozzle.

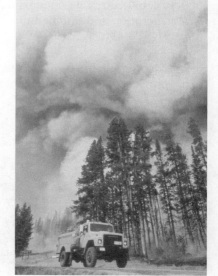

FIGURE 5.6 ◆ Brush trucks come in all shapes and sizes. (*Courtesy of Index Stock Imagery, Inc.*)

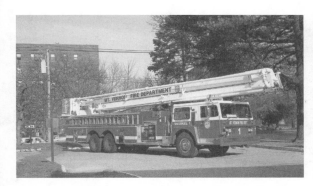

FIGURE 5.7 ◆ A snorkel has an articulating boom. (*Courtesy of Dorling Kindersley Media Library*)

Squirt. A smaller articulating boom, usually mounted on an engine. The main purpose is to have an elevated fire stream. This does not make an engine a quint or a quad. This gives the engine's deck gun more reach and versatility. This is not a Snorkel, although the Snorkel company did manufacture such devices in the 1960s and 1970s.

Quint. A piece of firefighting apparatus that can perform five of the major functions of fire apparatus. These include carry hose, carry water, pump water, and aerial ladder/water tower operations. It may also carry large amounts of ladders (Figure 5.8).

Aerial Truck. Also known as a ladder truck, aerial ladder, or just plain truck (Figure 5.9). A hydraulically powered ladder or articulating platform, mounted on a vehicle that also carries several different-length extension ladders, extrication gear, ventilation equipment, and lighting. Some trucks can reach as high as 200 feet.

Color Schemes. The color of fire apparatus is as broad a spectrum as the rainbow. Most people think of red when they think of fire engines. Stephen Solomon and James King (1995) have conducted psychological research on human visual and auditory perception. According to their findings, humans are most sensitive to greenish-yellow colors under dim conditions, which make the lime green fire truck easiest to see in dim lighting. Color schemes are important when designing a vehicle and should be taken into consideration for safety reasons.

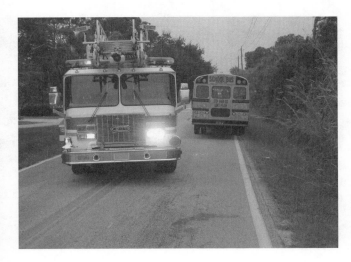

FIGURE 5.8 ◆ A quint can be used as a pumper or ladder depending on the needs.

FIGURE 5.9 ◆ An aerial can be a bucket truck or a straight stick ladder as pictured here. This is also a tiller, which requires a driver in the rear cab to steer the back portion of the truck.

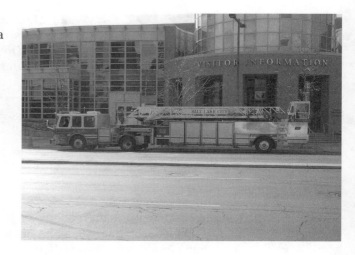

◆ OPERATION

Besides the limitations put on the vehicle by the weight restrictions, there are differences between driving a car and driving an emergency vehicle. These differences make an emergency vehicle harder to drive than a car. The driver needs to know these differences and understand how they affect the ability to operate the emergency vehicle safely.

SIZE

An emergency vehicle is larger than a standard car. It is wider, longer, and taller, which makes it harder to maneuver. The emergency vehicle's width and length affect turning; its height means the driver must be aware of height clearances; for example, parking garages, bridges or overpasses (Figures 5.10a and 5.10b), and covered entrances.

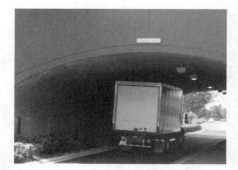

FIGURE 5.10A ◆ There are a number of overpasses that have height restrictions. It is important for emergency vehicle drivers to know the limitations of their vehicles including height and weight.

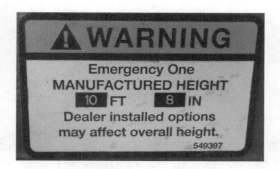

FIGURE 5.10B ◆ The emergency vehicle typically has the height of the vehicle on a placard near the driver as shown here.

> ### Points to Ponder
>
> What other problems can the size of the emergency vehicle cause?
> In your area, in what specific places is there a need to exercise extra caution because of the size of the emergency vehicle?

WEIGHT

An emergency vehicle typically weighs more than a car. This is important to remember because it takes longer to accelerate and brake. When pulling out into traffic, for example, an emergency vehicle does not move out as quickly as a car. When braking, the driver needs more room to come to a complete stop.

WEIGHT RESTRICTIONS

No matter what type of emergency vehicle drivers operate, they must know the vehicle's weight restrictions in order to operate safely during all driving conditions. When an emergency vehicle arrives at the facility from the manufacturer, it is labeled with a gross weight. Drivers can usually find this information on the weight/payload certification sticker mounted on the body in a conspicuous location.

The payload capacity is part of gross weight and represents the MAXIMUM safe weight of the emergency equipment, crew, and patients in ambulances. This capacity has already been determined at the facility and should be displayed on the vehicle.

The payload capacity is used to determine, after considering equipment weight, how many crew members and, with transport vehicles, how many patients it can safely transport. The national standard for determining the weight of one person is 175 pounds per person.

Each emergency service organization should have a current loading plan in the vehicle logbook. The loading plan should have the current payload, that is, how much the vehicle can carry. The loading plan should evenly distribute the weight of the patient (if an ambulance), crew, and equipment. Too much weight in one location can change the handling characteristics of the vehicle. As equipment is added to the emergency vehicle, the new weight should be figured and the loading plan updated. Remember that for each piece of equipment added, the passenger weight that can be safely carried decreases.

Knowing how many people you can carry and keeping an accurate loading plan will help you decide how to load your vehicle. Just because you have seats available does not mean that you can load a passenger into each one. And just because the ambulance is designed to carry only two patients does not mean that you leave a third patient at a crash scene rather than loading that person. Two children might actually equal one adult person.

The driver's good judgment is needed. If it is the only ambulance at a crash scene, there may be more weight than ideally recommended loaded on the vehicle. In this instance the driver needs to adjust his or her driving to accommodate the situation.

VISIBILITY

Because of the size and configuration of most emergency vehicles, blind spots along both sides are normal and to be expected. An emergency vehicle driver must be aware of these areas and recognize that side view mirrors often will not allow full visibility of these areas. Other crew members can assist the emergency vehicle driver in viewing these difficult areas.

Points to Ponder

Locate the gross weight information and the payload information on each of your organization's vehicles. Identify whether the weight creates issue for any of the roadways in your jurisdiction.

What are the weight/patient restrictions with only the ambulance operator and an EMT as crew?

With a crew of _____, our ambulances can safely carry _____ pounds or _____ patients.

What are the weight/patient restrictions with one operator and two EMTs as crew?

With a crew of _____, our ambulances can safely carry _____ pounds or _____ patients.

What are the weight restrictions with only the apparatus operator and a crew of two?

With a crew of _____, our apparatus can safely carry _____ pounds or _____ equipment.

What are the weight restrictions with one operator and three crew members?

With a crew of _____, our apparatus can safely carry _____ pounds or _____ equipment.

FOLLOWING DISTANCE

Total stopping distance consists of **perception time, reaction time,** and **braking time**. Most authorities recommend a 4-second rule as an acceptable following distance at speeds of 40 miles per hour or less, and 5 seconds for higher speeds (40 mph or greater). One rule of thumb for calculating following distance (seconds of safety cushion) is to note a stationary point that the vehicle ahead passes and then count 1,000 one, 1,000 two, and so on until your vehicle passes the same point.

A comparison of the safety cushions and total stopping distances at 40 mph, 50 mph, and 60 mph is summarized here for reference.

Speed	Safety Cushion	Distance Traveled	Distance Required to Stop (*)
40 mph	4 seconds	240 feet	210 feet
50 mph	4 seconds	320 feet	340 feet (**)
60 mph	5 seconds	400 feet	340 feet

(*): These stopping distances do not include perception distance.
(**): As illustrated, a 4-second safety cushion is not sufficient.

Rate of Closure. The emergency vehicle driver should be aware of his or her rate of closure on other vehicles and pedestrians at all times. This is to maintain a safe following distance as defined. There are many reasons people may not yield to emergency vehicles even when all warning devices are operating. Some examples include the following.

- Emergency vehicle drivers outrun the siren's effectiveness.
- Field of view is blocked.
- Direction of the sound of the siren is misinterpreted.
- Hearing impaired driver.
- Inattentive driver (loud music, cellular phone, kids, stress).
- The rate of closure by emergency vehicle driver is too fast and doesn't allow the civilian driver to perceive the presence of the emergency vehicle.

Traffic Closure from Behind. Another aspect of **space management** is to observe regularly the vehicles behind the emergency vehicle. Often, curious drivers will either follow the emergency vehicle or use the emergency vehicle to "break" traffic in an effort to move more quickly down the street or highway. In either case, the emergency vehicle driver must be aware of the presence of any vehicles and keep them under observation. Signaling any intent to turn, pass, or stop is extremely important to keep the civilian driver(s) from following too closely or colliding with the emergency vehicle.

SPEED MANAGEMENT

There are two primary rules regarding speed management. Although they may seem extreme, it is essential that an emergency vehicle not lose control because of excessive speed.

1. **Emergency vehicles must not be driven in excess of the posted speed limits regardless of any traffic law exemption.** Within urban areas, average response speed is less than 35 miles per hour. If speeds are increased to 45 mph, and the average response distance is one mile; a total of about 23 seconds is saved. In rural areas, if average response speeds are increased from 55 mph to 65 mph over a response distance of 5 miles, a total of about 51 seconds is saved in the response time.
2. **Emergency vehicles must not exceed cautionary speeds. Cautionary speeds** such as limitations on hills, curves, or ramps are designed for passenger cars. Emergency vehicles are typically heavier overall and more top heavy than cars. The posted cautionary speeds are an even more important consideration for emergency vehicles.

BASE MANEUVERS

Competent emergency vehicle drivers understand and properly complete all of the basic driving maneuvers necessary to operate the emergency vehicle they are certified to drive.

STEERING

Steering an emergency vehicle, whether driving nonemergency, responding to an emergency, or making an evasive maneuver, requires certain habits, which include

- Using both hands on the steering wheel. Exceptions include operating another device on the vehicle such as shifting or turning on the windshield wipers.
- Keeping arms inside the vehicle. Do not engage in other activities such as drinking, eating, and smoking.
- Maintaining hands in the two and ten o'clock position. (Nine and three o'clock with airbag.)

BRAKING AND STOPPING

Effective braking is essential to safe operation of an emergency vehicle. The intent is to stop the vehicle in as short a distance as possible without losing control.

In a vehicle with hydraulic brakes, this involves firmly pumping the brake pedal and releasing it prior to the locking of wheels. Air brakes require firm and steady pressure without pumping.

For vehicles equipped with an antilock braking system (ABS), whether installed in conjunction with a hydraulic or air system, proper procedures include the following.

- ❖ On vehicles equipped with air brakes, the brake pedal should be firmly pressed initially. The driver must ease up as the braking continues and ease the pressure on the brake pedal just before stopping to avoid a jerking motion.
- ❖ It is important to recognize that continuous braking over a period of time builds up a tremendous amount of heat.
- ❖ On vehicles equipped with a secondary braking system, apply the system in accordance with the directions of the manufacturer. Recognize that some applications of secondary braking systems can cause a reduction in tire traction.
- ❖ In areas where there is a high probability of braking, when passing through an intersection or traveling against traffic, the driver should place his or her foot over (cover) the brake pedal. This action will reduce reaction time.

BACKING UP

Although backing up usually occurs at slow speeds, it accounts for a disproportionate number of minor low-speed accidents and has the potential for serious consequences. Some guidelines for backing in an emergency vehicle follow.

Park as to Minimize the Need for Backing. If thought is given to the position necessary for a vehicle leaving its location, a simple adjustment in the final placement can minimize or even eliminate the need for backing.

Give Audible Notice That Backing Will Occur. If the vehicle is equipped with a backup alarm, shift the vehicle to reverse while applying the brakes. This will initiate most backup alarms. If the vehicle is not equipped with a backup alarm, touch the horn lightly three times before beginning the backup maneuver.

Use a Spotter. Locate a spotter at the left rear of the vehicle whenever backing (Figure 5.11). The driver must be able to see the spotter through the mirror and vice versa. The driver and the spotter must make mutual eye contact. If the spotter disappears from the mirror, the driver must immediately stop. If a spotter is not available conduct a walk around the vehicle first before backing.

Understand Hand Signals and Audible Signals. Standard hand signals are illustrated in Chapter 7 on communications. Be sure that all drivers and spotters have been trained in the meaning of the signals. When using an audible signal (buzzer), *one* means stop immediately, *two* means to go forward, and *three* means back up.

Use Side Mirrors Whenever Backing. The driver should not attempt to lean out to the mirror or turn around trying to see. Periodically check the right side mirror for objects in the path of the vehicle. Mirrors should be adjusted prior to leaving the station.

Check the Front Corners of the Vehicle. This is especially important if the vehicle is turning while backing. Either the right or left front may swing around and hit a fixed object that did not initially appear to be a potential problem.

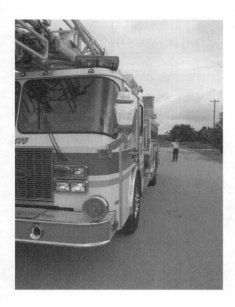

FIGURE 5.11 ◆ It is imperative that there is at least one spotter when backing an emergency vehicle.

Maintain Speed Control. Backing up should be done at an extremely low speed. It is imperative to maintain tight control on the speed of the emergency vehicle.

LANE CHANGING

Lane changing on multilane roads can usually be accomplished with little difficulty provided some basic rules are followed, such as:

- Plan ahead.
- Signal intention.
- Practice space management. (This is especially important in areas that have blind spots.)
- Make the change of lanes smoothly.
- Always signal before turning. Do not operate an emergency vehicle with its four-way flashers going. This prohibits the emergency driver from properly signaling the turn.

These principles should also be applied when merging onto a high-speed highway (entrance ramp) or leaving the highway (exit ramp).

TURNING

Two basic principles need to be followed but are often ignored or violated.

- **Always signal before turning.** Do not operate an emergency vehicle with its four-way flashers working. This prohibits the emergency vehicle driver from properly signaling a turn.
- **Whenever possible, turn from one proper lane into another proper lane.** If turning left, position the emergency vehicle in the left turn lane, or in the left lane. Avoid crossing lanes in order to execute the turn. Position the emergency vehicle into the proper lane after making the turn. This is especially important on multilane streets.

PASSING

It is often necessary for the emergency vehicle driver to pass other vehicles during an emergency response. At highway speeds (40 to 60 mph), a safe pass can be completed in about 10 seconds. The emergency vehicle will travel about 1/6 mile (825 feet) at 55 mph during that 10-second period. A rule of thumb for passing and visibility distance follows.

Starting Speed	Passing Distance	Visibility Distance
30 mph	450 ft	900 ft
35 mph	525 ft	1,050 ft
45 mph	675 ft	1,350 ft
55 mph	825 ft	1,650 ft
60 mph	900 ft	1,800 ft

Other considerations when passing vehicles include the speed of the vehicle, visibility limits (such as crests of hills), blind curves, or environmental limitations.

Passing should include the following steps:

- Check traffic both ahead and behind.
- Check sides and double-check blind spots.
- Signal before initiating the pass.
- Accelerate while changing lanes.
- Signal before returning to the driving lane.
- Check mirror before returning to the driving lane.
- Cancel directional signal and resume cruising speed.

One must be alert for vehicles planning to move into the passing lane.

NEGOTIATING INTERSECTIONS

Intersection procedures are extremely important. A large percentage of accidents involving emergency vehicles occur at intersections. Careful consideration should be given to establishing policies for addressing both controlled and uncontrolled intersections (Figure 5.12).

An intersection that does not offer a control device (stop sign, yield sign, or traffic signal) in the direction of travel of the emergency vehicle or when a signal is green for the emergency vehicle, is defined as an uncontrolled intersection. Emergency drivers should:

- Scan the intersection for possible hazards (right turns on red, pedestrians, vehicles traveling very fast, etc). Observe traffic in all four directions: left, right, front, and back.
- Slow down and cover the brake pedal with the foot.

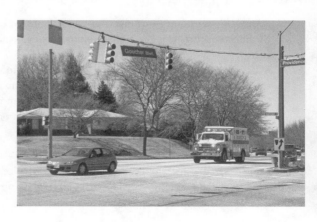

FIGURE 5.12 ◆ Emergency vehicle drivers need to utilize caution when proceeding through intersections. (*Courtesy of Pearson Education/PH College*)

- Change the siren cadence not less than 200 feet from the intersection.
- Avoid using the opposing lane of traffic, if at all possible.

Any controlled intersection requires a complete stop by the emergency vehicle driver. In addition to bringing the vehicle to a complete stop, these additional steps must be followed:

- Do not rely on warning devices to clear traffic.
- Scan the intersection for possible hazards as well as driver options.
- Begin to slow down well before reaching the intersection, and cover the brake pedal with the driver's foot.
- Change the siren cadence not less than 200 feet from the intersection.
- Scan the intersection for possible passing options (pass on right, left, wait, etc.).
- Avoid using the opposing lane of traffic, if at all possible.
- Come to a complete stop.
- Establish eye contact with the other vehicle drivers; have partner communicate all is clear; reconfirm all other vehicles are stopped.
- Proceed one lane of traffic at a time. Treat each lane as a separate intersection.

CRASH AVOIDANCE

Despite the best training and precautions, sometimes a crash may be unavoidable. If such an occurrence is seen as inevitable, there are several things an emergency vehicle driver can do.

Identify Escape Route. The emergency vehicle driver must scan ahead along the roadway, shoulders, and/or median to identify any potential escape routes that can be safely used to avoid a crash. Certain areas such as the crest of a hill or a curve can minimize identifying potential escape routes.

Brake Smoothly and Firmly. If there is enough room to stop or no escape route is available, emergency braking may be the only way to avoid a collision or minimize its consequences. The goal of emergency braking is to produce the shortest possible stopping distance without locking the wheel or losing control.

With hydraulic brakes, emergency braking is accomplished by hard pressure to the pedal without locking the wheels. If the vehicle does not have antilock brakes (ABS), this should be followed by quick, firm jabs that result in steady pressure. Air brakes should be applied with a steady pressure at the beginning and eased off as the vehicle slows. The foot pressure is eased just before the vehicle stops in order to avoid a jerk and rebound.

Air brakes should not be fanned (pumped). Finally, vehicles with ABS should have the brakes applied as hard as possible and held down until the vehicle stops.

Accelerate Smoothly and Rapidly. Evasive acceleration is making a quick burst of speed. This maneuver should be used to avoid a collision with side approaching vehicles, merging vehicles, or quickly closing vehicles.

Steer to Avoid a Head-on Impact. When one is sure that a collision is unavoidable, choose an object with which to collide. Always choose the course least likely to result in a serious accident. Head-on collisions are the most damaging. Attempt to sideswipe or brush another object. Impact-absorbing objects are better to choose than large, immobile items that will not "give." Examples of impact-absorbing objects are parked cars, brushes and shrubs, and small signs.

◆ ROAD CONSTRUCTION AND ENGINEERING

ROAD SURFACES

There are various road surfaces an emergency vehicle drives on. Although the road surface greatly influences the quality of the ride, the driver can't control it or change it. Drivers must learn how to adjust their driving to match the road conditions. When roads are built, the engineers plan each road to handle different kinds of traffic, and they use different materials to build each road.

Asphalt. Asphalt is not as durable as some other common surfaces and requires repair more often (Figure 5.13). Repairs normally consist of patching the surface with more asphalt material or with tar to fill in cracks. These patches then create bumps in the road. Asphalt is at its worst during the hot summer months. When it's very hot, the oils used to make asphalt bleed to the surface, making it slick, especially when it rains. An asphalt roadway can also become wavy with heavy use during extremely hot days. Not only is that very uncomfortable to ride over, but the driver does not have full control of the emergency vehicle because the tires are in contact with the road only half the time.

Concrete. During hot weather, concrete expands and may break up at its joints, leaving a hole in the surface. Concrete also settles more than other road surfaces. As the earth under it settles, the concrete sections develop severe dips, causing the emergency vehicle to bounce heavily between dips. Concrete road surfaces also glaze over very quickly in freezing conditions, much more so than asphalt.

Dirt/Gravel. Dirt and gravel roads are tricky to drive on if the driver is not used to them. Because of the irregular shape, size, and weight of the stones, they move about easily. This movement can cause a vehicle to go out of control with only a slight action by the operator. Braking on gravel can cause a vehicle to slide easily. When following another vehicle on dirt and gravel roads, stay back to increase visibility and to avoid flying stones (Figure 5.14).

Transitions Between Surface Types One of the most dangerous areas of a road surface is that place where the surface changes from one type to another, such as from hard

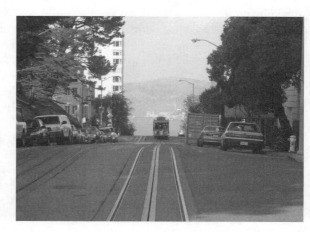

FIGURE 5.13 ◆ Asphalt roads typically need more repair work; however, it is very commonly used for roadway surfaces. This photo also shows how other factors such as trolley tracks may be part of the roadway.

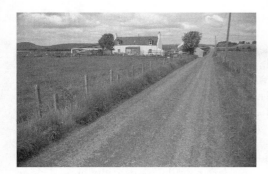

FIGURE 5.14 ◆ Dirt roads sometimes present challenges to emergency vehicle drivers. The surface may cause a rough ride and the width of the roads is typically narrow. (*Courtesy of John Serafin*)

surface to gravel. When this happens, drivers must change their driving style before moving onto the gravel road, or they could easily lose control of the emergency vehicle.

ROAD CONDITIONS

Bumps. One of the easiest ways to see a bump in the road ahead is to watch the vehicles ahead bounce as they hit the bump. This gives the driver time to slow the emergency vehicle and lessen the effects of the bump. Another way to see bumps is to look at the road surface itself. A clear path in the center of the roadway followed by a dark spot indicates a large dip or bump in the road. When vehicles hit the bump, loose oil and debris under the car fall off, creating the dark spot.

Mud. Mud on the roadway causes problems, first by creating a slick surface, and second, by filling the tread pattern of the tire and making the reaction ability of the tire very slow.

Potholes. Potholes are holes in the road surface, sometimes at the joint of a concrete road or, more commonly, where an asphalt surface has failed. Potholes cannot be easily fixed and keep returning, getting wider and deeper each time they reappear. Potholes cause two problems. First, they can destroy the emergency vehicle's tires or suspension system. Second, they can cause the driver to lose control as one corner of the emergency vehicle drops into the hole and the emergency vehicle frame twists. Both problems cause hardship for the personnel and increase the discomfort of the passengers.

During prerun route planning, the driver should be sure to select roads known to be free of potholes. And, if a pothole is discovered, the driver should pass this information on to the dispatcher so that the route information can be updated. The best way to handle a pothole is to try to drive around it. If you must drive through a pothole,

- ✦ Release the brakes just as you get to the pothole. If you hit a pothole with the brakes on, the front tire can actually stop as you cross the leading edge of the pothole. By the time you get to the other side, the wheel is no longer turning and the impact can tear the tire apart.
- ✦ Hit the pothole squarely, rather than on the side of the tire. The face of the tire can take considerably more impact than the sidewall.

Animals, Tree Limbs, and Miscellaneous Objects. Another problem a driver will encounter is objects in the road. These could be animals, tree limbs, or dropped debris. Everyone's natural reaction is to swerve to avoid hitting objects in the road, but this often causes more problems than the object itself. Instead of swerving:

- ✦ If it is a small object, hit the object head-on.
- ✦ Do not cause a larger collision by swerving into another lane or oncoming traffic.
- ✦ If it is a large animal or object, maintain control of the vehicle and attempt to avoid a head-on collision.

Bridges and Ramps. Bridges and ramps can cause control problems if the driver is not accustomed to driving on them. Bridges often have an open metal grating over the main expanse of the bridge. When the emergency vehicle's tires cross this grating, the tire tread tries to align itself with the grating, causing the wheels to jump and jerk. The best way to handle the grating is to slow while approaching the bridge and then hold the steering wheel firmly in both hands. There will still be some jerking of the wheel, but the driver should be able to control it by using both hands.

Bridges and ramps often have a reinforced concrete bed, which will freeze before the roadway on either side. This is because, as the temperature drops, the cold air circulates around the concrete bed of the bridge or ramp and the concrete becomes cold faster than the roadway that is built on the warmer ground. Use caution when driving on bridges and ramps during freezing temperatures.

Curves. When highway engineers design a new roadway, they use the natural contour of the land. Most of the time, they can re-form the land slightly and create comfortable roads. Sometimes, they can't. In hilly or mountainous areas, following the land's natural contour often results with roads designed with deep or multiple curves.

This means that the driver can never take a curve for granted. The driver must enter a curve carefully, following the posted recommended speed limit for the curve, and watch how the curve changes as the driver continues. If it gets tighter, the driver must slow down even more to retain control of the emergency vehicle.

Banking: Most curves that are created for today's highways are banked to help the driver maintain speed while going through the turn. This was not always true in the early days of road building when speed was not a problem. If a roadway is built so that the inside of the curve is lower than the outside edge, then it is banked properly. If the inside edge is level with or higher than the outside edge, you will have to slow down to complete the curve.

Posted Speed Limits: The speed limit posted at the beginning of most curves is the recommended speed that allows the driver to safely continue through the curve. This speed is often lower than the prevailing highway speed because of the amount of banking or because the curve is a compound curve.

Crown. Older roads and those in areas that receive a lot of rain often have a crown in the middle of the road. When a road has a crown, the center of the road is higher than both edges. Because the crown is normally not very high, it does not pose a problem on a straight road. But in a corner, the crown acts like improper banking and works against the vehicle going around the corner. Again, the driver must slow down to retain control of the emergency vehicle.

Water Drainage. Road crowns are essential for good water drainage during rainy periods. When water drains quickly from the road surface, the danger of hydroplaning is reduced. Some concrete roads accomplish drainage by cutting grooves into the road surface. Hopefully, the water will drain completely away from the road, thus eliminating the dangers of hydroplaning and possibly losing control of the vehicle. The driver must look ahead and remain clear of areas of standing water and water collected alongside the roadway.

ROADSIDE ENGINEERING

Roadside engineering consists of all the signs, guardrails, and barriers along the roadway. These include speed limit, no passing, and intersection signs, and the safety barriers beside deep ditches or bridges.

◆ **DRIVING SKILLS THAT INFLUENCE THE QUALITY OF THE RIDE**

Let's now look at some of the driving skills that influence the quality of the ride. These skills will permit the driver to meet any challenge of driving.

ADVERSE EFFECTS ON PATIENTS WHEN RIDING IN AN AMBULANCE

Both sick and injured patients may feel nauseated. When placed on the stretcher and put into the ambulance head first, they may become even more nauseated from motion sickness. If the ride is not smooth and comfortable, their nausea may increase and they may vomit, causing further complications. Also, patients will tense their muscles to counteract the pitching forces encountered in turns and while vehicles are braking and accelerating. When patients have broken bones or internal injuries, these muscle contractions will aggravate their condition.

ADVERSE EFFECTS ON PASSENGERS WHEN RIDING IN AN AMBULANCE

Patient care cannot continue if the medical team has to hold on. Patient care must continue uninterrupted while en route to the hospital. Several basic and advanced life support skills are difficult to perform in a moving ambulance, no matter how smoothly it is driven. These skills are impossible if the ambulance is bouncing and swaying as it is driven down the road. For example, studies have demonstrated that CPR is best performed in a moving ambulance that is being driven at speeds below 25 mph and not being driven in the emergency mode.

HOW DRIVING SKILLS INFLUENCE THE QUALITY OF THE RIDE

Suspension System.   Like most cars and trucks, the emergency vehicle is a body that is attached to the engine and wheels with a suspension system. The suspension system is designed to do two things: (1) to keep all four wheels firmly on the ground, no matter what the surface is like, so that the driver can steer, brake, and accelerate; and (2) to isolate the body and its occupants from the bouncing of the wheels when they hit bumps and uneven road surfaces.

Because of the design of the suspension system, when the driver speeds up, brakes, or takes corners, the body leans. You have felt the body lean when a driver brakes hard or goes around a corner too fast. Because an emergency vehicle is a heavy vehicle and crammed full of equipment, it has a stiff suspension and the amount of lean is not great, but it must still be taken into account when driving.

The four main driving skills are cornering, braking, accelerating, and maintaining appropriate speed.

Cornering.   The force that must be considered when going around a corner or a curve is called centrifugal force. It throws a body toward the outside of a curve as the vehicle goes around the curve. For example, if you travel down the highway at 55 mph and enter a curve to the left, you feel yourself being pushed toward the right side of the vehicle. You naturally lean to the left to counteract this push. That works fine for the passengers sitting upright in the seats, but if driving an ambulance, the patient strapped to the stretcher can't lean. And the medical team can't lean, and their equipment can't lean. So the driver has to reduce the force that they feel. And the force is reduced by slowing down and making smooth turns so that they can balance and stay balanced throughout the turn.

Braking. Body lean is a very important factor when the driver brakes or accelerates. When the driver brakes hard, the nose of the vehicle drops downward and all the weight of the vehicle, and its occupants, shifts toward the front. When the driver accelerates hard, just the reverse happens. Everything shifts toward the back. Just like when cornering, body lean is not a big problem for the driver who is sitting upright in a seat with a seat belt on, but the passengers and, if driving an ambulance, the patient aren't as fortunate. They are forced to lean forward and backward as the driver brakes hard and then accelerates. They can't see what's coming so that they can brace themselves. The driver has to protect them by braking no harder than necessary and by accelerating smoothly and steadily. When braking, the driver must take two factors into consideration: reaction time and braking time.

Reaction Time and Braking Time: Reaction time is a combination of the time it takes drivers to see and understand that they will have to brake and to actually move their foot to the brake pedal. Braking time is the time it takes the brakes to bring the vehicle to a complete stop. Total stopping distance, then, is equal to the reaction time plus the braking time.

Training can reduce reaction time. When the brain is under stress, as it is when you recognize a problem ahead, the body will react the way it was trained to react. Factors that can affect reaction time are illness (e.g., cold, flu), a physical injury that could affect the ability to maneuver the vehicle, medication(s), and lack of sleep. All of these factors influence the reaction time and ultimately determine whether the driver will be able to stop in the time (distance) available. The driver needs a way to maximize the time and distance available for braking by placing the vehicle in the safest position.

4-5-12 Rule: One recommended way to calculate where the driver should place the vehicle is called the 4-5-12 rule. It permits the driver to see what is happening well ahead of the vehicle and to take action early. The 4-5-12 rule states the following:

- Maintain a 4-second interval between your vehicle and the vehicle ahead for speeds below 55 mph.
- Increase the following distance to 5 seconds when speeds get above 55 mph to allow for increased stopping distances at higher speeds.
- Give yourself a 12-second visual lead time. In other words, look ahead for possible hazards and alternate paths of travel should an emergency arise.
- Use your 12-second visual lead time to constantly make speed and position adjustments. Simplify your choices as much as possible. Don't tackle more hazards than you absolutely have to.

For example, if drivers are looking 12 seconds ahead, they will see the traffic light almost a block away turn red. Drivers are able to respond by removing their foot from the accelerator and begin slowing early. Then by smoothly applying the brakes, drivers can bring the vehicle to a stop without having to slam on the brakes. When traffic clears and drivers can proceed forward, they can gently release the brakes and begin to accelerate at a steady pace. As drivers continue to look ahead, they begin slowing for that next corner and make a smooth turn that doesn't throw the passengers from one side to the other. Look ahead, see what is happening all around, and begin actions early. Driving will improve and the driver will begin providing a smooth ride for the crew and the patient.

> **Point to Ponder**
>
> If two emergency vehicles are going down the same road, one at 55 mph and one at 35 mph, which one do you think is providing the smoother ride?
>
> *Answer: The one at 35 mph.*

Accelerating. To reduce body lean and strain on the passengers, accelerate smoothly and steadily. Steadily does not mean to push the accelerator down quickly and hold it there. Instead, drivers can provide a more comfortable ride by using a smooth, slow rate of acceleration. This method requires that drivers initially apply a feather touch to the accelerator and then continue to move the accelerator pedal downward gradually but steadily. As drivers approach the desired speed, they hold the accelerator still for a moment. The driver then begins to ease up on the accelerator to the point where they are using just enough engine power to maintain the selected speed.

To practice, drivers can do two things: (1) Pretend there is a raw egg between their right foot and the accelerator pedal. Try not to break the egg. (2) Practice the following but not do it on a response. Place a half-full cup of water on the dash and try to accelerate (and brake and take corners) without spilling any of the water.

Speed. Of course, the emergency vehicle doing 35 mph is providing a smoother ride. High speed makes the ride rougher than lower speed does. The faster an emergency vehicle goes, the more it bounces. Each turn of the steering wheel throws the emergency vehicle harder from side to side.

When dealing with ambulances transporting patients, high speed normally makes the patient's ride so much worse that it is actually detrimental to the patient, not beneficial. The unit may get to the hospital faster, but the ride may have made the patient's injuries worse just from the bouncing. And the medical team hasn't been able to work because they had to hold on to counteract the effects of a less than smooth ride. Most patients are stabilized and on life support, if necessary, before the ambulance leaves the emergency scene. Therefore, speed is not as necessary when transporting the patient to the medical facility.

Slow down for curves and corners and take them smoothly. Brake smoothly and no more than is required. Accelerate smoothly and steadily and go no faster than necessary. There is a delicate balance between the operator, the machine, and the environment:

- The machine, or emergency vehicle, is the most reliable and is responsible for only 1 percent of crashes.
- The environment is constantly changing and is responsible for approximately 10 percent of the crashes.
- That leaves the driver. The driver is responsible for a large percentage of emergency vehicle crashes. The driver is also responsible for the successful merging of the three-part relationship.

Preventable Collisions. Most collisions are preventable. The key to preventing collisions is called **situational awareness.** This means that drivers must be constantly aware of their situation by remaining alert at all times, knowing what's going on all around the emergency vehicle, and driving defensively. There is no time to relax while driving. To begin talking about situational awareness, let's discuss defensive driving.

Point to Ponder

What do you think is meant by "maintaining a safety cushion"?

Answer: Driving so that drivers position their vehicle in relation to other vehicles and possible hazards so that drivers have a cushion of empty space completely surrounding the emergency vehicle.

Defensive Driving: Defensive driving means doing everything reasonably possible to avoid being involved in a preventable crash, regardless of what the law is, what the other driver does, or adverse driving conditions. Defensive driving requires continual exercise of good judgment and good driving habits with an awareness that all other drivers cannot be relied on to drive properly and safely. When the driver is driving an emergency vehicle, the driver is operating a lethal weapon on a crowded, public roadway. The driver has to expect the unexpected and be prepared to act. It is vital to have a plan of action at all times. The driver has to have the final responsibility for his or her safety and that of the passengers.

Maintaining a Safety Cushion: Drivers want to allow enough room around the emergency vehicle so that they can identify possible hazards, decide on a course of action, and react by either bringing the emergency vehicle to a controlled stop or maneuvering to avoid the hazard. In a road emergency, drivers don't want to get boxed in without an escape route. Maintaining a safety cushion around the emergency vehicle reduces the chances of being involved in a crash. Obviously, the safest position for the emergency vehicle is as far away from any possible collision hazard as possible. It's easy to be involved in a crash with the vehicles in front, beside, and behind.

Tailgaters: Tailgaters are people who follow too closely behind the vehicle in front of them. Normally, they are so close that if the driver has to stop suddenly, they don't have time to stop or prevent running into the back of the emergency vehicle. Drivers should not allow other drivers to tailgate them. Use any method to make them pass or fall back. If necessary, slow and pull to the right of your lane to encourage them to pass. Tailgaters are safer for the driver if they are tailgating the vehicle in front of you. The driver at least can see them and plan his or her action if they run into the other vehicle.

Multiple Responding Units: Emergency units responding along the same route should maintain 300 to 400 feet of distance between them. To make sure the other motorists know there is more than one emergency unit in the area, the driver should use a different siren tone than the vehicle ahead of it. Change tones at intersections and allow the siren to partially wind down prior to the intersection so that both you and the other motorists will be alerted that there are multiple emergency vehicles in the area.

Communication: To get the maximum advantage from proper positioning, the safety cushion, and defensive driving, the driver must communicate with other drivers. Remember: Always expect the unexpected from the other drivers. Don't assume that they see or hear you. And even if they do see and hear you, don't assume that they will give you the right-of-way.

◆ **PRECRASH PLANNING**

Sometimes a crash is going to happen even though the driver has done everything possible to avoid it. The driver needs to plan ahead for that situation and think about how to handle it. There are three things to do to reduce the effects of a crash.

1. Keep the doors locked. A locked door will withstand many times more strain in a crash than an unlocked door. You typically won't fly out of a locked door, and you are generally better off staying inside your vehicle during a crash rather than being thrown from it.
2. Always wear your seat belt. It's the best protection you have in a collision. Seat belts must be worn in all positions in the vehicle, both front and back of vehicle. Provide guidance on local regulations for seat belt use.
3. Good housecleaning habits also can prevent serious injury. Keep loose items, such as clipboards, secured. Properly secure your equipment to reduce the number of potential missiles inside your vehicle.

◆ **BASIC MANEUVERS**

BRAKING AND STOPPING

Braking is very effective in stopping the emergency vehicle if it is done properly, but it can be hazardous if done improperly. If the driver applies too much pressure and locks the brakes, the wheels will skid and the driver will lose steering control. If all four wheels skid, the rear end of the vehicle may slide to the side and the driver will lose control of the vehicle. To avoid these problems, the driver must keep the wheels turning.

Apply pressure on the brake pedal with the upper half of the right foot, preferably with the heel contacting the floor. Try to pivot on the heel for greater sensitivity on the pedal. This involves fewer leg muscles and reduces unwanted "pumping" or "lockup" of the brakes. In a straight line, the most efficient way to brake to a stop on any surface is by gently but firmly pumping the brakes. Braking, when properly done, involves firmly pressing the brakes to the point before lockup, then gently releasing them so that there is a minimum amount of front-end weight change and bounce. The main point is never to lock up the brakes. Remember, ABS brakes work differently; refer to Chapter 8 for additional information on ABS brakes.

- Avoid staring at the front of the vehicle while braking.
- Check the conditions to the rear to avoid being hit from behind.
- Check conditions to the side in an effort to find an escape route.
- Search 12 seconds ahead to see whether the conditions that forced your braking actions have changed.

MAKING LANE CHANGES

When making lane changes on a multilane road, the driver must plan ahead. Using the 12-second method, plan the lane change well in advance. Signal the intentions and look for reactions from the other drivers. If the new lane remains clear, gently steer into the new lane and continue straight ahead. A properly executed lane change should be smooth, and the passengers should never feel the change in the position of the vehicle.

When changing lanes for passing on multilane highways:

- Check other lanes for problems and a clear path.
- Check your mirrors to find an opening in the adjacent lane.
- Signal intentions by having the signal lever in the "on" position for at least three seconds before changing lanes.
- Check blind spots by making a quick glance over your shoulder in the direction the vehicle is to travel.
- Slightly turn the wheel for a smooth, gradual, accurate movement.
- Control speed with a slight increase in speed, if required.
- Time vehicle arrival into the adjacent lane to avoid interfering with other traffic.

PASSING

Passing on Two-Lane Roads. When on two-lane roads, the driver will sometimes have to pass a slower vehicle ahead. If the vehicle refuses to pull over or if there is no space beside the road for it to pull over, then the driver will have to plan and execute a pass. Passing on a two-lane road is a very dangerous maneuver because, for several moments, the driver is in the lane of approaching traffic. The closing speed on the approaching vehicle is the total of your speed and its speed. When passing at 55 mph, your vehicle and the oncoming vehicle will be about a half mile closer at the end of the passing maneuver than when you started. The driver has to ask him- or herself whether there is the space and if the risk is worth the few seconds saved. To pass a slower vehicle on a two-lane road, the driver must visually clear the oncoming lane, change lanes, accelerate past the slower vehicle, and smoothly pull back into his or her lane in just a matter of a few seconds.

Passing Stopped Traffic. Attempting to pass stopped traffic is a hazardous situation. The driver should pass stopped traffic only when able to determine the reason for the stopping. While the driver is passing stopped traffic, part of the escape route has been eliminated. If oncoming traffic suddenly appears or one of the stopped drivers suddenly pulls in front of the vehicle, the driver may have nowhere to go.

BACKING UP

The driver might be surprised to learn that Childs and Ptacnik, in *Emergency Ambulance Driving* (1986), report that backing accidents account for 85 percent of all single-vehicle crashes involving ambulances. This is normally a very slow maneuver, but remember that the area directly behind the vehicle is not visible to the operator. If backing is going to be necessary, it is best to do the backing when first arriving at the scene.

The driver should always use a ground guide positioned at the left rear of the vehicle to help. Position the guide so that you can see the guide in the side view mirrors and so that the guide can see all the obstacles behind the vehicle. Use agreed-on hand signals and, if there is any confusion, stop and clear up the confusion before continuing. When backing, the driver will either back in a straight line or make turns while backing.

For straight-line backing:

- Position your body so that you can properly use the side view mirrors.
- Position both hands on the wheel at nine and three o'clock.

- Make sure that you have a clear view to the rear.
- Begin to accelerate slowly.
- Keep hand movement on the steering wheel to a minimum.

For turning while backing:

- Position your body so that you can properly use the side view mirrors.
- Position both hands on the wheel at nine and three o'clock.
- Frequently check the front corners of the vehicle—remember that, as you turn, it is the front end that moves sideways.
- Begin to accelerate slowly.
- Turn the steering wheel while maintaining firm control, always keeping your hands on the wheel.
- Maintain speed control; in close quarters, creep the vehicle.

PARKING

Correct parking of the emergency vehicle prevents it from being hit by other vehicles at the scene of a crash or at other locations. Parking in an urban setting is the toughest parking problem. The driver has to search for a place to park and then squeeze the vehicle into a tight space while trying to keep from impeding other traffic or getting the vehicle hit by other vehicles. Provide guidance on local policy on parking at crash sites and other locations

Perpendicular or Stall Parking. Backing into a perpendicular parking space is highly recommended. The driver can get into and out of a tighter area than if parked forward in. When a vehicle is backed into a space, the driver is able to move it quicker in case of an emergency. To park in a perpendicular space:

- Use a ground guide.
- Position the vehicle two to three feet from the parked vehicles on the right.
- Stop the vehicle when the driver's body appears to be lined up with the center of the parking space.
- Select a 45-degree target—use the left corner post blind spot of the windshield as a target guide.
- Creep forward while rapidly turning the steering wheel—check for traffic. Aim for the 45-degree target. Set the tires straight.
- Shift into reverse.
- Line your vehicle up with the space and, looking over your right shoulder, aim the vehicle for the space.
- Back to the rear pivot point.
- Creep backward and turn the steering wheel.
- Get the vehicle straight in the space.
- Creep backward and straighten the wheels.
- Back to the rear parking line.

Angle Parking. Angle parking is used when there are 30- to 45-degree angle parking spaces. This type of parking is designed for head-in parking. To park in an angled space:

- Before parking, check the side view mirrors and check the parking space.
- Position the vehicle at least six to eight feet away from the side of the parked vehicles.

◆ **94** CHAPTER 5 *Emergency Vehicle Characteristics and Driving*

- See the center of the space without your line of sight curving across the parking line.
- Creep forward and turn the wheel.
- Line up with target in center of space.
- Straighten the wheels.
- Stop at front parking line.

To back out of the angle parking space:

- Use a ground guide.
- Back slowly.
- Check the traffic as you back up.
- Check all corners of the vehicle.
- Clear the fender of the car on the left, then turn the steering wheel hard.
- Straighten the wheels.
- Shift to drive and move forward.

TURNING

There are several turning maneuvers that need to be covered. The simplest turns are the right and left corners. In a left turn, the driver must cross the near lane before turning into the travel lane. The vehicle is exposed in the intersection longer than when making a right turn. The driver must give oncoming traffic more time.

U-Turn. The U-turn also leaves your vehicle exposed to both oncoming and ongoing traffic. To make a U-turn on a road without a median strip:

- Slow the vehicle.
- Pull to the extreme right of lane or onto the shoulder.
- Check traffic in both directions.
- Signal your intent to turn.
- Turn the steering wheel hard in the direction of the turn.
- When traffic is clear in both directions, move forward and complete the turn as quickly as possible.
- Do not accelerate until after the turn is completed.
- And if the turn cannot be completed in one motion, back only as far as necessary for completion of the turnabout.
- To turn around by using the right side of the roadway or by backing into a driveway requires a two-lane roadway.

Back-Around. To complete such a back-around:

- Use a two-lane roadway.
- Use the same method as backing into a perpendicular parking space.
- Check roadway for traffic before and during the maneuver.
- Avoid driving head-in into a driveway, as this reduces maneuverability when exiting the driveway.

URBAN DRIVING

Urban driving can be one of the most challenging experiences an emergency vehicle driver will face. In urban traffic, the vehicle is surrounded by others being driven closer together than is considered safe. Traffic is constantly changing speed, some traffic may be stopped, and vehicles are entering and exiting the traffic flow from all

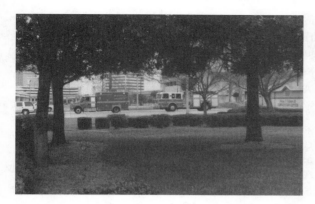

FIGURE 5.15 ◆ Emergency vehicle drivers need to pay attention to traffic, pedestrians, and a multitude of other factors when responding in an urban environment.

directions. Provide guidance on specific areas of concern in a local urban area, including agreements when entering other jurisdictions.

Obviously, the driver must be at peak alertness to drive safely in heavy urban traffic. In order for the emergency vehicle driver to drive a safe emergency response in heavy urban traffic, he or she must first understand and be able to drive routinely in heavy traffic. Urban driving requires that the driver be observant and learn to fit well within traffic.

When operating in congested city traffic, there are usually a lot of things happening. It is most helpful to have a second pair of eyes assist the driver. Because the most critical part of the response is getting to the scene and the primary duty is to drive the vehicle safely, have the officer/passenger sitting in the passenger seat help navigate and watch the traffic. This individual should also use the radio to request alternate routes from dispatch should you encounter stopped traffic or unforecasted road repairs. When it is not possible to have two people in the cab of the vehicle, slow down and always look twice. This is critical when proceeding through busy intersections.

Large buildings will limit visibility at intersections. Large buildings also limit the range of the siren and confuse people about which direction the siren is coming. The siren may get lost in all the other city noises unless the driver changes modes often, such as from wail to yelp. In urban settings—be alert for traffic entering the roadway from alleys, parking lots, driveways, and intersections. Also be alert for children playing in the streets, people exiting delivery vehicles, drivers opening doors to exit parked vehicles, bicyclists, and pedestrians at school crossings and crosswalks (Figure 5.15).

RURAL DRIVING

- ❖ Be alert for loose livestock and pets.
- ❖ Be alert for bicyclists, school buses, and children waiting for buses.
- ❖ At the higher speeds of driving in rural areas, drivers may have their windows up and the radio on and will not be able to hear the siren until you are close to them.
- ❖ Be alert for slow-moving vehicles, such as tractors, farm equipment, trucks, and horses and buggies.

TWO-LANE HIGHWAY DRIVING

Two-lane highways are dangerous because it is difficult to maneuver around other vehicles, making the driver contend with slower traffic. Do not take unwarranted chances in the hopes of getting to the destination faster. Studies have shown that the chances taken are not worth the few seconds saved by passing a slower vehicle. Remain calm and patient, and allow the other drivers sufficient time to slow and pull over so that you may pass without endangering yourself, your passengers, or the other drivers.

HIGHWAY/INTERSTATE HIGHWAY DRIVING

The special challenges of highway or interstate driving are directly related to the increased number of vehicles on the road and the increased speed of those vehicles (Figure 5.16). Use the 12-second rule to read constantly the subtle changes that occur in traffic. This includes vehicle brake lights, vehicles maneuvering for an exit, or a line of vehicles entering the highway. Always try to be at least two steps ahead of the other drivers on the road and three steps ahead of traffic.

Sudden moves, such as quickly changing lanes to get to an approaching exit or the reflex to brake after a driver misses an exit, are the cause of many interstate crashes. Know the exit you're supposed to take by at least one exit preceding it. Be aware of how other drivers may respond to the emergency vehicle. Abrupt lane changes or stops by other drivers are especially hazardous in crowded and fast moving traffic.

When exiting an interstate roadway, maintain the present speed until the emergency vehicle is completely off the interstate. Use the exit ramp for decelerating. Obviously, some common sense comes into play. If it's rush hour and the ramp is congested, the driver should not be traveling at 55 mph! The driver looking 12 seconds ahead will see the congestion and plan the highway exit accordingly. Also, shorter ramps will require a greater rate of deceleration, so be aware of this.

When entering an interstate roadway, use the entrance ramp to accelerate to the speed of traffic. Once on the interstate, progress lane by lane to the extreme left or "fast" lane. The siren should be in the yelp mode when making lane changes as this promotes vehicle recognition. Many agencies have set policy to turn their sirens and some instances their lights off when traveling on interstates. Nonetheless, use extreme caution while on the interstate. Most people mean well and are really trying to clear

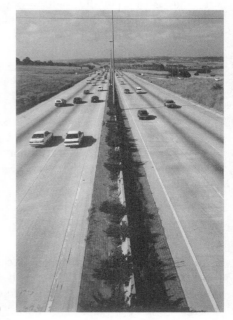

FIGURE 5.16 ◆ Interstate highways present challenges to responders. (*Courtesy of Dorling Kindersley Media Library*)

the path for the vehicle. A little patience will help keep the driver in good stead with the public and out of potential crash situations.

◆ CASE STUDY RECAP

NIOSH investigators concluded that, to minimize the risk of similar occurrences as noted in the case study, fire departments should do the following.

- Develop comprehensive apparatus maintenance programs in accordance with manufacturer's specifications and instructions that include regularly scheduled inspections, documentation, and procedures for removing apparatus out of service until major defects are repaired.
- Develop, implement, and enforce standard operating procedures (SOPs) on the use of seat belts in all emergency vehicles.
- Ensure all drivers of fire department vehicles receive driver training at least twice a year.

◆ SUMMARY

This chapter discussed the simple physics and inertia of vehicles. It is important to remember that a top-heavy vehicle such as a tanker or ambulance is inclined to tip over if the driver suddenly turns the wheel in effort to bring the wheels back onto the road. According to VFIS of York, Pennsylvania, only after the vehicle has been slowed to a safe speed, should it be gently steered back onto the road. The most common causes for skids are driving too fast for road conditions, oversteering, failing to properly appreciate weight shifts of heavy emergency vehicles/apparatus, overbraking, and failing to anticipate obstacles. The physical dynamics of operating an emergency vehicle are important for the emergency driver to understand in order to operate the vehicle in a safe manner.

Review Questions

1. Besides the type of road surface, what road conditions might affect your ride?
2. Are you more likely to have control problems going from concrete to gravel, or from gravel to concrete?
3. Just before you get to the mud, a small tree branch falls into the roadway in front of you. What would you do?
4. What problems might you have on asphalt in August when the temperature is 101 degrees?
5. What are the four main driving skills to improve?
6. What is the best way to improve these driving skills?
7. What does total stopping distance equal?
8. Why would a driver want to maintain a safety cushion of empty space around the emergency vehicle?
9. Why should you be concerned about vehicles behind you?
10. Why would multiple responding units be a problem behind your emergency vehicle?
11. On two-way streets, which takes more time and space to accomplish, a right turn or a left turn at a corner?
12. The best way to back the emergency vehicle is with the aid of what?
13. After stopping and visually clearing a controlled intersection, you accelerate normally and begin a right turn toward the medical facility. You notice that it is taking a lot of effort to turn the steering wheel. What is the probable failure and what do you do to recover?

■ ■

References

Childs, B. J., and Ptacnik, D. J. 1986. *Emergency Ambulance Driving*. Englewood Cliffs, NJ: Brady Publishing.

Fire Apparatus Manufacturers' Association. August 2004. *Apparatus definitions for statistics reporting.* Retrieved November 16, 2005, from http://www.fama.org/Committees/Technical/F04Apparatus Definitions.pdf.

NFPA. 2003. *NFPA 1901, Standard for Automotive Fire Apparatus*. Quincy, MA: National Fire Protection Association.

NFPA. 2006. *NFPA 1906, Standard for Wildland Fire Apparatus*. Quincy, MA: National Fire Protection Association.

NIOSH. September 12, 2002. *Volunteer Fire Fighter Dies When Tanker Crashes into Boulder and Tree—Oregon.*

Solomon, S. S. 1990. "Lime-yellow color as related to reduction of serious fire apparatus accidents: The case for visibility in emergency vehicle accident avoidance." *Journal of the American Optometric Association, 61,* 827–831.

Solomon, S. S., and King, J. G. 1995. "Influence of color on fire vehicle accidents." *Journal of Safety Research, 26,* 41–48.

Operations

6 CHAPTER

Objectives

After completing this chapter, you should be able to:

- Describe the SIPDE acronym as it relates to controlling the emergency vehicle.
- Describe how to select an appropriate route to respond to an incident.
- Discuss the various components associated with an emergency response.
- Describe the various types of adverse conditions.
- Discuss the use of seat belts.
- Describe the use of preemption systems.
- Explain the use of black box technology in emergency vehicles.
- Discuss GIS and GPS systems.
- Explain how to avoid crashes.

Case Study

**Motor-Vehicle Incident Claims the Life of a Volunteer Firefighter
and Injures a Lieutenant and Another Fire Fighter—South Carolina**

A 34-year-old male volunteer firefighter (the victim) died after the engine he was driving veered off the road and rolled two times before coming to rest. The incident occurred while the victim, a lieutenant, and another firefighter were responding in Engine 11 to a motor vehicle incident involving injuries. While en route, the tires on the engine's right side dropped off the road surface. As the victim attempted to bring the engine back onto the roadway, he overcompensated, causing the engine to cross the oncoming lane of traffic. The engine crossed a small ditch, rolled across another roadway, crossed another ditch, and rolled again before coming to rest in a resident's yard. The lieutenant and firefighter were thrown from the engine and the victim was killed instantly. The lieutenant and firefighter were taken by ambulance to a local hospital where they were treated and released. The victim, who was entrapped in the vehicle, was removed one hour later.

FIGURE 6.1 ◆ The driver has a critical responsibility in safely maneuvering and operating the emergency vehicle.

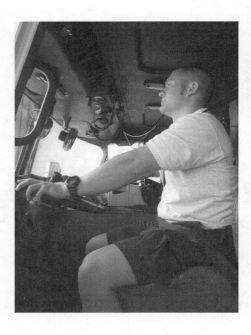

◆ INTRODUCTION

The ability to control and maneuver emergency vehicles safely is one of the most critical aspects of a driver's responsibilities (see Figure 6.1). While driving, the operator should be in control of the vehicle and take into consideration the vehicle characteristics, capabilities, and limitations (e.g., speed, road conditions, auxiliary braking systems, and weight transfer). Operating and controlling the vehicle at a speed from which the vehicle could be safely slowed or stopped could decrease the potential for a skid and loss of control.

◆ MORE THAN JUST DRIVING

Whenever emergency vehicle drivers operate emergency vehicles, they must adhere to the principles of defensive driving. These include:

- Predict the unpredictable.
- Expect the unexpected.
- Handle any unexpected problems.

One of the methods for accomplishing the principles of defensive driving is to apply the **SIPDE** system (scan, identify, predict, decide, and execute).

- *Scan.* The driver needs to continuously scan the surroundings and not have tunnel vision.
- *Identify.* A key component for identifying is to scan ahead. See the big picture, and detect relevant occurrences.
- *Predict.* Prediction makes judgments of space and time relationships relating to other highway users and travel features. These judgments are then projected into possible future options.
- *Decide.* Using the identification and prediction process, the emergency vehicle driver must decide on the appropriate course of action.

◆ *Execute.* Using approved techniques, the emergency vehicle driver then executes the necessary maneuvers within the time frame allowed.

Five visual habits that are of assistance in driving defensively follow:

1. Aim high in steering.
2. Get the big picture.
3. Keep eyes moving, scan.
4. Make sure the other drivers see the emergency vehicle.
5. Identify an escape route.

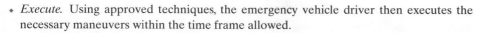

◆ **ROUTE SELECTION**

Route selection is a key decision for urban, suburban, and rural area driving. Each time drivers prepare to leave for a run, they must decide on a route that is quick and avoids potential hazards or delays. This section presents general information to help drivers decide which route to take to an incident scene. The necessary procedures for route selection are discussed.

PROCEDURES

Effective route selection considers procedures such as route planning, predetermined routes, and driver familiarization.

Route Planning. Safety is the most important factor when driving to the scene. Drivers must have a route plan if they want to get to the emergency scene quickly and carefully. Route planning involves learning the geographic and local conditions, the individual characteristics of the area, and the organization's procedures to map out the most efficient route to the emergency scene (Figure 6.2).

Geographic and Local Conditions: When planning a route, drivers should think about the geographic and local conditions affecting the roads they will be using. Be

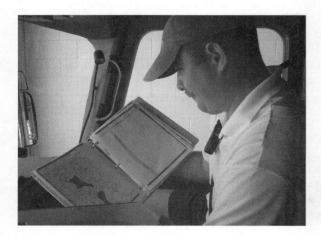

FIGURE 6.2 ◆ The officer or passenger needs to assist the driver in planning the route of response. A well-developed map book should be available.

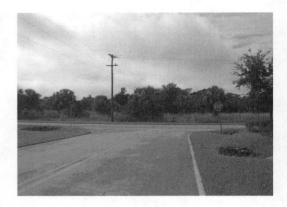

FIGURE 6.3 ◆ Rural intersections may not be properly marked or have adequate lighting. It may also be difficult to see approaching traffic.

aware of and prepare for the conditions in the type of area driving. Special considerations must be made when planning a route in a rural area (Figure 6.3).

Street and road signs in rural areas may be limited, and directions are often given in reference to buildings, gas stations, race tracks, or other past or present landmarks. Farms are commonly referenced because farm names never change. When responding to an emergency in a rural area, the distance driven is usually greater. The road conditions may not always be known, and law enforcement may not even get a call on the incident. When the driver responds to the emergency scene, communicate with dispatch or directly with the first responder. In rural areas, a first responder may get to the scene before the ambulance. The first responder will have information about the patient, incident, road, and weather conditions.

Choose Routes: The driver should plan ahead so not to waste time on a response. The driver needs to make sure to stay within the speed limit! Choose routes that:

- Minimize stops and turns.
- Avoid intersections.
- Take in consideration time of day.
- Avoid residential streets—the posted speed limits will be slower; the driver must be careful of pets, children, cars backing out, and so on.

Organization Procedures: The driver can use a variety of resources to help with route planning. Each organization should have a procedure for updating special events, road conditions, and other factors on a daily basis. The shift supervisor should conduct a briefing at the shift change. This briefing must cover any special events, route problems, personnel assignments, and so on. Volunteer organizations that do not have shift supervisors can note the same information on a board in the bay so the driver can take

> ### Point to Ponder
>
> What conditions could you expect in a rural area?
> *Answer: While driving in rural conditions, you may have to drive on two-lane, dirt, or gravel roads that are poorly marked.*

note prior to responding to an incident. Provide guidance on local resources available. Possible resources include detailed maps, the **preemption system**, helicopter assistance, and **automatic vehicle locators**.

Predetermined Route Procedures. Predetermined routes are standard response routes that are prepared in advance. These routes have been selected to avoid potential problems. Routes should be developed and maintained by the organization or coordinated with other emergency services in the area. Route planning includes the best way to get to the emergency scene AND the best way to get from the scene to the medical facility.

On the way to the emergency scene, the driver and your crew should communicate and navigate the route together. It is a good idea to have at least one experienced person on the crew who knows the area.

In transport units, after the crew picks up the patient and is on the way to the medical facility, the patient care provider will be busy caring for the patient and will not be able to help the driver navigate. The driver needs to make sure he or she knows the route from the scene to the medical facility before the patient care provider begins attending to the patient.

The driver needs to follow the organization's standard procedures so any two members can work together and understand what to do. Take every opportunity to practice communicating as a crew.

> **Example: The driver calls out road conditions, railroad crossing, other bumps on the route. Patient care providers in the patient compartment call out what they are doing to alert the ambulance driver. The operator should tell the patient care providers of any conditions that will limit medical attention.**

A good time to practice is during a practice response or when returning from a response and returning to the station.

Primary and Alternate Routes: When planning routes, primary and alternate routes should be identified. Alternate routes must be available in case of bad road conditions, weather, or other situations that affect primary routes. Navigation at night can be difficult, especially if the driver can't see the street signs, hazards, or other problems. Communicate as a team and follow the organization's standard procedure for giving directions.

To make it easier to choose an alternate route, map out the local areas commonly used and refer to these maps when deciding which way to go to the scene.

- Use a grid system to show any shortcuts, one-way streets, expressways, and so on.
- Add useful information that is not included on the map, such as dirt roads, dangerous intersections, very steep grades, and roads or lanes on roads that change direction according to the time of day.

Driver Familiarization

Know Your Area: Driver familiarization involves the awareness of daily route information, procedures to identify local information, height restrictions, and map reading. When the crew gets a call from dispatch, the driver is responsible for knowing how to get to the scene safely and without taking unnecessary risks. If the driver doesn't know the streets and the area, the responders could easily get lost.

Your area has buildings that the driver needs to pay particular attention to every day. Think of types of buildings that may have scheduled activities of which the driver needs to be aware.

Some considerations: schools, hospitals, auditoriums, concert halls, stadiums, factories, churches, shopping centers, downtown businesses.

Daily Route Information: Become familiar with the area to prevent getting lost.

- Review the primary and alternate routes.
- Find out if there are new developments and buildings under construction.
- If in an area with limited road and street signs, learn the local references, such as buildings, farms, gas stations, and so on.
- Review and learn about different activities that may affect the traffic flow of the route each day.

Keep in mind the approximate busy times for the buildings listed in the activity. Expect delays in high-traffic building areas during these times:

- Beginning and end of normal work and school day (Figure 6.4)
- Shift-change times for large factories, hospitals, and so on

The daily route can be affected by the weather and other environmental reasons:

- Emergency snow routes
- Roads closed due to flooding

Watch for changes in the condition of local roads and streets. Just think how uncomfortable it would be to ride in the back of an ambulance, while injured, and to go

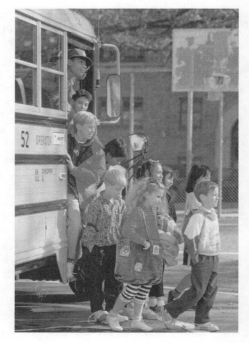

FIGURE 6.4 ◆ Emergency vehicle drivers need to be aware of school hours and potential routes that may be affected by buses and school children. A different route may be advisable during these time periods. (*Courtesy of Photo Researchers Inc.*)

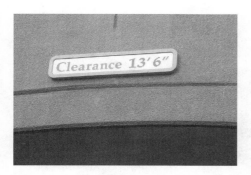

FIGURE 6.5 ◆ It is important for the emergency vehicle driver to heed clearances at overpasses and weight limits at bridges.

over a pothole or a huge bump in the road. Be aware of the following conditions of local roads and streets:

- Damage, potholes, badly rutted roads
- Expressway utilization policies during rush hour or construction
- Detours, closed roads
- Speed bumps, dips, bumps
- Areas of standing water

Dispatch can help when it is absolutely necessary; however, it is the driver's responsibility to know the conditions of the area before leaving the station.

Procedures to Identify Local Information

Height Restrictions: The driver should know the height of the vehicle (including the warning lights) in case the vehicle must go through or under a height-restricted area (Figure 6.5). There could be a bridge, tunnel, or parking ramp on the route. Many fast-food drive-through areas have a height restriction; don't leave the light bar and antennas in the drive-through! Keep the height posted in the vehicle where the driver can quickly see it during the run. The dashboard and visor would be good places to post the vehicle height.

If the crew were on the way back to the station after a response and had to pass under this overpass, could the vehicle pass under this height obstacle?

Point to Ponder

How to Read a Map

Obtain and select a section of a local map with which you are familiar. Prepare a list of factors that must be considered when planning a route. Use a local map to plan a route from an emergency site to various landmarks. Use the names of real roads, streets, and buildings. Factors to consider when planning your route:

- Indicate the road or street where the entrance to your local medical facility is located. (*Example: The entrance to the hospital is on Main Street.*)
- Indicate the road or street where the entrance to the emergency site is located. (*Example: The entrance to the mall is on Oak Road.*)
- List any special conditions, street closings, detours, and other factors that would affect the route to the emergency site. (*Examples: Highcliff Road is closed in the area of River Park. Oak Road is a heavily traveled road with several schools on it. It is 4:30 P.M.*)

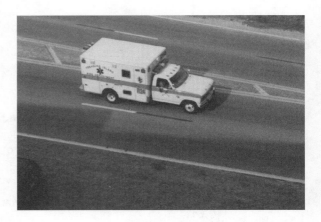

FIGURE 6.6 ◆ Every response is considered different. There will be different circumstances on each response.

◆ RESPONSES

Each emergency you respond to will be unique (Figure 6.6). The weather conditions will change, the nature of the response will change, and the traffic conditions will change. All these changes can easily lead to the emergency vehicle being involved in a traffic crash.

EMERGENCY DRIVING

How would you define **emergency driving**? The emergency mode of emergency vehicle operation is specifically defined by each individual state and refers to the use of emergency vehicles, equipment, and operations. Emergency driving, in general, is defined as using clearly defined procedures in the operation of an emergency vehicle when responding to an emergency, including the use of emergency signaling devices, such as lights and siren.

Emergency vehicle driving and high-speed driving are two distinctly different activities. You may think that high-speed driving is required in a desperate attempt to save a life or property. However, high-speed driving is dangerous for the patient, the crew, and everyone else on the road.

EMERGENCY SIGNALING DEVICES

An emergency vehicle driver has a responsibility to ensure that the emergency lights and/or siren on an emergency vehicle are utilized properly when it is responding to an emergency incident. If drivers expect to use one or more traffic law exemptions legally, they must adhere to the requirements for allowing the exemptions. Although there are no guarantees that members of the public will yield to an emergency vehicle, operation of the lights and siren are simply safety devices for increasing visibility, not an authorization to violate sound safety practices. The use of emergency warning equipment signals has two basic concepts:

- ◆ They notify other drivers that an approaching emergency vehicle is operating in an emergency mode; and
- ◆ They require other drivers to yield the right-of-way to the emergency vehicle in accordance with state and/or local law.

Emergency vehicle drivers should be aware of some information regarding emergency lights. Essentially, effectiveness is dependent on their intensity, color, and flash rate. Most state laws require at least one warning light to be displayed when the emergency vehicle is blocking a moving lane.

Light color recognition and reaction are based on a number of items involving more than just emergency vehicles. A summary follows:

- *Red.* Stop. May attract drivers who are fatigued or under the influence (drugs or alcohol).
- *Blue.* Emergency vehicles (fire or police). Good visibility day or night. Use by either fire and/or law enforcement varies state by state.
- *Amber.* Danger/caution. Viewed by many experts as the best warning light, especially for the rear of emergency vehicles. It provides improved visibility in fog or other hazy conditions; however, it should not be used as an emergency light on the front of the vehicle.
- *Clear.* Caution. Good visibility, but should be capable of being shut off at scenes and should not be used on the rear of the vehicle.

Some limitations involving emergency lights include:

- Low sun or glare can greatly reduce their effectiveness.
- At night, red beacons can be confused with traffic lights and neon signs.
- Lights on emergency vehicles may pass over motorists if the emergency vehicle is close to the rear of the passenger car ahead.

Vehicles are typically visible at 2,500 feet during the daytime on the open road. With their headlights on, they become visible at 4,700 feet under similar conditions. Based on this fact, it might be advantageous to consider a policy requiring all emergency vehicles to operate with headlights on during the daylight hours.

When parking emergency vehicles on the highway, it should be remembered that too many emergency lights on stationary vehicles create a carnival effect and cause confusion. Within this context, emergency vehicles should be safely parked at emergency scenes with most of the emergency warning lights off (Figure 6.7). The placement of warning triangles should create a safe lane between the emergency incident and the flow of traffic on the highway. Flares should be avoided due to potential flammable hazards.

Many emergency vehicle drivers overly rely on the use of sirens to alert drivers in the path of the emergency vehicles. Studies have indicated that the motoring public

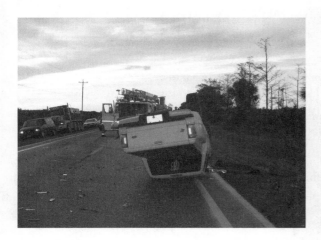

FIGURE 6.7 ◆ Emergency vehicle drivers do not always have the ability to park the vehicle along a curb as pictured here. Extra precaution needs to be taken when positioning vehicles at the scenes of incidents.

FIGURE 6.8 ◆ Emergency vehicle drivers need to approach intersections with utmost caution. (*Courtesy of J. Lindsey*)

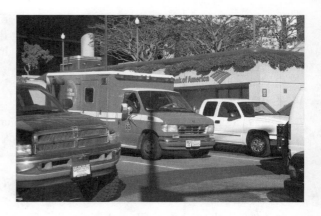

does not understand the different siren modes. Therefore, although changing the siren does increase the ability to attract attention, it does little to impact reaction. The use of a preemption system is another alternative that has proven to clear intersections for emergency vehicles.

A variety of studies indicates that the effective distance of sirens range from 30 feet to 150 feet. In some urban locations, the effective distance can be as little as 15 feet.

Emergency vehicle drivers should still follow several basic procedures:

- Utilize the siren whenever responding to an emergency.
- Change the mode of the siren from wail to yelp at least 200 feet from entering an intersection.
- Studies have indicated that the high–low mode is the least effective siren mode.
- Use another audible device, if so equipped, to alert vehicles or otherwise clear traffic that fails to hear the siren. If using an air horn, use short, repetitive blasts.

Emergency signaling devices (lights and siren) are used during emergency driving for two reasons:

- To notify other drivers that an emergency vehicle is approaching
- To request that the other drivers yield the right-of-way to the emergency vehicle

The driver has to ask for the right-of-way; he or she cannot demand it (Figure 6.8).

OTHER DRIVERS' RESPONSES TO EMERGENCY DRIVING

Most drivers will yield the right-of-way to an emergency vehicle if:

- They realize the emergency vehicle is there.
- They have sufficient time to make a decision as to what to do.
- They have sufficient time and space to carry out that decision.

Even during an emergency response, there is time for courtesy. If drivers take the time to let a motorist make a rational decision as to how to help them, the crew will arrive at the destination quickly and safely. It takes panicked drivers longer to overcome their panic and react properly than it would if they weren't frightened by the blaring siren of an emergency vehicle behind them. The use of the emergency lights and siren cannot guarantee safe, clear passage. Although most drivers will yield the right-of-way, some won't be able to see and/or hear the emergency vehicle because of visibility restrictions in the vehicle or because of other noise or radio interference. And some drivers, even though they see and hear the emergency vehicle, will refuse to yield the right-of-way. Emergency vehicle drivers must be prepared to respond to them.

The use of lights and siren actually increases the danger of a collision. Other drivers are suddenly placed under stress when they look in their rear-view mirrors and see an approaching emergency vehicle with lights and siren on. People under stress do not always act as the driver would expect. The driver needs to give them plenty of warning, approach them with reasonable speed, give them time to react, and, if needed, give them time to counteract any inappropriate response they might make.

RESPONSE TIME

Although there is a need to respond to an emergency as quickly and efficiently as possible, some time-saving methods can have harmful effects and, in the majority of cases, the few minutes saved will probably not matter. Even in those rare cases when minutes matter, the time saved does not justify exposing the public to the jeopardy of a high-speed response by the emergency vehicle.

SPEED LIMITS

Speed limits are based on the quality of the road and the normal traffic conditions (Figure 6.9). Traffic conditions do not remain normal when an emergency vehicle approaches. First, the emergency vehicle is larger than most of the vehicles on the road. Second, it has emergency lights flashing and siren wailing. And third, most vehicles are trying to get out of the way of the emergency vehicle. It is very dangerous for emergency vehicle drivers to think that they can go faster than the posted speed limits and not become involved in a crash. Sirens do not give sufficient warning to drivers of vehicles approaching head-on or traveling on converging roads.

The difficulty in projecting the siren sound around corners in urban areas, or ahead of emergency vehicles traveling at higher speeds in rural areas, can cause the warning time to be too short to allow other drivers to yield the right-of-way. In a rural environment, a person in a closed car proceeding at 55 miles per hour (mph), with the radio playing, may not be aware of a penetrating electronic siren (wail) until it is as close as 33 feet away. In city traffic, a driver with the car windows open and no radio playing might not detect the siren more than 123 feet away.

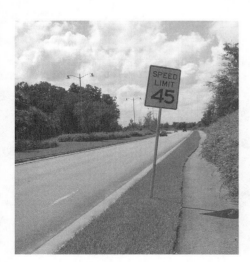

FIGURE 6.9 ◆ The emergency vehicle driver needs to be aware of the posted speed limit. In most states it is only courtesy that emergency vehicle drivers responding with lights and sirens can exceed the posted speed limit. They still must operate the vehicle with due regard.

The effectiveness of the siren warning system to vehicles on crossroads is only about one-third of that for a vehicle straight ahead of the siren and traveling in the same direction. The driver can still drive quickly, but must do so within the speed that the road and traffic conditions will safely allow and not count on the lights and siren providing a clear path ahead.

Even when operating in the emergency mode, follow the state statute concerning speed. It is always better to stay within the posted speed limit. The local regulations governing the use of lights and siren follow.

- Provide local criteria for use of lights and siren.
- If appropriate, provide local regulations when they authorize the driver's ability to exceed posted speed limits.

CONTROLLED INTERSECTION PROCEDURE

What is a *controlled intersection*? It is an intersection with traffic control equipment, such as pavement markings, stop or yield signs, or traffic lights (Figure 6.10).

Dangers. The New York State Department of Health reported in the Ambulance Accident Prevention Seminar that 60 percent of ambulance crashes occur at intersections with stop signs or traffic lights. If the intersection is controlled, why would ambulances have so many crashes? The following are possible answers: ambulance driver running red light, other drivers running red light while trying to get out of the way of the ambulance, crossing vehicles not seeing approaching ambulance.

At an intersection controlled with traffic lights, who has the right-of-way, the approaching ambulance or the cars with the green light? The cars with the green light have the right-of-way. The lights and siren do not automatically grant the right-of-way to the emergency vehicle. Remember, by using the emergency lights and siren, the emergency vehicle driver is asking the other drivers to yield the right-of-way to the emergency vehicle. Until they grant the emergency vehicle the right-of-way, the driver of the emergency vehicle cannot proceed.

Due Regard. As discussed in Chapter 3 on legal aspects, one of the laws that applies to emergency vehicle crashes, especially when they occur at controlled intersections, is the law of due regard. The law of **due regard** says that "a reasonably careful person, performing similar duties and under similar circumstances, would act in the same

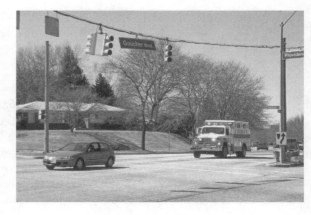

FIGURE 6.10 ◆ A controlled intersection typically has traffic lights and signs to define street names and direction of travel. Never assume you have the right-of-way at these intersections. It is always good to come to a complete stop and be prepared to stop as you progress through the intersection. (*Courtesy of Pearson Education/PH College*)

manner." This means that the driver must drive the emergency vehicle with due regard for the safety of the passengers and patients, and all other persons and drivers using the streets, highways, and freeways, and to protect them from the consequences of the actions when operating the emergency vehicle.

As you can see, due regard is not a hard and fast rule, such as "the speed limit is 55 mph." Instead, it requires that the courts look at each collision and determine whether the emergency vehicle driver was abiding by the law of due regard at the time a traffic crash occurred. To do so, they must get answers to questions such as the following:

- Was it necessary to use the emergency warning system under the circumstances of the call you were responding to and the medical condition of the patient you were transporting?
- Did the emergency vehicle driver give enough warning of the vehicle's approach to allow other motorists and pedestrians to clear the way for the emergency vehicle?
- Was the emergency warning system activated and operating prior to the crash?
- Was the emergency vehicle driver using the emergency warning system in the manner for which the system was designed to be used?
- Was the driver of the emergency vehicle operating the vehicle at a speed greater than necessary to allow the complete control of the emergency vehicle in relation to traffic, road, and weather conditions?

The performance of the emergency vehicle driver is going to be closely looked at in relation to the nature of the emergency and the traffic, road, and weather conditions. With a law such as this, rules cannot be written that cover all situations.

The National Voluntary Consensus Standard. The standards have used the American Society for Testing and Materials (ASTM) guideline as a reference. The standards for controlled intersection management during emergency response mode follow.

- The siren should be in the wail mode 300 feet prior to the intersection.
- Switch the siren to the yelp mode 150 feet prior to the intersection.
- Remove your foot from the accelerator to cover the brake pedal and allow compression to slow the vehicle. Start applying the brake to bring the emergency vehicle to a complete stop at the crosswalk line.
- If the emergency vehicle has an air-driven air horn, give two short blasts on the air horn.
- Make a complete stop. Look to the left, look to the immediate front, look to the right, and then again to the left. Then proceed through the intersection under 10 mph if traffic is stopped in all lanes to the left, in front of, and to the right of the emergency vehicle. After making eye contact with all stopped vehicle drivers, you may proceed through the intersection exercising the highest degree of care.
- Continue with the siren in yelp mode and proceed through the intersection exercising the highest degree of care.
- When there are vacant lanes to the left or right, complete the previous steps of clearing each lane of traffic prior to crossing that lane.
- Expect that any vacant lane to the left or right may become occupied by another vehicle that did not see or hear the emergency vehicle's warning systems.
- Be aware that other emergency vehicles may be approaching the same intersection that you have taken control of. Do not enter the intersection until the other vehicles have stopped or proceeded through the intersection.

- Turn right at the intersection only after all vehicles have stopped and drivers on the right are aware of the emergency vehicle.
- Expect that any vehicles in front may make an unexpected left turn in front of the emergency vehicle after it has started to enter the intersection.
- Be aware of other hazards at the intersection, for example, pedestrians, road hazards, and defective traffic control systems.

DRIVING AGAINST TRAFFIC

Occasionally, emergency vehicle drivers try to save time by driving in traffic against the normal flow of traffic. Although this is seldom recommended, there are times when it may be necessary. On a multilane highway, do not enter an opposing traffic lane until it is safe to do so and all other oncoming vehicles are aware of the emergency vehicle's presence. Similarly, do not enter a one-way street against traffic until all opposing traffic is aware of the emergency vehicle's presence and has yielded the right-of-way.

◆ ADVERSE CONDITIONS

One of the goals of the emergency driver is to provide a smooth, uneventful ride for the crew, not the fastest ride possible. Commercial aircraft pilots face the same goal as they fly through all types of weather conditions. Because drivers can't change the weather conditions, they must learn how to adjust the driving style to the existing conditions. Another goal is to remember that smooth driving keeps the emergency vehicle balanced. In Chapter 5 on emergency vehicle characteristics and weight, when an emergency vehicle is balanced, its weight is distributed evenly to all four wheels, the suspension is stable, and steering and braking are most effective.

The two types of adverse conditions to discuss affect:

- Traction
- Vision

CONDITIONS AFFECTING TRACTION

Rain. Rain affects traction in three ways.

- When it rains, a layer of water forms over the road. As a rolling tire moves over this layer of water, it loses contact with the road surface. This is called hydroplaning. **Hydroplaning** is especially dangerous because the driver loses steering and braking control. As little as one-sixteenth of an inch of water on the road surface can cause hydroplaning.
- Driving through large areas of water can affect brake performance because the brakes become wet and less effective. In older vehicles, splashing water can short out the vehicle's electrical system and stall the engine.
- If the water is concentrated on one portion of the road and only one side of the vehicle goes through the water, the vehicle will tend to pull in that direction. The force of the pull is dependent on the depth of the water and the speed of the vehicle.

By understanding the effects of rain and by taking the following precautions, the driver can lessen the effects of the rain and standing water:

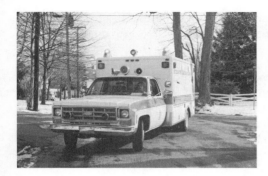

Figure 6.11 ◆ Ambulance driving in snowy conditions. (*Courtesy of Pearson Education/PH College*)

- Slow down before hitting water. This will lessen the splashing and reduce the effects of hydroplaning, giving the driver more control of the vehicle.
- Gently apply the brakes for a few moments when exiting the deeper puddles to heat the brake shoes and dry them.

Until the brakes are dry, the driver will notice that it takes more foot pressure to stop the vehicle.

Snow and Ice. Snow and ice form an extremely slick barrier between the vehicle's tires and the roadway; this includes black ice. Extreme caution must be taken when driving on snow and ice to avoid sliding when turning, braking, and accelerating (see Figure 6.11). Remember that in cold weather, bridges and shaded roadways freeze first. Often this freezing is nearly invisible, and all bridges and shaded areas must be approached with caution.

When driving through deep snow, proceed slowly and shift into a lower gear before entering the snow, and attempt to keep the vehicle moving through the snow.

High Winds. Although the emergency vehicle is a heavy vehicle, it is tall, and the large flat-sided body acts like a sail, making the vehicle very susceptible to the effects of the wind. Crosswinds can blow the vehicle off the road or across the center line, particularly at curves and corners and especially when it's raining, snowing, or icy and traction with the road is already reduced.

Wind shifts occur as the vehicle passes buildings, travels through underpasses, or passes large trucks. These shifts toss the vehicle first one way and then another. Reduced speed will lessen the effects of these wind shifts.

Leaves. Wet leaves on the roadway can become as slick as ice or snow. If the driver cannot avoid driving through areas of wet leaves, slow down and treat them as a large patch of ice.

Increasing Traction with Traction Devices. When it starts to rain, the driver cannot pull to the side of the road and put on a set of "antihydroplaning" or "wet-leaf" tires. Reduced speed and smooth steering, braking, and acceleration are all the driver can do to retain control of the vehicle. However, during the winter months, certain traction devices can be installed on or carried in the emergency vehicle.

Snow Tires: Organizations located in areas where it snows often and where the snow remains for weeks at a time often install snow tires in the fall and remove them in the spring. Snow tires have a tread pattern that is different from that of normal highway tires. This open, deeply grooved tread pattern increases the tire's grip on the snow and is designed to clean itself as the tire rotates.

Chains: Chains are convenient in that they can be carried in the vehicle and installed by the driver when needed. Chains bite into the snow or ice and greatly increase traction. When using chains, the driver must reduce the vehicle speed to keep from banging against the vehicle. Because chains will dig into asphalt surfaces as they do into ice, they should be removed before driving on bare roads, if possible. New technology has allowed for the chains to be automatically put into place.

CONDITIONS AFFECTING VISION

The driver's vision can be affected in three ways. First, the environment may give the driver problems. Second, the vehicle and the way the driver cares for it may affect the way the driver is able to see things. Finally, the driver's physical condition and preparation for duty will affect the eyes' ability to see.

Driving at Night. Even under the best of weather conditions, visibility is decreased at night. Because there is less light, a person's eyes work differently and see things differently than in the daytime. Because of the way the eyes are designed, there is a small blind spot right in the center of where a person looks, or right in the center of one's field of vision. During the daytime, this is not a big problem because different parts of the eyes are at work and there is a lot of light. At night, this small blind spot comes into play because it may hide small, poorly lit objects if a person looks directly at them or tries to stare at them. To compensate, a person must constantly scan the different parts of the area ahead.

Here are some other problems a driver may encounter when driving at night:

- Darkness conceals hazards and the driver must make decisions based on incomplete information.
- It is more difficult to judge the speed and position of another vehicle because the driver does not have distinct shadows and other objects as reference points.
- The driver's peripheral vision is reduced if he or she smokes. This makes it more difficult to judge the speed and position of other vehicles, especially at night.
- Adequate highway lighting is limited.
- Glare from roadside lighting and oncoming vehicle headlights impair the driver's visibility (Figure 6.12).

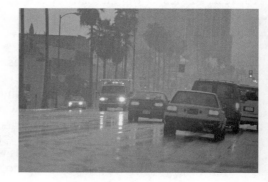

FIGURE 6.12 ◆ Ambulance responding to an emergency in inclement weather. (*Courtesy of PhotoEdit*)

Night Driving Techniques: Even with these problems, driving at night is possible and, with careful attention, does not have to be dangerous. A few night driving techniques will help:

- Keep dash and panel lights dim for better vision, but always have enough light to read the speedometer.
- Reduce speed so that you can stop within the visible distance.

Remember, the act of braking begins with the recognition that something ahead requires that the driver slow or stop. Drivers can't begin stopping if they can't see ahead, so drive within the range of the headlights. By driving within the range of the headlights, drivers are able to begin braking as soon as the vehicle headlights reveal an object. When drivers overdrive the range of the headlights, they may not see the object in time to stop.

- Increase sight distance by keeping the headlights clean and properly aimed and the windshield clean.
- Watch beyond the headlights on or near the roadway for slow-moving or unlighted vehicles, curves, T intersections, road obstructions or defects, trains, pedestrians, and animals.
- Keep your eyes moving so that your blind spot does not hide objects ahead.

Maintaining Night Vision: There are several things drivers can do to increase their ability to see at night:

- Don't move immediately from a brightly lit room to a dark vehicle and begin driving. Give your eyes a chance to adjust to the darkness.
- Avoid looking directly into glaring headlights of oncoming vehicles. The human eye takes about 7 seconds to recover fully from being blinded by a bright light. At 60 mph, the vehicle would travel 616 feet in 7 seconds.
- Don't smoke.
- Don't wear sunglasses at night.

Rain and Fog. Rain and fog affect visibility in two ways:

- *Reduced Visibility.* Rain and fog shorten the distance a driver can see. In addition, other vehicles on the roadway may splash water and mud onto the windshield and headlights. Fog also reduces the range of the siren. The visibility and warning capabilities are reduced.
- *Glare.* The sun and headlights will reflect off the many drops of moisture in the air with both rain and fog. Not only is the random light reflected back into a driver's eyes, but a large portion of the light from the headlights is reflected and never reaches the roadway.

Emergency lights, including strobes, are especially prone to reflect off of fog and mist. Use caution in checking outside mirrors when it is raining. Rain can distort or obliterate the images in the mirrors.

The Vehicle

Windshield/Wipers: If the windshield is cracked or broken, the light rays are scattered improperly and a driver's vision will be obstructed. Have cracked or broken windshields fixed or replaced, and keep the windshield clean and the wipers operative so that the windshield can be cleaned. Don't let dead bugs and trash accumulate under the wipers.

Visors: Use the visors mounted above the windshield to prevent looking directly into the sun. Move the visors to the side to reduce glare and the hypnotic effect of the sun flashing through trees as you drive down the road.

Bug Screens: Plastic bug screens mounted on the front of the hood on certain vehicles are very effective in deflecting bugs, and even light rain and snow, up and over the windshield.

Headlights: Keep the headlights clean and operative to provide maximum lighting at night and in adverse weather conditions.

Side View Mirrors: Keep the side view mirrors clean and properly adjusted so that you are able to see down both sides of the vehicle (Figure 6.13). If necessary, adjust a mirror slightly to prevent glare when the sun is behind the vehicle. It is important to keep in mind that convex mirrors should not be used to judge clearance. Convex mirrors distart distance and are specifically resigned to view objects in immediate surroundings. They should be adjusted to see out of the side and the ground.

The Driver

Compensating for Visibility Problems: There are several things that a driver can do to compensate for visibility problems. A few specific items have already been discussed, but here are a few more general ones:

- Prepare yourself. Get enough sleep and do not drink alcohol before going on duty. Smoking also reduces night vision.
- Turn on low-beam headlights and the wipers, if needed. Never drive with only the parking lights on. As their name implies, they are for use when the vehicle is parked, not when driving. If the conditions are such that a driver needs to use the wipers, turn on the headlights.

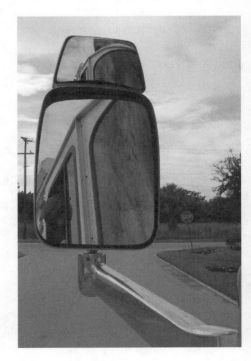

FIGURE 6.13 ◆ The driver should be very familiar with the type of mirrors on the vehicle. Various styles of mirrors work in different ways.

- Headlights should be on at all times.
- Watch for slow-moving and stopped vehicles.
- Check the side view mirrors frequently for vehicles approaching quickly from the rear.
- Be alert for patches of fog in valleys and low-lying areas.
- Drive slowly, but keep moving.
- If conditions are too bad to continue, pull over as far as possible, stop, leave lights on, and activate hazard lights.

Do not create another emergency by continuing at all costs. Hydroplaning occurs when it rains and a layer of water forms between the tire and the road surface.

◆ SEAT BELTS

The emergency vehicle driver is responsible for the safety of all passengers in the vehicle. This includes making sure that restraints are being used properly, that all equipment and other objects have been secured, and that only safe behavior is tolerated within the vehicle.

RESTRAINTS

All passengers, the crew, patients, and driver, must wear a seat belt when the vehicle is in motion (Figure 6.14). If a child is transported as a nonpatient passenger, the driver should properly restrain the child in a safety seat. All patients must be secured at all times when the vehicle is in motion.

SECURE EQUIPMENT

Secure all equipment in the driver and passenger compartments to prevent an injury if the vehicle has to stop suddenly or swerve (Figure 6.15). When leaving the scene, all equipment used on the scene should be secured in the vehicle. This includes such things as clipboards, portable radios, and flashlights.

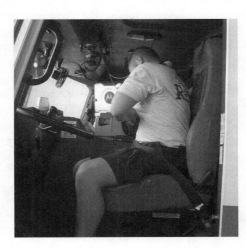

FIGURE 6.14 ◆ Emergency vehicle drivers need to utilize their seat belts every time they are driving a vehicle.

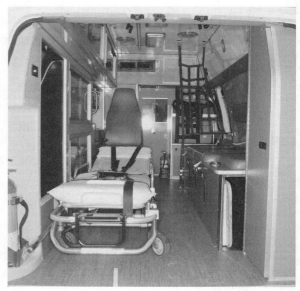

FIGURE 6.15 ◆ Equipment should be secured in the emergency vehicle to prevent objects from becoming projectiles in an accident or when the driver may need to stop quickly. (*Courtesy of Stockbyte*)

UNSAFE BEHAVIOR

While the vehicle is in motion, if the driver notices unsafe behavior in the vehicle, it is his or her responsibility to stop it. If someone is interfering with patient care or vehicle operation, demand that it stops. If necessary, pull the vehicle over until the unsafe behavior has stopped. Do not allow unsafe behavior to threaten patient care or passenger safety.

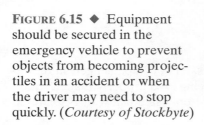

◆ TECHNOLOGY

TRAFFIC PREEMPTION SYSTEMS

Traffic signals can disrupt the progress of emergency vehicles by causing them to slow or stop. Because other vehicles in cross traffic often have the right-of-way when the emergency vehicle reaches the intersection, hazardous situations can occur. Preemption involves switching the appropriate signal at a signalized intersection to green, allowing traffic to clear the intersection safely and to grant an approaching emergency vehicle right-of-way regardless of the normal signal-phasing pattern. Preemption creates a green light in the direction of travel while all other lights turn yellow, then red.

Various types of preemption systems are in use in urban areas across the nation. The solution described next is an example of a low-cost siren-activated system.

There are siren detectors that detect the sirens of emergency vehicles up to half a mile away from an equipped intersection. This activates a signal preemption phase, giving a green light to the oncoming emergency vehicle and switching all pedestrian crossings to the Don't Walk message. The green light can be held for a preset time of between 5 and 45 seconds. A visual verification system consisting of a white light and a blue light is installed next to the regular traffic signal. When the white light is activated, this confirms to the driver of the emergency vehicle that it has been given the right-of-way. The blue light indicates that the intersection is being controlled by an emergency vehicle approaching from another direction.

Benefits:

- ◆ Emergency vehicles activating a traffic signal preemption system can negotiate an intersection more safely.
- ◆ Traffic in the direction of the emergency vehicle clears intersection safely.
- ◆ Traffic approaching an intersection where preemption has been activated by an approaching emergency vehicle is safer.
- ◆ Patients transported in emergency vehicles will reach their destinations in a more timely and safe manner.
- ◆ More timely response to emergency calls results.

Low-powered wireless communication devices in vehicles, similar to garage door openers, could also be used to trigger receivers mounted on the signaled intersections to give oncoming vehicles a green phase. In addition, systems using infrared technology could perform this function. In noise sensitive operations or environments, a non–siren-based system should be considered. New technology permits preemption without direct sight lines. Signals can preempt from around corners and buildings.

Institutional Issues: As no special equipment on the emergency vehicle is required, equipped vehicles could cross jurisdictional boundaries and activate the signals of neighboring cities or counties if the same siren-based system is also deployed there.

Implementation Issues: In one instance, shortly after implementing a siren-activated signal preemption system (manufactured by another vendor), local drivers discovered that signals could be preempted by activating their car alarms. Depending on the frequency of the siren technology, this may occur with other implementations as well.

THE BLACK BOX

Smooth vehicle accelerations, decelerations, and cornering are key components to driving safely and efficiently. They come easily to the driver who is not under stress. Drivers sometimes confuse getting on scene quickly and safely with getting there at any cost. The problem is compounded by the adrenaline rush many experience while "running hot." Add to this a false sense of security created when running emergency lights and sirens that other drivers either don't see, don't hear, or just ignore, and you have a crash waiting to happen. These are some of the factors that contribute to crashes that are both predictable and preventable!

Black box technology is an excellent behavior modification system. Management needs to realize that any system that is dependent on corrective action, days or even weeks later, will not change inappropriate driving behavior and achieve compliance with company policies. With the Road Safety On-Board Computer system (Figure 6.16), driving parameters such as speed, rate of acceleration and deceleration, and how the vehicle is driven while cornering are all part of the SafeForce™ driver grading system. If drivers operate their vehicles outside acceptable ranges of these parameters, they hear an immediate audio warning to take corrective action. This gives drivers a clear understanding of what management expects and allows them to monitor and instantly correct their own driving performance.

The Road Safety On-Board Computer system records each second and each mile of operation of every vehicle in the fleet. Active driver identification enables the system to evaluate driver performance based on the amount of miles drivers cover and how safely they operate their vehicles.

FIGURE 6.16 ◆ Black boxes are installed in emergency vehicles as a means of behavior modification. Research has demonstrated that they are successful in changing the behavior of drivers. (*Courtesy of Road Safety International*)

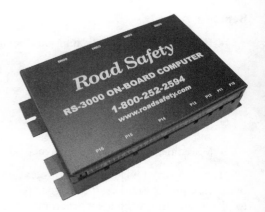

Examples of unsafe vehicle operations include speeding, hard braking, rapid acceleration, and hard cornering. When the driver begins to operate the vehicle in an unsafe manner, the SafeForce system produces an audible warning tone, much like a Geiger counter. This warning tone alerts the driver that he or she is approaching an unsafe vehicle operating condition and gives ample time to correct the mistake before a crash occurs. If this warning is ignored and the driver continues to push the vehicle into a dangerous condition, the system produces a steady tone. This tone alerts the driver that the system has started recording the occurrence into the driver grading system, further encouraging the driver to correct the unsafe action.

The ABCs of SafeForce Driving. The SafeForce driver grading system logs each second the driver operates the vehicle in an unsafe condition. The system converts these seconds into mathematical "counts." A level of performance grade is computed based on the Average (miles) Between Counts (ABCs).

A Level 10 driver has a greater number of safely driven miles between counts than does a Level 6 driver. Figure 6.17 shows how many safely driven miles the driver needs to average between counts to achieve each performance level. Many fleets

SafeForce™ Driving System Level Requirements	
ABC Miles	**Level**
250 ⟶	10
125 ⟶	9
64 ⟶	8
32 ⟶	7
16 ⟶	6
8 ⟶	5
4 ⟶	4
2 ⟶	3
1 ⟶	2
<1 ⟶	1

FIGURE 6.17 ◆ The following chart depicts the report of safe miles driven. (*Courtesy of Road Safety International*)

consider Level 6 as their standard for minimum safe vehicle operation. Drivers below this standard receive additional training or performance review by supervisors.

The Road Safety SafeForce driving system is easy to install and can be configured with a wireless RF data transceiver for automatic downloading. No driver or administrator intervention is required. All vehicle and driver information, including the driver's ABC performance, is downloaded to the system administrator's desktop computer. Database reports allow the administrator to look at driver performance individually or in comparison to others. Driver performance data can also be viewed for emergency driving, nonemergency driving, and total driving.

Figure 6.18 is an example of the Driver Grading Summary Report.

In addition to ABC reports, the SafeForce system will produce many other reports that can be used to ensure the safe and efficient operation of vehicles. These exception

---

Road Safety International

Summary File: dayshift.que   From: 3/1/2006
Reported: 9/2/2006   To: 3/31/2006

Driver Safety Summary (Emergency & Non-Emergency Driving)

Driver ID	Driver	Distance	Force Total	Counts High	Over Total	Speed High	Counts Counts	Seatbelt Reverse	Unsafe ABC Miles	Level
00091	Dillard, Mike	1,818.9	0	0	0	0	0	1	1,818.920	
00103	Rome, Jeni	1,338.9	1	0	0	0	0	0	1,338.929	
00169	Issel, Nathan	1,268.4	0	0	0	0	0	1	1,258.408	
00175	Volpe, Oscar	1,732.8	2	0	0	0	0	0	866.414	
00064	Erwin, Charles	1,433.5	2	0	0	0	0	0	716.727	
00181	Cornier, Jenus	2,772.6	14	0	0	0	0	0	198.039	
00090	Allen, Dale	976.8	4	0	0	0	0	1	195.357	
00052	Menge, Alexander	3,056.4	20	0	0	0	0	0	152.819	
00062	Bensen, Thomas	2,279.8	15	0	0	0	0	0	151.990	
00126	Lord, Britiany	1,220.1	0	0	10	0	0	0	122.012	
00057	Olindyke, Andrew	1,503.2	12	0	0	0	1	0	115.628	
00176	Walker, Julianna	2,031.2	4	0	0	0	1	14	106.904	
00011	Simonson, Mark	1,107.5	10	0	0	0	0	2	92.289	
00076	Carrera, Alexis	2,033.4	29	0	11	0	0	0	50.834	
00056	Anderson, Terry	2,579.1	58	0	0	0	0	0	44.467	
00010	Rollins, Darren	696.4	15	0	1	0	0	1	40.964	
00088	Cartright, Ben	2,328.2	48	0	10	0	1	6	35.819	
00060	Hedge, Josh	1,673.6	55	0	0	0	0	0	30.430	
00063	Iverson, Richard	3,449.8	63	3	23	0	2	0	21.164	
	S T A N D A R D L I N E									
00087	Prichard, Martin	2,239.9	16	2	30	2	3	10	14.087	5
00073	Sibmann, Francis	1,838.3	86	2	33	0	1	0	10.814	5
00079	Uberoff, Hank	1,219.4	31	3	3	0	0	18	9.601	5
00130	Cunningham, Lauren	272.9	12	0	0	0	6	11	9.410	5
00046	Keen, Paul	1,045.1	9	3	8	2	0	5	7.109	4
00133	Silk, Courtney	1,387.6	68	6	0	0	1	22	5.757	4
Total Drivers:	25									
Fleet Totals:		43,293.6	574	19	129	4	16	92	31.236	6
Average Driver:		1,731.7	23	1	5	0	1	4		7

FIGURE 6.18 ◆ Sample Driver Grading Summary Report. (*Courtesy of Road Safety International*)

reports include failure to wear seat belts, unsafe vehicle backing, failure to use turn signals consistently, code violations, and detailed second-by-second reporting and analysis.

Rewards for Learning the ABCs: While using ABCs to mean Average Between Counts, it could also be thought of as "A Bunch of Carrots." Using the ABCs of Safe-Force driving, management has the opportunity to reward top performers and foster teamwork, rather than forcing people into submission. Although some might say that any reward system is manipulative, it remains one of the most proactive ways to create permanent behavior change and eliminate unsafe driving habits.

The Database Reports Do the Work for You: With the power of the SafeForce database, reports ranking groups of drivers, including supervisors, are easily created. Competition has always been a strong motivator and now the organization can use it to its advantage. For example, any group of drivers obtaining a driving level score above the standard line could be presented with a commendation letter posted on the bulletin board, pizza, patches, certificates, or any other affordable reward. Teamwork, group pressure, and the undeniable fact that everybody wants to beat the supervisors, can all contribute to creating safer drivers in a positive working environment.

Identifying Those Who Need Help: The ABCs of SafeForce driving reports quickly identify those in need of driver training or driver refresher courses. Helping drivers improve may save a life and will significantly reduce vehicle maintenance costs. ABCs will then document and quantify the improvements as they are made. Unfortunately, there are still a small percentage of people who refuse to improve, even when opportunities and incentives are provided. The SafeForce driving system objectively points these people out. Sometimes, encouraging people to pursue a new career path works to the benefit of all parties concerned.

Road Safety Advanced Technology Partnership: Many new opportunities are available by adding the power and flexibility of the onboard computer that is the backbone of the SafeForce system. Road Safety system data can be integrated with GPS, AVL, CAD systems, video cameras, pen pads, maintenance management, and intelligent defibrillator/ monitors. Significant enhancements to dispatch, patient care, transport documentation, billing, and much more are now affordable and within the reach of every fleet.

SafeForce Driving Makes Dollars and Sense: SafeForce driving prevents costly crashes and drastically lowers fleet maintenance expenses. This in turn lowers the insurance costs. Lower operating costs, increased vehicle availability, extended vehicle life, and improved utilization all contribute immediately and positively to the profitability of the operation.

If you consider employees to be the company's most valuable asset, then providing a system that effectively trains drivers, reduces on-the-job stress, and allows them to perform their primary mission of assisting the injured and saving lives, makes total financial sense. Failure to make a comprehensive driver safety commitment eventually results in vehicular crashes, which almost always leads to unnecessary injuries and, possibly, fatalities. As is said, "frequency breeds severity." The longer ineffectively trained drivers operate your vehicles, the more frequent and severe the crashes will be.

GIS, AVL, GPS, AND OTHER TECHNOLOGY

Geographic Information System (GIS). **GIS** is a computer-based tool for visualizing, mapping, analyzing, and processing data that has a geographic component

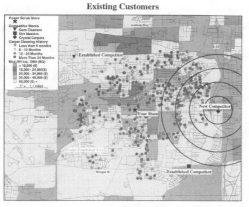

Existing Customers

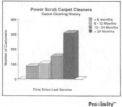

FIGURE 6.19 ◆ GIS devices are being utilized in many systems. The map illustrates the output from a GIS system. (*Courtesy of Decisionmark Corporation*)

(Figure 6.19). GIS technology integrates common database operations such as query and statistical analysis with the unique visualization and geographic analysis benefits offered by maps. These abilities distinguish GIS from other information systems and make it valuable to a wide range of public and private enterprises for explaining events, predicting outcomes, and planning strategies. GIS can be used to integrate mapping analysis into decision support for network planning and analysis, vehicle tracking and routing, inventory tracking, and route planning and analysis. GIS combined with AVL can be utilized to track vehicles visually, to plan their routes, and to signal an alert if vehicles go off schedule. In this application, GIS can also be used to view actual routes taken.

Benefits:

- Better analysis of road network to prioritize congested or potentially hazardous areas for road improvements.
- Improved analysis tool to prioritize funding for certain areas.
- Improved fleet management.

Opportunities: Opportunities for GIS in rural areas include nearly every area, with particular emphasis on those that require real-time mapping to location databases. As an example, accidents, construction, or heavy vehicle permit restrictions can be tied to GIS in order to allow automatic consideration and display by numerous response agencies.

Institutional Issues: GIS software can be used for a wide range of situations, from static network analysis to dynamic, real-time tracking of vehicles. Any organization utilizing GIS will recognize the benefits it has to offer soon after the software is installed. GIS software is mature and is readily used by numerous public and private agencies.

Issues associated with GIS are few; however, GIS software can be difficult to install, set up, and maintain, and therefore requires adequately trained personnel to run it. To ensure the maximum utilization of the GIS software, an information technology position should be created, at least on a part-time basis, to maintain the GIS software.

Implementation Issues: Initial costs may be large. Agencies must consider the various opportunities for other applications when investing in GIS systems and potential issues involving integrating the new GIS with legacy systems. Also, ongoing support or licenses may be required to continue to operate GIS software. Agencies should be aware of and consider any such costs.

Automatic Vehicle Locator (AVL). The majority of Automatic Vehicle Locator (AVL) technologies use the **Global Positioning System** (GPS) to pinpoint the location of various vehicles equipped with a GPS receiver. GPS is a free service provided by the U.S. government that allows the use of a constellation of 24 satellites in orbit 10,900 miles above the Earth. Vehicles with GPS receivers have their positions determined by a space/time triangulation of three or more of the 24 satellites. AVL also incorporates a wireless communications system to communicate the vehicle location back to the control center. Some options for this communications link are existing radio frequency system, cellular communications, cellular digital packet data (CDPD), or satellite communications. The goal of implementing AVL on vehicles is to track vehicle locations to incident sites for fleet management, for special applications to provide communications, both voice and data, between agency vehicles and dispatch centers.

Combined with GIS software or mapping database, and road/weather information systems, this technology can ensure the most cost-effective use of resources and deploy the closest emergency vehicles to the incident. AVL has been utilized heavily in the commercial vehicle industry in fleet management, and the U.S. government uses GPS regularly for the deployment of ships, airplanes, and missiles. It should be noted that, in order to protect GPS from being used against the United States, the U.S. government builds a degradation into the signal, resulting in less accurate location. However, depending on the accuracy needed, for additional ongoing fees agencies can also use differential GPS (DGPS) to gain extremely accurate locations.

Public Vehicle Fleet Management Systems. The widespread use of new technologies such as Global Positioning Systems (GPS) and handheld computers with wireless capability allows for many new and innovative ways of improving operational efficiency in many transportation-related areas. With regard to fleet management, GPS can be used to locate vehicles and deploy them to incident sites for congestion mitigation, or for special applications. Handheld computers allow vehicle inspectors in the field to enter information on site and then synchronize it with their office PCs. This process eliminates the redundancy of reentering information and also allows for onsite comparison with data from prior years.

Benefits:

- Vehicle maintenance operations become more streamlined.
- Accuracy of data entered can be improved due to on-site entering of information and the availability of previous years' information.

The cost of GPS systems for fleet vehicles varies widely; thorough research of available systems will need to be conducted before equipment and software are chosen.

Some municipalities and private companies use a magnetic key system for dispensing fuel. The user takes the vehicle to a fueling station, inserts the key for that vehicle, enters the mileage, and the fuel dispenses in the vehicle. Hence, the record keeper has an automatic record of fuel usage by every vehicle in the fleet. This information may then be downloaded to a handheld computer.

Simple technologies to enhance fleet management have few, if any, institutional issues. Challenges with such a system are low.

Implementation Issues:

- Training on how to use the handheld computers may be necessary.
- Consideration interaction with numerous vendors and examination of numerous products are needed to ensure technology is feasible in the appropriate environment and to ensure cost-effectiveness.

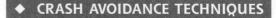

◆ CRASH AVOIDANCE TECHNIQUES

What do you think of when someone says, "crash avoidance"? You should think of driving to keep the emergency vehicle out of a situation where a crash is unavoidable.

JUSTIFICATION

In *Emergency Ambulance Driving*, Childs and Ptacnik (1986) point out that one in four drivers will be involved in a major motor vehicle crash. Emergency vehicle drivers are not left out of that statistic just because they are driving a big vehicle equipped with flashing lights and screaming sirens. Crashes don't have to be caused by the emergency vehicle. In their panic to get out of the way, other drivers may cause a crash that eventually involves the emergency vehicle.

TECHNIQUES

A crash's severity can almost always be lessened if the emergency vehicle driver continues to drive the vehicle. When faced with an impending crash, most drivers panic. They either slam on the brakes and grip the steering wheel until the crash is over, or they close their eyes and hope for the best. These drivers have stopped driving and are doing nothing to help lessen the severity of the crash.

PLAN AHEAD TO AVOID A CRASH

Planning ahead for a crash does two things:

- It physically prepares the vehicle for the effects of a crash.
- It prepares the driver mentally by making him or her think about avoiding the crash.

Secure Equipment. Because of the quantity of equipment the vehicle carries and the fact that much of the equipment will be in use while traveling, especially in an ambulance when involved in a crash, there will be many missile hazards to contend with. The more items that can be stored in cabinets or tied down, the fewer things there will be flying forward during a crash.

Check the vehicle for items that may come loose and doors or drawers that may open. Try to find ways to fasten them so that they remain closed or tied down when not in use. Use padding to cushion sharp corners and prevent injury.

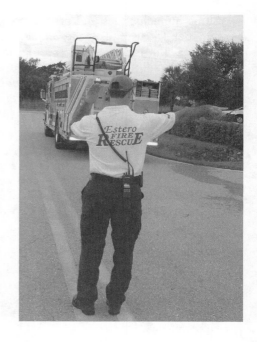

FIGURE 6.20 ◆ A spotter should be used to assist the driver in backing the vehicle. If a spotter is not available, the driver needs to do a 360° walk around the vehicle to look for any obstacles.

Wear Seat Belts. Always wear your seat belts and have your passengers wear theirs. Keep the patient belted to the stretcher and the stretcher secured to the chassis on transport units.

Mentally Prepare Yourself. While driving down the road, plan an escape route from every situation around you. The driver should avoid a head-on impact at all costs. Think about how to avoid a crash if it happened in front of you, or to the right or left, or even right behind. Decide which item to hit if a crash is unavoidable. The driver has two choices, but always hit at an angle rather than head-on. Sideswiping a parked car is preferable to colliding with one head-on. Choose to hit items that will absorb the impact rather than solid objects. It is better to hit a utility pole than a concrete bridge abutment.

Maintain Rear and Side Space Cushion. The farther other vehicles are from the vehicle, the more difficult it is to be involved in a crash with them.

Space Management. Establishing a cushion of safety on all sides of an emergency vehicle is essential for safe operation. Following distance, rate of vehicle closure, blind spots, and traffic closure on an emergency vehicle are major areas of concern in maintaining this cushion.

Back Up with a Ground Guide. Use all the help you can to avoid backing into other vehicles or items on the ground. Back up with a ground guide (Figure 6.20).

MULTIPLE RESPONDING UNITS/MULTIPLE AGENCIES

Response. Anticipate other units responding to the same emergency or to other emergencies in the vicinity. Look out for their lights. The driver should change the volume of the siren to be able to hear the sirens of other units.

Clearing a Controlled Intersection. We've talked about how to cross controlled intersections. Imagine that there is a crash hidden in the next intersection and you must eliminate it before crossing the intersection. The driver can eliminate some of these just by warning other drivers of the approach with the lights and sirens. The driver can eliminate others by slowing and stopping before having a chance to start the crash. But, the only way to eliminate the potential crash is to look each of the other drivers in the eye and see that they have acknowledged your presence and have agreed to yield the right-of-way to you. Then, and only then, are you safe to proceed toward the next intersection. Or are you? Is there another driver hidden behind that truck beside you or around the corner? Always be alert and never get careless.

Sometimes, despite all the planning a driver can do, crashes are going to happen. Faced with the certainty of a crash, there are three things a driver can do: brake, accelerate, or turn to avoid it or lessen the impact.

Braking: Braking is the normal reaction of most drivers when faced with a crash. Remember that braking takes time and distance to be effective. If brakes are required, apply them smoothly and firmly. Do not lock the brakes. With locked brakes, the driver loses steering control and braking distances are increased.

Acceleration: If, when crossing an intersection, the driver realizes that the emergency vehicle is about to be hit from the side or rear, the driver may be able to avoid a crash by accelerating as smoothly and rapidly as possible without spinning the wheels.

Steering Out of the Way: There are many times where steering out of the way is the only way to avoid a crash. To do so, the vehicle must be moved sideways as far as required and as quickly as possible to clear the hazard. The driver may be afraid that the vehicle will tip over, but this is seldom the case because most vehicles will slide before tipping. Even if the driver only partially clears the object, the driver will hit it with a glancing blow instead of head-on.

Steering quickly to avoid a crash cannot be done if drivers must move their hands on the steering wheel. Drivers should practice driving with their hands at the ten and two o'clock or nine and three o'clock position so that they are always prepared to execute a smooth, but rapid, turn.

VEHICLE RECOVERY TECHNIQUES

Sometimes, the driver may be able to avoid a crash by driving off the road, or, for some reason, the driver has driven off the road and needs to recover by returning to the road without causing a crash. At other times, the driver may have a vehicle malfunction and needs to respond to the malfunction and then safely pull off the road.

Running Off the Road Recovery Techniques

Initial Reaction: The most common reaction when leaving the road surface is to try to get back onto the road quickly. This reaction frequently causes a head-on crash or rollover because the driver overcorrects and crosses the center line into the oncoming lane.

Control: To avoid overcorrecting, immediately remove your foot from the accelerator and continue to drive the vehicle. Do not brake heavily or you may be pulled farther from the road. If no obstacles are directly ahead, continue to slow and regain steering control in preparation for pulling back onto the road.

Pulling Back onto the Road: Check the side view mirrors and signal drivers behind you that you plan to return to the road. Smoothly turn the steering wheel and drive back onto the road. In the event that an additional hazard (such as a pole or guardrail) is directly ahead on the shoulder of the road, the driver may have to drive immediately back onto the road, even though he or she may not be fully prepared to do so.

To do so, smoothly turn the steering wheel toward the road and then immediately straighten it as the front tire makes contact with the edge of the roadway. The brief period between the steering input and the resulting action should allow the rear tire also to climb onto the road. This rapid maneuver will allow the steering to be corrected before the vehicle is driven into oncoming traffic.

Responding to Vehicle Malfunction. When drivers experience a vehicle malfunction, they must respond to the malfunction and then move the vehicle out of the flow of traffic.

Tire Blowout: Tire blowout seldom occurs with today's tires. A blowout occurs when the tire is damaged to such an extent that it instantly deflates, often disintegrating in the process. If a front tire blows out, the vehicle immediately swerves in the direction of the destroyed tire, causing the driver to whip the steering wheel in the opposite direction. If a rear tire is involved, the back of the vehicle sways back and forth, making it difficult for the driver to maintain control.

In either situation, hold the steering wheel firmly and steer enough to maintain lane position. Ease off the accelerator, but do not brake. Rapid deceleration or braking may make steering control more difficult. Once speed has been reduced to the point where you can steer, slowly begin braking, signal your intentions, and move off to the side of the road.

Brake Failure: Brake failure seldom occurs in today's vehicles. If brake failure occurs, try the brakes again. If pumping the brakes does not work, shift into a lower gear and use the engine to brake. Carefully apply the parking brakes. The parking brakes work only on the rear brakes and stopping distances will be much longer. Continue to steer and maneuver to where you can safely leave the road.

If brake failure occurs while going down a hill and engine braking and use of the parking brake are not effective, the driver may have to sideswipe parked cars, guardrails, small trees, or dirt banks to slow sufficiently.

Steering Failure: Today's emergency vehicles are equipped with power steering. In these vehicles, steering failure occurs whenever the engine quits. It may also occur if all power steering fluid is lost. In either case, the vehicle can still be steered, but it will take more physical strength because the driver has to overcome the failure of the hydraulic system.

If steering failure occurs, slow the vehicle and pull off the road. Do not brake heavily in case the vehicle pulls to one side; the driver does not have the strength to overcome this extra force.

Stuck Accelerator: The seemingly obvious solution to a stuck accelerator is to turn off the ignition. In today's vehicles, drivers cannot do this or they will lose power steering, power brakes, and possibly lock the steering wheel. The best response in today's vehicles is to shift the transmission into neutral and get the vehicle off the road and stopped as quickly as possible. Understand though, that once the resistance of the drive train is released by the transmission, the engine will rev up quickly. If the engine is not shut off quickly, it will probably fail, resulting in the loss of steering control and brakes.

Released Hood: Although this may sound comical, it is very serious. If the hood releases and breaks the driver's vision, try to find a small gap through which you can look at the base of the hood and pull the vehicle off the road. If all forward visibility is blocked, quickly get your head out the side window and drive the vehicle to the side of the road and stop.

Techniques for Pulling off the Road: Once drivers have responded to the immediate threat of the vehicle malfunction, they still have to get the vehicles safely off the roadway and parked where further damage will not occur.

Planning: Plan the exit with the time available. Signal your intentions and use the first available parking area.

Braking: Most vehicle malfunctions require rapid deceleration. Remove your foot from the accelerator and begin smooth, firm braking. The driver may have to release some of the braking pressure if it becomes difficult to control the steering. Continue to drive the vehicle and do not just jam on the brakes.

Parking: Once the driver has driven off the roadway, stop the vehicle where it will not be hit by other traffic. Turn on the emergency flashers and turn off the emergency lights and siren.

◆ CASE STUDY RECAP

NIOSH investigators concluded the following to minimize the risk of similar occurrences:

- Fire departments should establish, implement, and enforce standard operating procedures (SOPs) on the use of seat belts in all emergency vehicles. The SOPs should apply to all persons riding in all emergency vehicles and state that all persons should be seated and secured in an approved riding position any time the vehicle is in motion.
- Fire departments should ensure that drivers of fire apparatus do not move vehicles until all occupants in vehicles are secured with seat belts.
- Drivers of fire apparatus should ensure that vehicles are not moved until all persons riding in them are secured with seat belts. The apparatus involved in this incident was equipped with seat belts; however, all occupants, including the driver, were not wearing them at the time of the incident. The use and wearing of seat belts could greatly reduce injuries to the driver and passengers in the event of a wreck.
- Fire departments should ensure all drivers of fire department vehicles are responsible for the safe and prudent operation of the vehicles under all conditions.
- Fire departments should ensure driver/operators of fire service vehicles are responsible for the safe and prudent operation of the vehicles under all conditions. The state allows emergency vehicles responding to an incident to exceed the maximum speed limit if the driver does not endanger life or property; however, drivers of fire apparatus should reduce their speed when traveling on hazardous routes (e.g., insufficient shoulder). Drivers should always maintain a safe speed to avoid losing control of the vehicle.

INVESTIGATOR INFORMATION

This incident was investigated by Kimberly Cortez, Occupational Health and Safety Specialist, and Richard Braddee, Project Officer/Team Leader, Surveillance and Field Investigations Branch, Division of Safety Research, NIOSH.

◆ SUMMARY

Route selection is necessary for the driver to get to the scene quickly and carefully. Route planning, predetermined route procedures, and driver familiarization all contribute to effective route selection. Choose a route to arrive at the emergency in the most efficient way. Minimize travel time, minimize crash exposure, and allow the driver to focus attention on driving. When planning a route:

- Consider geographic and local conditions.
- Utilize your organization's procedures.

Use predetermined routes to avoid potential problems on the road. If primary routes are not in good condition, use alternate routes. The driver should be familiar with:

- Daily route information
- Procedures to identify local information
- Height restrictions
- How to read a map

To review, when the driver is in the emergency mode of vehicle driving, the driver is using emergency signaling devices while responding to a medical emergency. Emergency driving is not a clearance to engage in high-speed driving, which puts everyone on the road in serious jeopardy. Safe, controlled driving will normally get the crew to the emergency scene and the medical facility (if applicable) without endangering the driver, the crew, or the patient.

Emergency signaling devices are used during emergency driving for two reasons:

- To notify other drivers that an emergency vehicle is approaching
- To request that the other drivers yield the right-of-way to the emergency vehicle

When approaching other drivers with lights and siren on, always expect the unexpected. Even when operating in the emergency mode, there is no reason for the driver ever to exceed the posted speed limit. The controlled intersection is the most dangerous part of any run the driver makes. The driver must approach each intersection slowly and carefully and thoroughly ensure that he or she has been granted the right-of-way before proceeding through the intersection.

Adverse weather conditions affect traction and the driver's vision. To improve traction, slow down. Remember that wet leaves on the roadway are just as slick as snow and ice. To improve the driver's vision, make sure the windshield and mirrors are clean and the driver needs to be well rested and not under the influence of drugs or alcohol.

Before a crash occurs, the driver can prepare the emergency vehicle so that the equipment does not become missile hazards. The driver can prepare mentally by thinking about the escape paths and, when faced with two choices, selecting the one that minimizes injury and damage.

When faced with an impending crash, the driver can sometimes brake, accelerate, or steer to avoid the crash. Most vehicle malfunctions require that the driver go slow, continue to maintain control of the vehicle through careful steering and braking, and exit the roadway.

The law of due regard puts the burden on drivers, to ensure that their actions are necessary and appropriate for the situation.

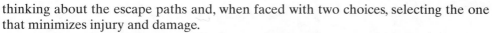

Review Questions

1. Why is route planning important?
2. When you plan a route, what factors should be considered?
3. Who must wear restraints?
4. Why should all equipment be secure?
5. What are some examples of unsafe behavior?
6. There are two reasons to use emergency signaling devices. What are they?
7. Three hundred feet prior to approaching a controlled intersection, the siren should be in which mode? And, 150 feet prior to the intersection, you should change the siren to which mode?
8. How can your vision be affected by the vehicle? What things might you do that affect your own vision?
9. Why is hydroplaning dangerous?
10. After it has rained and there are puddles of standing water, how can you reduce the effects of hydroplaning?
11. What is the problem associated with high crosswinds?
12. What things improve your night vision?
13. What are some of the things you can do to mentally prepare yourself to avoid a crash?
14. As you are moving through a controlled intersection, you suddenly notice a car moving rapidly toward you from your left side. What is probably the best way to avoid a crash?

References

Cook, John Lee Jr. 1998. *Standard operating procedures and guidelines*. Saddle Brook, NJ: Penn Well.

Federal Highway Administration. October 1997. *Technology in rural transportation "simple solutions."* FHWA Publication No. FHWA-RD-97-108.

Federal Highway Administration. *Commercial vehicle fleet management and information systems.* Electronic Document Library.

NFPA. 1997. *NFPA 1451, Standard for a fire service vehicle operations training program.* Quincy, MA: National Fire Protection Association.

NFPA. 1997. *NFPA 1500, Standard on fire department occupational safety and health program.* Quincy, MA: National Fire Protection Association.

NYSDOT. *ITS Toolbox for rural and small urban areas.*

U.S. DOT. *Rural ITS Toolbox.* Retrieved, from http://www.its.dot.gov/JPODOCS/REPTS_TE/13477.html

U.S. DOT booklet on signal preemption. Electronic Document Library. *Technology in rural transportation "simple solutions."* October 1997. FHWA Publication No. FHWA-RD-97-108.

Virginia Department of Transportation, Northern Virginia District. December 1997. *Automated vehicle location system pilot project.*

CHAPTER 7

Communications

Objectives

After completing this chapter, you should be able to:

- Define the emergency vehicle operator's roles and responsibilities involving communications pertaining to emergency vehicle operations.
- Define proper communications including radio etiquette and hand signals.
- Relate the technology and role of communications in emergency vehicle operations.

Case Study

The tones activate the station's alerting system with the dispatcher's voice echoing the information of the emergency call. It is a possible stroke at a local nursing home. You are familiar with most nursing homes in your response district, but this one is new to you. The street sounds familiar, but you recall it to be a residential section of the town. You and your crew take your position in the ambulance and begin your emergency response to the location. You arrive in the area of the call but are not able to locate the facility. Neither you nor your crew has ever been to this location and really do not know what you are even looking for. Over the next ten minutes you communicate with the dispatcher, who is very familiar with the location and has been to it many times in the past. A few minutes later the dispatcher advises you to cancel; another unit from your agency was in the area and is familiar with the location. They are on the scene with the patient.

◆ INTRODUCTION

Communication is a vital aspect of everything we do in life. You can walk into just about any organization or business in this country, and many times the number-one issue cited is communication or a lack thereof. Emergency vehicle operations are no different. In virtually every aspect of operating the vehicle, some form of communication needs to take place.

It begins from the time an incident occurs until the unit is back in the station and the ignition has been turned off. An incident begins by a caller recognizing there is a situation he or she cannot handle. The call is made to the dispatch center and the dispatcher begins the interrogation to determine as much information as possible in the shortest amount of time. The information needs to contain everything from the location to the event that is occurring. In turn, the dispatcher determines through local protocols who to send and how to send them. If proper communication is not determined from the beginning, the wrong unit or the wrong equipment will be sent and potentially to the wrong location. Communication is essential in time critical events to get the right equipment to the right location in the right amount of time. This chapter covers some of the issues surrounding effective communications and the emergency vehicle operator.

◆ COMMUNICATION RESPONSIBILITIES

The entire crew is responsible for communications involving your vehicle (Figure 7.1). Each member of the crew has specific responsibilities involving communications. Teamwork is essential. As with other aspects of the call, understanding the other crew members' expectations and in turn their understanding of your expectations is a vital link for a successful call and shift.

At various points of any response, reporting is a normal requirement. They include the following:

- Prior to the start of the call
- When you are dispatched on a response
- When you arrive at the scene of an incident
- At-patient on medical calls or other key trigger points such as water on the fire
- Incident choreography
- When the fire is under control or the patient has been extricated
- When transporting patients, notifying dispatch you are en route to your destination
- Arrival at destination such as a hospital in EMS situations
- When available

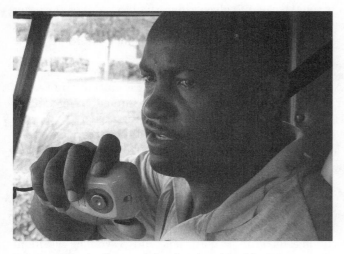

FIGURE 7.1 ◆ Communication is critical in emergency vehicle response.

PRIOR TO THE START OF THE CALL

Prior to any response it is imperative to ensure that equipment is checked and ready to use. The portable radios should be checked for battery power, the onboard equipment checked as part of the routine daily vehicle check, and all findings documented. You need to be sure dispatch knows the status of your vehicle.

DISPATCHED ON A RESPONSE

Critical Information

- ◆ Address (location)
- ◆ Nature of call

When alerted for a response, it is essential to get to your vehicle as quickly as possible and begin your response. Prior to leaving the station or your starting point, you must be sure of the address and the safest route to reach the incident. When discussing reduction of response times, this is where time should be made, and not during the response by driving faster than posted speed limits.

The passenger in the cab should find the location in a map book of the area. In many agencies technology is becoming more advanced; hence GPS may allow the passenger or the driver to punch in the address, and detailed directions are given in order to reach the scene of the incident. The map or grid book is an important resource for all departments to have on their vehicles regardless of whether advanced technology is available. Dispatch should also notify you of any route problems you may encounter to the call. There are a number of dispatch centers that notify local agencies of road construction or various other traffic situations units may encounter in their district.

> **Example: There is major construction at an intersection you would need to travel through en route to the scene or Main Street is blocked due to a parade.**

These items are essential for a safe response. In turn, you need to communicate any findings you may encounter on the call. It is always important to know of any other emergency vehicles that may be traveling in the same direction as you are. Phoenix Fire produced a video in which Engine 9 and Ladder 9 literally meet en route to the same call.

Nationally recognized protocols have been established to evaluate and dispatch incidents for police, fire, and EMS calls. If your dispatch center is currently not using such a nationally recognized protocol, it is essential that it look into adopting and implementing such a protocol. These protocols can be obtained from such agencies as the National Association of Emergency Medical Dispatch and the American Public Communications Organization. There are no known successful lawsuits regarding using such protocols. Notice the word *successful*. Anyone can sue anyone for any reason; however, not everyone is successful in the litigation attempt. Acknowledgment needs to be made by the dispatch center with pre-arrival instructions and response mode advised as per the local protocol. Any information regarding hazards should be relayed to the vehicles responding.

A vehicle accident involving hazardous materials and a vehicle accident involving multiple vehicles and patients are examples of important information that needs to be relayed to responding vehicles. In cases of scene safety, it is crucial

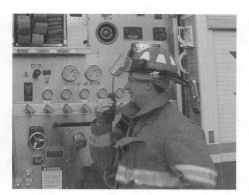

FIGURE 7.2 ◆ Communication is an ongoing process.

that dispatch relays scene safety and that crews stage with their vehicles until law enforcement can secure the scene.

INCIDENT ARRIVAL

When the first unit arrives on the scene, a proper size up should be given over the radio in a short, concise manner; yet give enough detail to advise incoming units what you are encountering (Figure 7.2).

> **Fire example: "Engine four is on scene. Single story structure. Heavy smoke and fire showing from sides one, two, and four. Engine four is attacking the fire."**

This gives an accurate picture of the incident, what you have, and what you are doing. A few key points to remember are to establish written standard operating procedures and guidelines (SOP/SOG), the labeling of building sides, how incident command is to be established, and what your agency wants established as an incident size up. SOGs should also be flexible enough to include the judgment of the company officer or person in charge of the incident.

> **Another example of an incident size up of a motor vehicle collision: "Rescue four-two is on scene, car versus pickup truck, heavy damage, occupants still in vehicle, rescue four-two investigating."**

AT-PATIENT ON MEDICAL CALLS OR OTHER KEY TRIGGER POINTS

A number of times when emergency personnel respond to medical calls, they arrive on the scene to find the patient is on the fifth floor of a high-rise or on the opposite side of a 200,000-square-foot factory. The on-scene time does not adequately reflect when responders reach the patient's side. The "at-patient" time is noted when they actually reach the patient and make contact. In the same instance, if it is a fire, a key factor to record through communication is water on the fire. These benchmarks and others are important for the emergency responder to communicate and the dispatch center to record for record keeping and future statistical analysis. Benchmarking is an important concept and component in order for the emergency service industry to progress forward into the twenty-first century.

INCIDENT CHOREOGRAPHY

When emergency personnel are at the scene of an incident, it is important that communication is accurate and concise. This will afford other responders, dispatch personnel, and incident commanders the ability to hear and understand what the crew is encountering.

Establishing incident command at small incidents or major incidents is critical to its success at the major events. The small incidents will allow you to practice your incident command structure so that when a major event occurs, it should be second nature.

FIRE IS UNDER CONTROL OR PATIENT HAS BEEN EXTRICATED

Additional benchmarks that are valuable to communicate are when the fire is under control or the patient has been extricated from the vehicle. Some emergency service organizations also verbalize the delivery of their first shock to patients who are in v-fib or pulseless v-tach when they arrive on the scene.

WHEN EN ROUTE TO DESTINATION

Notification should be made to dispatch when you leave the scene and begin transporting patients to the medical facility and/or destination. Dispatch should also notify you of any destinations not accepting patients. New technology has capabilities to transmit this information to the PDA or laptop computer in your vehicle.

ARRIVAL AT DESTINATION

When arriving at your destination, such as a hospital in EMS situations, notification needs to be made that your vehicle has successfully arrived at the intended destination.

WHEN AVAILABLE

The vehicle should be made ready to respond and then placed available with your dispatch center as soon as possible after completing your call.

Keeping your dispatch center informed of the different parameters and benchmarks provides invaluable data for future reference. Lawsuits and data analysis are two prime examples that will benefit from the benchmarks communicated and recorded.

◆ PERSONNEL

Various personnel are involved in a successful response. These include:

- ◆ Crew chief/officer
- ◆ Driver/operator
- ◆ Dispatcher
- ◆ Medical director
- ◆ Medical facility

CREW CHIEF/OFFICER

The crew chief/officer's responsibility is overall incident control in most organizations. Individuals in this position are responsible for communicating on the radio in most organizations. The crew chief/officer can be an additional set of eyes and ears for the driver/operator. The driver/operator may not see or hear a hazardous condition during the response or operation of the vehicle. The crew chief/officer must not assume the driver/operator sees or hears everything and so warns the latter of what he or she may see or hear. As the individual in charge of the crew and the unit, you will potentially be held to the same standards as the vehicle operator should a negative effect occur. The legal term for this is vicarious liability, which is covered in Chapter 3.

DRIVER/OPERATOR

The driver/operator should not be responsible for radio communications, especially when the vehicle is in motion. The driver/operator's main concern is to get from point *A* to point *B* in a safe manner. The driver/operator cannot maintain two hands on the steering wheel as advocated in a safe driving environment, by using one hand to talk on a microphone and the other trying to steer a large vehicle. The potential for the cord from the radio microphone getting wrapped around an object such as the steering wheel is an additional hazard that should be avoided.

DISPATCHER

Communication centers around the dispatcher (Figure 7.3). After all, if there isn't anyone to take the information, give the unit the proper information, and maintain constant communication with the units, the system will fail. Therefore, the dispatcher has one of the more important roles in the whole communications aspect of a response. Dispatchers are intimately involved from the beginning to the end. They initially need to obtain the appropriate information from the caller, send the proper vehicles to the proper location, and monitor the call until it is complete. They will need to assist crews in making contacts to other services and agencies as requested. This may include utility companies or medical receiving facilities. The dispatcher is the cog that keeps the communications wheel turning. In most communities, emergency service personnel depend on the communication center to be the resource center for all their needs when on the scene of an incident. It coincides with the old adage "I may not

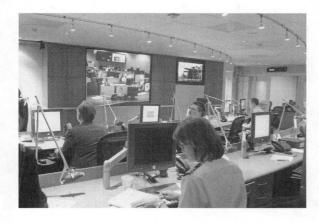

FIGURE 7.3 ◆ The dispatcher is key to communication. (*Courtesy of Getty Images, Inc.—Liasion*)

know everything, but I know whom to call." The dispatch center resembles this remark. Dispatchers may not have all the answers, but they do know whom to call for resources or additional help.

MEDICAL DIRECTOR

Many systems require their EMS personnel to make on-line communications with the medical director for additional medication or advanced orders. In these situations the radio operator needs to paint a vivid picture of what the crew is seeing, feeling, hearing, and smelling with the patient. The operator is now the senses for the medical director, because the medical director cannot experience any of these.

MEDICAL FACILITY

The medical facility needs to be informed that a patient is en route to it. In most instances these facilities are interested only in the overall impression of the patient. With staff cuts and patient loads increasing, they are not interested in a long dissertation of the patient findings.

> **Example: "This is rescue 456 en route to your location with a 56-year-old male with a possible fractured ankle. Vitals are stable, leg is splinted, and ETA [estimated time of arrival] is 5 minutes." Wait for the receiving facility to acknowledge before you clear your channel.**

Remember that local protocol governs your actions and needs to be followed.

In addition, new technology offers the means to send an electronic report through satellite communications to the receiving facility. Technology is available whereby the patient report can be completed on a PDA and then beamed to the hospital before the patient ever leaves the scene. This not only allows the emergency department staff to prepare for the patient but also gives them more information in an organized manner that typically cannot be communicated effectively over the radio.

◆ RADIO COMMUNICATIONS

RADIO FREQUENCIES

Communications has grown into a monstrous complexity. Agencies use a variety of frequencies to communicate and different means to communicate. It is essential that you know the frequencies of the various agencies in your community plus those of the surrounding communities. You also must have the capabilities to communicate to mutual aid departments whether they are responding to your incident or you are responding to theirs. You will need to ascertain the various radio frequencies and communication devices neighboring agencies have the capability of using and when to use the designated frequency or communication device. In an incident that arises in which you respond in an area and do not have the designated frequency, you will need to rely on your dispatch center to relay the information. This is not always the best method because the dispatcher will be facing the normal volume of calls, plus direct communication is always best to avoid miscommunications.

HEADSETS

Protecting our crew from loss of hearing is a safety priority. A number of regulations and standards, including NFPA 1500, recommend personnel wear hearing protection when responding with sirens. Headsets are one means to protect crews from potential hearing loss as a result of siren noise. Headsets also allow personnel to communicate in the vehicle to all crew members regardless of where they are riding in the vehicle. Different states have some restrictions on the use of these devices. The driver of the vehicle may be affected the most pertaining to these rules. You need to check your state's laws governing the use of headsets while operating a motor vehicle.

MOBILE VERSUS PORTABLE RADIOS

When transmitting, you must remember the transmit and receive capabilities of your device. A mobile device can typically transmit over a longer distance than can a portable radio. Most systems have placed fixed repeaters throughout their service area. In various areas communication may be impossible due to "dead spots," areas where radio signals cannot be sent or received. There are usually buildings and geographical locations in your response area that you may be aware of prior to an incident occurring. A repeater may be of value in these situations; it is a device that receives a transmission from a low-power portable or mobile radio on one frequency and retransmits it at a higher power on another frequency.

Certain buildings create a significant life hazard for fire and rescue personnel during a fire event. Part of preplanning a building should be to check communication capabilities in that building and note any potential problems that may be associated with transmitting and receiving in that particular building. Many firefighters lose their lives in a burning structure because of poor or a lack of communication.

RADIO ETIQUETTE

Most radio communications can be heard by anyone who has a radio or scanner with that frequency. An SOP/SOG needs to be implemented to govern radio communications. Confidentiality is essential to patients. Off-the-wall comments are not appropriate at any time, and when transmitted across the radio, everyone with a radio or scanner will hear the comment. Keep conversations to what is necessary and professional.

Think about what you are going to say before you say it. Remember to identify your unit designation and whom you are calling. Keep your transmissions brief and to the point. Use plain English and speak distinctly and clearly.

Example: "Headquarters from district four-one."

Examples of plain English follow.

Use	*Instead of*
Affirmative	Yes or yea
Negative	No or nay
Four-two	Forty-two
One-four	Fourteen

Always confirm by repeating the message back to the person sending the message, especially if there is any doubt of what that person is trying to say. When spelling words, use the phonetic alphabet, which is a universal, standardized to be used when communicating over a two-way radio system.

Phonetic Alphabet	
A—Alpha	N—November
B—Bravo	O—Oscar
C—Charlie	P—Papa
D—Delta	Q—Quebec
E—Echo	R—Romeo
F—Foxtrot	S—Sierra
G—Golf	T—Tango
H—Hotel	U—Uniform
I—India	V—Victor
J—Juliet	W—Whiskey
K—Kilo	X—X-ray
L—Lima	Y—Yankee
M—Mike	Z—Zulu

Some departments like to use ten-code or a special collection of codes to communicate. Many departments are trying to get away from the ten-codes and limit the number of special codes used. Codes can be difficult to remember, and the wrong code could be transmitted in the wrong situation resulting in the wrong response.

Examples of some codes may include:

Signal 7	Death
Code H	Crew in trouble
Code B	Bomb threat

HOW TO USE THE RADIO EQUIPMENT

There are a number of rules you should consider when speaking on the radio. They include the following.

1. Listen to the channel before transmitting to assure that it is not in use.
2. Press the transmit button for one second before speaking.
3. Speak at close range, approximately two inches, directly into or across the face of the microphone.
4. Speak slowly and clearly. Pronounce each word distinctly, avoiding words that are difficult to understand.
5. Speak in a normal pitch, keeping your voice free of emotion.
6. Be brief. Know what you are going to say before you press the transmit button.
7. Do not waste airtime with unnecessary information.

The emergency services industry utilizes a variety of other communication devices. Some vehicles have a system whereby pressing a button sends a signal to the dispatch center. Inside the communication center a system decodes the signals and records the vehicle's status. This allows minimal verbal radio communications. Technology is exploding almost daily. Certain computerized devices that are installed in the cab allow the dispatch center to generate and send all the pertinent information directly to the responding units. With the development of GPS, units can have a mapping system within their units to get clear and concise directions to the scene of the incident. They can also follow their response on the computer screen and identify potential delays and other factors that may hamper their response.

Cellular phones have become very popular and may be used by your agency. Cellular phones can still be monitored by the public if they tune to the frequency you are speaking on. You need to use caution during your conversation and by no means should the driver of the vehicle be utilizing the cellular phone while the vehicle is in motion. As noted earlier, individual states may have laws governing the use of cell phones in a moving vehicle. Emergency service providers are by no means exempt from the law. We are given certain privileges. However, should something go wrong, not only will you probably be held to the same standard as anyone else; in most instances you will be held to a higher standard.

◆ **HAND SIGNALS**

Hand signals are an important communication tool for both the driver and the spotter(s) (Figure 7.4). Hand signals will assist in directing the drivers of emergency vehicles to maneuver the vehicles in areas where they may not have a clear vision of their entire surroundings. Remember to keep the signals uniform, use signals that everyone can understand. Your organization should adopt a set of hand signals. The hand signals in Figure 7.4 are commonly recognized in the industry and may be adopted for your agency to use.

◆ **CASE STUDY RECAP**

Communication is important for all organizations. It is imperative in the emergency service business to have effective communication because it may mean the difference between life and death. In this case, the patient's outcome was not affected by the lack of the crew being able to reach the facility.

Signal Number 1: Come Ahead

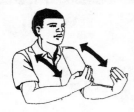

Day
Extend arms in front of your body, palms facing up. Move arms toward your body, bending at the elbows.

Night
When using conventional flashlights, direct lights forward.

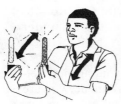

Signal Number 2: Slow Down

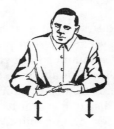

Day
Turn palms facing downward with thumbs toward your body at waist level. Move hands down and up.

Night
When using conventional flashlights, direct lights forward.

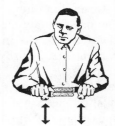

Signal Number 3: Stop or Halt

Day
Extend right arm forward with palms facing outward.

Night
Light in right hand pointed upward, blinking. When using conventional flashlights, direct light in right hand forward, blinking.

FIGURE 7.4 ◆ Hand signals need to be standardized.

Signal Number 4: Move in Reverse

Day
Extend arms in front of you, palms facing forward. Move hands forward and back.

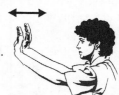

Night
When using conventional flashlights, direct lights forward.

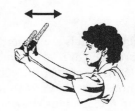

Signal Number 5: Turn Left

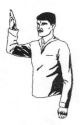

Day
Facing the vehicle, raise right arm to your side, bending at the elbow. Face palm outward and move hand to your right.

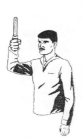

Night
When using conventional flashlights, direct light in right hand forward.

Signal Number 6: Turn Right

Day
Facing the vehicle, raise left hand to your side, bending at the elbow. Face palm outward and move hand to your left.

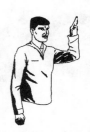

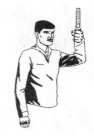

Night
When using conventional flashlights, direct lights forward.

Signal Number 7: Turn Off Engine

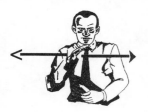

Day
Place right hand above chest level, with elbow at your side, and palm facing downward. Move hand from right to left.

Night
When using conventional flashlights, direct light in right hand forward.

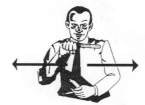

Signal Number 8: Increase Speed

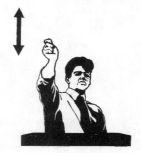

Day
Extend right arm above you with a closed fist, palm forward. Move arm up and down in front of your body.

Night
When using conventional flashlights, direct light in right hand forward.

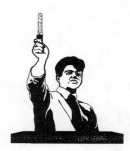

FIGURE 7.4 ◆ (*continued*)

Signal Number 9: Start Engines

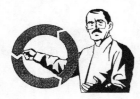

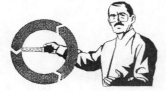

<u>Day</u>
Circle right arm clockwise in front of your body.

<u>Night</u>
When using conventional flashlights, direct light in right hand forward.

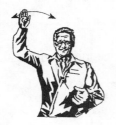

Signal Number 10: As You Were

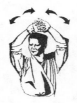

<u>Day</u>
Extend arms above your head; cross and uncross your hands at the wrists.

<u>Night</u>
When using conventional flashlights, direct lights forward.

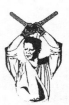

Signal Number 11: Attention

<u>Day</u>
Extend right arm above you, palm facing outward. Wave hand right and left above your head.

<u>Night</u>
When using conventional flashlights, direct light in right hand forward.

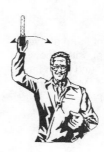

FIGURE 7.4 ◆ *(continued)*

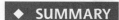
◆ SUMMARY

As an emergency vehicle operator, your first priority is to operate the vehicle in a safe manner. The crew chief/officer in the passenger seat should be the communicator and use the radio, especially when you are driving the vehicle. The dispatcher is the cog of the communications wheel. Spend a day in the communication center to understand that side of the communications process.

It is imperative that you know the address of the call and have preplanned a safe route to respond, prior to leaving the station. Limit your radio transmission to what is essential and be professional. You don't know who may be listening. Remember the adage, "If you can't say something nice, don't say anything at all"; the same philosophy goes when communicating on the radio.

When you are transmitting:

1. Plan what you are going to say.
2. Identify your vehicle and whom you are calling.
3. Be brief.
4. Use plain English.
5. Pronounce your words clearly.
6. Spell confusing words phonetically.
7. Repeat directions and medical orders.

Remember how to use the radio equipment:

1. Listen before you speak.
2. Depress the microphone key for one second before speaking.
3. Talk with the microphone close to your mouth.

Review Questions

1. Define the emergency vehicle operator's role in communicating.
2. List three main points relevant to radio etiquette.
3. Describe a role that technology plays in communication.
4. Describe why benchmarking should be an important part of communications.
5. List the essential components of communication during an incident.

References

NFPA. 2002. *NFPA 1500 Standard on fire department occupational safety and health program.* Quincy. MA: National Fire Protection Association.

NHSA. 1995. *Emergency vehicle operator course* U.S. Department of Transportation. Washington, DC.

CHAPTER 8 ◆ Maintenance

Objectives

After completing this chapter, you should be able to:

- Identify the major mechanical components of a vehicle.
- Define the types of preventive maintenance.
- Discuss the characteristics of an emergency vehicle.

Case Study

This case study gives an example of negligence related to vehicle inspection. Think about the operator's role in the situation.

Background.   A crew was taking a patient to a hospital in the next county. The ambulance maintenance log, which contains information about previous inspections and work requested and completed, was kept in a room upstairs from the vehicle. The crew was in a hurry, so they did not review the log before they left, contrary to the organization's procedures. They also did not perform a Quick Check.

Midway through the trip, the oil pressure warning light came on, and the engine temperature rose. The crew pulled over and called for a replacement vehicle.

Investigation.   The follow-up inquiry included a review of the ambulance maintenance log. The two most recent vehicle checks each noted a slow oil leak. The maintenance log contained a note to the operator to check the oil level before each trip. The log showed that repairs were scheduled for the following Monday, when the regular mechanic returned from vacation.

How might the operator be judged negligent in this situation?
How might the organization also be found at fault?

◆ INTRODUCTION

Each year a percentage of firefighter/EMS injuries and deaths are the result of mechanical problems and apparatus failure. In these cases, the public and legal systems are increasingly inclined to look to the organization's adherence to maintenance standards.

In an ongoing attempt to minimize risks and fatalities, several groups have been working together to establish and implement standards, training and education, and certification programs supporting the safety of emergency vehicle equipment.

In August 2000, NFPA 1071, *Standard for **Emergency Vehicle Technician** Professional Qualifications,* was issued. This standard establishes a set of professional qualifications that can be used to develop educational requirements and corresponding certifications for emergency vehicle technicians and mechanics. In addition, NFPA 1915, *Standard for Fire Apparatus Preventive Maintenance Program,* provides guidance for creating and maintaining a comprehensive maintenance program. Together, these standards can be used to ensure that a department's staff has skills adequate to service and maintain the full spectrum of emergency vehicles. Although NFPA standards are not legally binding unless formally adopted by the authority having jurisdiction (AHJ), many departments, companies servicing emergency equipment, and original equipment manufacturers have adopted NFPA 1071 and NFPA 1915 as part of their internal policies and operating procedures.

In an ongoing effort to ensure vehicle safety, the Emergency Vehicle Technician (EVT) Certification Commission was established to write and administer tests that would demonstrate proficiency in established standards. The tests resemble those used by the Automotive Service Excellence (ASE) organization, applying its high "blue seal of excellence" standards to fire equipment. Technicians who receive all of the EVT and ASE certifications are recognized as master certified EVTs. The EVT certification program presently has two certification tracks, one for technicians who service and maintain fire apparatus and another for technicians who service and maintain ambulances. The levels of fire apparatus certification are shown in Figure 8.1. The levels of ambulance certification are shown in Figure 8.2.

Today, there are approximately 60,000 emergency vehicle technicians and mechanics in the United States (Figure 8.3). It is estimated that less than 25 percent have

Emergency Vehicle Technician Fire Apparatus Certifications

Fire Apparatus Technician Level Requirements—Level I

ASE Exams:
• T-7 or A-7, Heating and Air Conditioning
• T-2 Truck, Diesel Engines
• T-4 Truck, Brakes
• T-5 Truck, Suspension and Steering

EVT Exam:
• F-2 Design and Performance Standards and Preventive Maintenance of Fire Apparatus

Fire Apparatus Technician Level Requirements—Level II

ASE Exams:
• T-3 Truck, Drive Train
• T-6 Truck, Electrical Systems

EVT Exams:
• F-3 Fire Pumps and Accessories
• F-4 Fire Apparatus Electrical Systems

Fire Apparatus Technician Level Requirements—Master Level III

ASE Exams:
• T-1 Truck, Gasoline Engines

EVT Exams:
• F-5 Aerial Fire Apparatus
• F-6 Allison Automatic Transmissions

FIGURE 8.1 ◆ The levels of fire apparatus certification.

Emergency Vehicle Technician Ambulance Certifications

Ambulance Technician Level Requirements—Level I

ASE Exams:
- A-4 Automobile, Suspension and Steering
- A-5 Automobile, Brakes
- A-6 Automobile, Electrical Systems
- A-8 Automobile, Engine Performance

EVT Exams:
- E-1 Design and Performance and Preventive Maintenance of Ambulances

Ambulance Technician Level Requirements—Level II

ASE Exams:
- A-1 Automobile, Engine Repair
- A-3 Automobile, Manual Drive Train & Axle
- A-7 Automobile, Heating and Air-Conditioning
- T-2 Truck, Diesel Engines

EVT Exams:
- E-2 Ambulance Electrical Systems
- E-3 Ambulance Heating, Air-Conditioning, and Ventilation

Ambulance Technician Level Requirements—Master Level III

ASE Exams:
- A-2 Automobile, Automatic Transmission and Transaxle
- T-4 Truck, Brakes
- T-5 Truck, Suspension and Steering

EVT Exams:
- E-4 Ambulance Cab, Chassis, and Body

FIGURE 8.2 ◆ The levels of ambulance certification.

received certification meeting the requirements outlined in NFPA 1071. It is a common belief that increasing the number of certified emergency vehicle technicians will assist in reducing the number of emergency worker injuries and fatalities related to equipment failure. Ensuring that quality educational opportunities are readily available is central to increasing the number of certified EVTs.

Point to Ponder

How can you ensure that an emergency vehicle is in safe operating condition?

- Inspect the vehicle according to established procedures.
- Check that all scheduled maintenance has been performed.
- Check that all needed repairs have been made. If a vehicle is NOT in safe operating condition, the operator has the responsibility to take the vehicle out of service until the problems have been fixed.

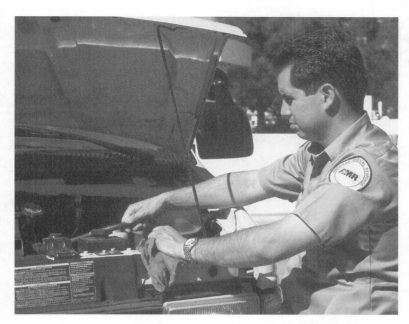

FIGURE 8.3 ◆ Emergency vehicle technicians are becoming more standard as part of the emergency service organization team.

More information about the EVT Certification Commission is available online at http://www.evtcc.org. Additional information about the ASE is available online at http://www.ase.com.

◆ MAJOR MECHANICAL SYSTEMS

Before the discussion about inspection of the vehicle, it is important to cover the major mechanical systems, such as engines, drive trains, and cooling systems. Because most emergency vehicles are specialized bodies added to truck frames, there are many similarities between different makes and models.

ENGINE/DRIVE TRAIN

The weight of the vehicle and its installed auxiliary systems require most emergency vehicles to have a large engine, either diesel or gasoline powered. To provide the smoothest ride possible, these power plants are most often connected to automatic transmissions.

Point to Ponder

Spend some time with the maintenance officer of your organization or a local emergency service organization. Discuss with this officer the problem areas that you can cover in the lesson that will help the organization do a better job.

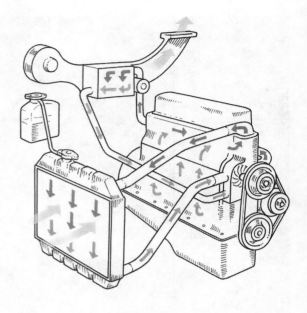

FIGURE 8.4 ◆ Cooling system.
(*Courtesy of Dorling Kindersley
Media Library*)

COOLING SYSTEM

Heavy duty vehicles, such as ambulances and fire engines, require heavy duty engine cooling systems (Figure 8.4). It is critical that the driver checks the fluid level of the cooling system every day, especially in hot weather. It is essential to follow the correct procedures for the vehicle. Severe burns can be the result of doing this check wrong. Transmission fluid cooling systems are installed in many emergency vehicles to maintain proper operating temperatures and to help prevent breakdown of the transmission fluid.

BRAKING SYSTEM

A variety of types of brake systems are in use today. The older **drum brakes** are still used extensively in trucks. Many of the newer vehicles use the more reliable disc brakes. These two types are often used together, with the **disc brakes** installed on the front wheels, where most of the braking effort occurs, and the drum brakes on the rear. Antilock braking systems are available from some truck manufacturers and are especially efficient on snow and ice.

Operators must understand that if the vehicle is not equipped with an antilock braking system (ABS) and goes into a skid, the proper response is to release the brakes and allow the wheels to rotate freely while gradually letting up on the accelerator. The steering wheel should be turned so that the front wheels face in the direction of the skid. If using a standard transmission, the clutch should not be released until the vehicle is under control. Another key factor for skid prevention is proper maintenance of tire air pressure and adequate tread for tires. Operators need to be aware that while operating a tanker, the weight shifting of baffled water can have a serious effect on the ability of the operator to steer, brake, and maintain control of the vehicle.

Antilock Brakes. Stopping an emergency vehicle in a hurry on a slippery road can present a challenge for the driver. An antilock braking system (ABS) equips the vehicle so the emergency vehicle driver can accomplish such a feat.

The theory on how antilock brakes work is very simple. There is less traction when the vehicle begins to skid. The portion of tire that contacts the road begins sliding on the road surface. A great example of this is when a vehicle slides on ice. Essentially the tire is touching the surface; however, there is virtually no traction. Antilock brakes benefit you in two ways: The vehicle will stop faster and the driver will be able to steer while stopping.

The four main components of an ABS system (Figure 8.5) are the speed sensors, pump, valves, and controller.

Speed Sensors: The ABS needs to know when a wheel is going to lock up. Each wheel has a speed sensor, or in some cases it is the differential that provides this information.

Pump: Because the valve is able to release pressure from the brakes, there has to be some way to put that pressure back. That is what the pump does; when a valve reduces the pressure in a line, the pump is there to get the pressure back up.

Valves: Each brake controlled by the ABS has a valve in the brake line. The valve has three positions on some systems. In position one, the valve is open; pressure from the master cylinder is passed right through to the brake. In position two, the valve blocks the line, isolating that brake from the master cylinder. This prevents the pressure from rising further should the driver push the brake pedal harder. The valve releases some of the pressure from the brake in position three.

Controller: The controller is a computer in the vehicle. It watches the speed sensors and controls the valves. The speed sensors are monitored by the controller. The controller is looking for decelerations in the wheel that are out of the ordinary. There

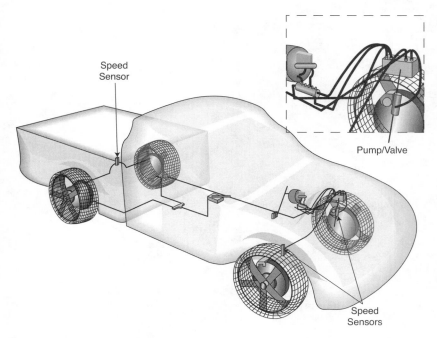

FIGURE 8.5 ◆ Diagram of ABS.

will be a rapid deceleration right before the wheel locks up. The ABS controller realizes that such a rapid deceleration is impossible and reduces the pressure to the brake until it detects an acceleration. It then increases the pressure until it detects the deceleration again. This occurs rather quickly before the tire can actually change significant speed. The result is that the tire slows down at the same speed as the car with the brakes maintaining the tires very close to the point at which they will start to lock up.

It is important that you do not pump antilock brakes. The ABS system when operating will feel like a pulsing sensation in the brake pedal. This is a result of the rapid opening and closing of the valves. When stopping a vehicle with an ABS system, apply the brake firmly and hold it while the ABS does all the work.

Brake Basics. There are three basic principles to braking: leverage, hydraulics, and friction.

Leverage: The brake pedal is designed in such a way that it can multiply the force from your leg several times before any force is even transmitted to the brake fluid.

Hydraulics: The hydraulic system works by applying force at one point and transmitting the force to another point by using an incompressible fluid, which is typically an oil of some sort (Figure 8.6).

Friction: Friction is measured by how difficult it is to slide one object over another. The type of material has a bearing on how difficult it is to slide a material between another material. For example, it is more difficult to slide rubber against rubber than to slide steel against steel. The coefficient of friction is determined by the type of

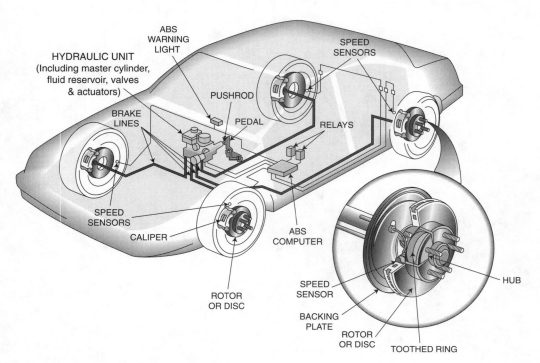

FIGURE 8.6 ◆ Diagram of how brakes work.

material. If the coefficient of a material is 1.0 and the material weighs 100 pounds, then it would take 100 pounds of force to slide the material. If the coefficient were 0.1, then it would take 10 pounds to slide the 100-pound object. It is all proportional; the more the weight the greater the force to stop it. This can be illustrated with brakes: The more force that presses on the pad, the greater the stopping force.

Drum Brakes. The drum brake has more parts than the disc brake and is typically more difficult to service. The drum brake has two brake shoes and a piston. There is also an adjuster mechanism, an emergency brake mechanism, and a lot of springs. The brakes work when the driver pushes on the brake pedal; then the piston pushes the brake shoes against the drum. The multitude of springs is to create the wedging action that pulls the shoes away from the drum when the brakes are released. The remainder of the springs help hold the brake shoes in place and return the adjuster arm after it actuates.

Changing the brake shoes is the most common service requirement for drum brakes. The brake shoe should be replaced when the friction material has worn to within 1/32 inch (0.8 mm) of the rivets. If the brake shoes are not changed and grooves are in the drum, then the drum will need to be refinished.

Disc Brakes. The main components of a disc brake are (Figure 8.7)

- ◆ The brake pads
- ◆ The caliper, which contains the piston
- ◆ The rotor, which is mounted to the hub

A disc brake works by the brake pad squeezing the rotor, and the force is transmitted hydraulically. The friction between the pads and the disc slows the disc. The most common service required for disc brakes is changing the pads. A disc brake typically has a wear indicator on it. When the material is worn away, the metal wear indicator will contact the disc and make a squealing sound. If a deep score is worn into the brake rotor, it will need to be turned to restore the rotor to a flat, smooth surface.

Air Brakes. Air brakes are used in many emergency vehicles. These units are drum type. Air enters the chamber when the brakes are applied. The push rod moves out, turning the slack adjuster, which rotates the S cam and forces the shoes into the drum.

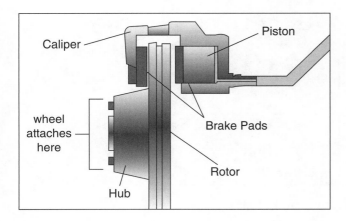

FIGURE 8.7 ◆ Parts of a disc brake.

Exhaust Brakes. The biggest factor in favor of the diesel engine is the high torque/displacement factor. The biggest factor against the diesel is its inherent lack of retarding power. Take your foot off the throttle and a diesel virtually free wheels. Add a 6 to 8 percent grade hill to the equation, and the result is overheating brakes, brake fade, and a good chance of a runaway. An **exhaust brake** traps cylinder compression pressure, creating back pressure.

Exhaust brakes can help save money. They are designed so that the vehicle will require less use of the service brakes.

Brake Fade. **Brake fade** occurs when the brake linings get hot (Figure 8.8). The friction provided by the linings decreases. At this point the linings no longer offer the same resistance to the rotation of the drums and get slick.

ELECTRICAL SYSTEM/AUXILIARY POWER

With the additional demand of emergency lighting systems, sirens, and installed medical support systems on ambulances, the electrical system is a vital component of the emergency vehicle. These heavy duty systems require careful attention and monitoring to ensure that they retain peak efficiency. To provide electrical power while parked, without drawing from the vehicle's battery or batteries, many units have auxiliary power systems installed. An auxiliary power system is a small, engine-powered generator, such as a portable generator. It is independent of the vehicle's electrical system and is used during heavy electrical load conditions.

Most ambulances are equipped with a DC to AC inverter to provide AC power. The inverter provides a constant 115 volt AC power source for onboard AC systems. The patient compartment has AC outlets for using AC systems. Some of the vehicle's lighting is also powered by AC. The crew will select AC power when needed to supply certain systems in the ambulance. When activating the inverter, a red light indicator will be illuminated.

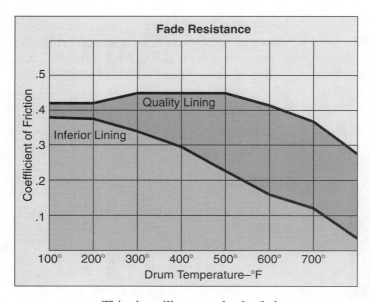

FIGURE 8.8 ◆ This chart illustrates brake fade.

ENVIRONMENTAL CONTROL SYSTEMS

Environmental control systems are the heating and air conditioning systems. Some vehicles may have separate units for the cab and the patient compartment.

◆ **TIRES**

TREAD WEAR

The tread wear grade is a comparative rating based on the wear rate of the tire when tested under controlled conditions on a specified government test course. For example, a tire graded **150** would wear one and a half times as well on the government course as a tire graded **100.** The relative performance of tires depends on the actual conditions of their use, however, and may depart significantly from the norm due to variations in driving habits, service practices, and differences in road characteristics and climate.

TRACTION

AA, A, B, and C. The traction grades from highest to lowest—AA, A, B, and C—represent the tire's ability to stop on wet pavement as measured under controlled conditions on specified government test surfaces of asphalt and concrete. A tire marked C may have poor traction performance.

> **WARNING: The traction grade assigned to this tire is based on braking (straight ahead) traction tests and does not include cornering (turning) traction.**

TEMPERATURE

A, B, and C. The temperature grades are A (the highest), B, and C, representing the tire's resistance to the generation of heat and its ability to dissipate heat when tested under controlled conditions on a specified indoor laboratory test wheel. Sustained high temperature can cause the material of the tire to degenerate and reduce tire life, and excessive temperature can lead to sudden tire failure. The grade C corresponds to a level of performance that all passenger car tires must meet under the Federal Motor Vehicle Safety Standard No. 109. Grades A and B represent higher levels of performance on the laboratory test wheel than the minimum required by law.

> **WARNING: The temperature grade for this tire is established for a tire that is properly inflated and not overloaded. Excessive speed, underinflation, or excessive loading, either separately or in combination, can cause heat buildup and possible tire failure.**

TIRE PRESSURE AND LOADING

Tire information placards and vehicle certification labels contain information on tires and load limits (Figure 8.9). These labels indicate the vehicle manufacturer's information including

- Recommended tire size
- Recommended tire inflation pressure (usually given in PSI cold)

Tire Size Designation

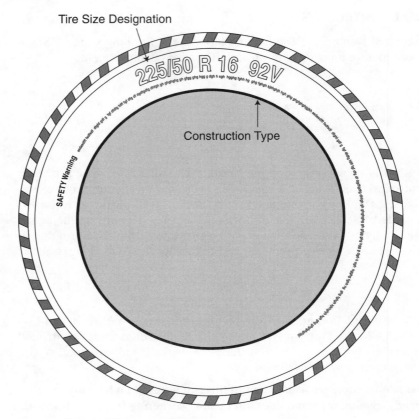

Construction Type

SAFETY Warning

225/50 R 16 92V

FIGURE 8.9 ◆ Diagram of a tire.

- **Gross vehicle weight rating** (GVWR)
- The maximum occupant and cargo weight a vehicle is designed to carry
- **Gross axle weight ratings** (GAWR) for front and rear axles
- The maximum weight the axle systems are designed to carry
- The recommended tire pressure and load limit for your vehicle in the vehicle owner's manual
- Understanding tire pressure and load limits

Tire inflation pressure is the level of air in the tire that provides it with load-carrying capacity and affects the overall performance of the vehicle. The tire inflation pressure is a number that indicates the amount of air pressure—measured in pounds per square inch (psi)—a tire requires to be properly inflated. (You will also find this number on the vehicle information placard expressed in kilopascals [kPa], which is the metric measure used internationally.)

Remember, the correct pressure for your tire is what the vehicle manufacturer has listed on the placard, NOT what is listed on the tire itself. Because tires are designed to be used on more than one type of vehicle, tire manufacturers list the **maximum permissible inflation pressure** on the tire sidewall. This number is the greatest amount of air pressure that should ever be put in the tire under normal driving conditions.

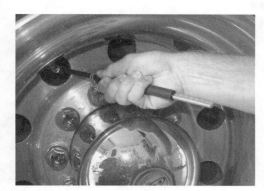

FIGURE 8.10 ◆ Tire pressure should be checked on a regular basis.

Checking Tire Pressure. It is important to check your vehicle's tire pressure (Figure 8.10) at least once a month for the following reasons:

- Most tires may naturally lose air over time.
- Tires can lose air suddenly if you drive over a pothole or other object or if you strike the curb when parking.
- With radial tires, it is usually not possible to determine underinflation by visual inspection.

Purchase a tire pressure gauge to keep in the vehicle. Gauges can be purchased at tire dealerships, auto supply stores, and other retail outlets. The recommended tire inflation pressure that vehicle manufacturers provide reflects the proper psi when a tire is cold. The term *cold* does not relate to the outside temperature. Rather, a cold tire is one that has not been driven on for at least three hours. As you drive, the tires get warmer, causing the air pressure within them to increase. Therefore, to get an accurate tire pressure reading, measure tire pressure when the tires are cold or compensate for the extra pressure in warm tires.

Steps for Maintaining Proper Tire Pressure

Step 1: Locate the recommended tire pressure on the vehicle's tire information placard, certification label, or in the owner's manual.

Step 2: Record the tire pressure of all tires.

Step 3: If the tire pressure is too high in any of the tires, slowly release air by gently pressing on the tire valve stem with the edge of your tire gauge until you get to the correct pressure.

Step 4: If the tire pressure is too low, note the difference between the measured tire pressure and the correct tire pressure. These "missing" pounds of pressure are what you need to add.

Step 5: Add the missing pounds of air pressure to each tire that is underinflated.

Step 6: Check all the tires to make sure they have the same air pressure (except in cases in which the front and rear tires are supposed to have different amounts of pressure).

If after driving the vehicle the tire still feels underinflated, fill it to the recommended cold inflation pressure indicated on the vehicle's tire information placard or certification label. Although the tire may still be slightly underinflated due to the extra pounds of pressure in the warm tire, it is safer to drive with air pressure that is slightly lower than the vehicle manufacturer's recommended cold inflation pressure than to drive with a significantly underinflated tire. Because this is a temporary fix, don't forget to recheck and adjust the tire's pressure when you can obtain a cold reading.

FIGURE 8.11 ◆ Another method for checking tread depth is to place a penny in the tread with Lincoln's head upside down and facing you. If you can see the top of Lincoln's head, you are ready for new tires.

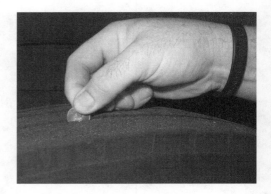

The tire tread provides the gripping action and traction that prevent the vehicle from slipping or sliding, especially when the road is wet or icy. In general, tires are not safe and should be replaced when the tread is worn down to one-sixteenth of an inch. Tires have built-in treadwear indicators that let a driver know when it is time to replace the tires. These indicators are raised sections spaced intermittently in the bottom of the tread grooves. When they appear "even" with the outside of the tread, it is time to replace the tires.

Another method for checking tread depth is to place a penny in the tread with Lincoln's head upside down and facing you (Figure 8.11). If you can see the top of Lincoln's head, you are ready for new tires.

BALANCE AND ALIGNMENT

To avoid vibration or shaking of the vehicle when a tire rotates, the tire must be properly balanced. This balance is achieved by positioning weights on the wheel to counterbalance heavy spots on the wheel-and-tire assembly.

A wheel alignment adjusts the angles of the wheels so that they are positioned correctly relative to the vehicle's frame. This adjustment maximizes the life of the tires and prevents the vehicle from veering to the right or left when driving on a straight, level road.

These adjustments require special equipment and should be performed by a qualified technician.

ROTATION

Rotating tires from front to back and from side to side can reduce irregular wear (for vehicles that have tires that are all the same size). Look in the owner's manual for information on how frequently the tires on the vehicle should be rotated and the best pattern for rotation.

Figure 8.12 shows examples of common rotation patterns (for vehicles with tires that are the same type and size).

REPAIR

A plug by itself is not an acceptable repair. The proper repair of a punctured tire requires a plug for the hole and a patch for the area inside the tire that surrounds the puncture hole. The repair material used—for example, a "combination patch and plug" repair—must seal the inner liner and fill the injury to be considered a permanent repair.

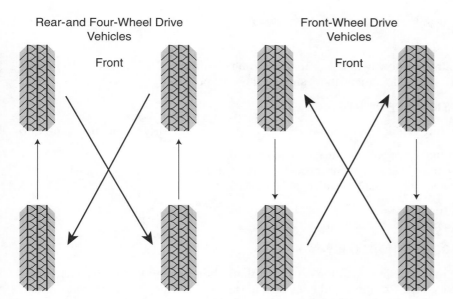

Rear-and Four-Wheel Drive Vehicles

Front

Front-Wheel Drive Vehicles

Front

FIGURE 8.12 ◆ Examples of common rotation patterns (for vehicles with tires that are the same type and size).

Punctures through the tread can be repaired if they are not too large, but punctures to the sidewall should not be repaired.

Tires must be removed from the rim to be properly inspected before being plugged and patched.

◆ SUPPORT EQUIPMENT

All ambulances have similar basic medical support equipment installed by the manufacturer. Each organization may customize its vehicles with additional equipment, often outfitting vehicles to meet specific requirements. So, not all vehicles will carry the same equipment.

When the typical ambulance leaves the factory, it is designed to carry a driver and an EMT at 175 pounds each, two patients at 175 pounds each, and the following medical support equipment:

- Main and portable oxygen cylinders
- Stretchers, cots, and patient handling equipment
- Portable, removable medical devices
- Durable and disposable medical items
- Optional vehicle equipment such as battery charger, inverter, or auxiliary power unit
- Communications equipment
- Extrication and rescue equipment

The driver/operator will be responsible for inspecting the vehicle and for properly operating the mechanical systems. The driver/operator may also be responsible for providing routine servicing and preventive maintenance for each system and its components.

◆ VEHICLE INSPECTION

The most important way to check the operating condition of the vehicle is to inspect it regularly and to document the results of those inspections.

SYSTEMATIC INSPECTIONS

By conducting regular, systematic vehicle inspections, the driver/operator is able to

- Find and report problems that need to be fixed.
- Keep track of preventive maintenance requirements.
- Document the overall condition of the vehicle.

The driver/operator will evaluate the results of the inspection before deciding whether to place the vehicle into service.

INSPECTION METHODOLOGY

To ensure that vehicle inspections are consistent, thorough, and accurate, each emergency service organization should develop specific vehicle inspection procedures and checklists to meet its needs. The completed checklists should then be kept on file and used to document the condition of the vehicles. Examples of these procedures and checklists will be discussed later in this chapter.

IMPORTANCE OF MAINTAINING RECORDS

If an emergency vehicle were involved in a crash, and there is the possibility that a mechanical malfunction was the cause, the courts would be very interested in reviewing the maintenance records of the emergency vehicle. If the operating organization knew in advance of the malfunction and continued to operate the vehicle, it might be found negligent and held liable for all damages resulting from the crash.

Maintenance organizations must be able to document in writing the servicing, maintenance, and repair of the vehicles and equipment (Figure 8.13). A good general

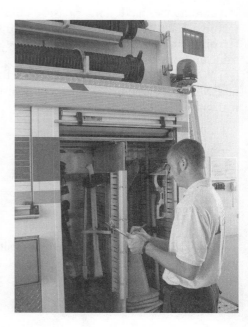

FIGURE 8.13 ◆ The emergency vehicle driver needs to document vehicle checks.

guideline for documenting inspections and maintenance actions is "If it's not in writing, it did not happen."

INSPECTION SCHEDULE

Whether the vehicle is inspected by number of runs per week, by hours of operation, or by specific days of the week, the important thing is that the vehicle is inspected according to a specific schedule that is strictly adhered to.

Recommended Inspection Schedule. An organization's inspection schedule should be determined by a number of factors, including vehicle age and mileage, insurance requirements, and past experience.

INSPECTION TYPES

There are two types of vehicle inspections recommended for emergency vehicles:

The **Quick Check** covers those systems that should be checked most often.
The **Full Check** covers all vehicle systems that can be checked without special equipment or facilities.

Quick Check

Checklist: Let's review a sample checklist for the Quick Check. An organization's checklist may not look exactly like this one, and it may include different items arranged in a different order.

The first thing that should be completed is the unit number, the station where it is located, and the date and time of the inspection. This important information is included because the form may be reviewed by someone not from the driver's organization and at a much later date. The driver may not be present to explain the entries.

When you conduct the inspection (Figure 8.14), you should:

◆ Inspect each item and place a check mark in the column labeled OK if there are no problems. By checking off an item as OK, the driver verifies that he or she (1) inspected it and (2) found no problems with it.

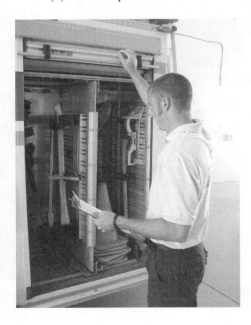

FIGURE 8.14 ◆ A vehicle check is part of the driver's responsibility.

- Fix any problems found, if the driver is capable and authorized to do so, and document that he or she did so in the Work Completed block, OR file a work request for the problem(s) found.
- Note that any starred (*) problems must be fixed before the vehicle is placed in service.
- Decide whether to place the vehicle in service, and document the decision by circling the appropriate word in the printed statement above the signature.
- Sign and date the checklist.

This is how to document that you have properly completed the inspection; according to your judgment, the vehicle is or is not in safe operating condition.

Remember that all starred (*) problems must be fixed before the vehicle is placed in service.

Point to Ponder

Suppose a vehicle you have inspected has one cracked turn signal lens and a slow oil leak. Based on the organization guidelines and other circumstances, you may or may not place the vehicle in service. Before making your decision, you may want to talk to a supervisor and/or maintenance. How would you handle this situation?

Checklist Format: The inspection is divided into specific areas of the vehicle. The driver will have several items to inspect in each area. The sequence is designed so that the driver inspects all the listed items in one area before moving clockwise around the vehicle to the next area. Because all the items to be inspected are listed by area, there is less chance that the driver will forget an item that was checked in a previous area.

For example, if, in area three, the driver were directed to "inspect the tires," then he or she would have to either break off the inspection of the left front of the vehicle or inspect all four tires, or would have to hope that he or she didn't forget to inspect the other three tires in continuing around the vehicle.

Preparation: To prepare for performing the Quick Check, you need to do three things:

- Arrange for another crew member to help check the lights.
- Place wheel chocks where they can be quickly retrieved if required.
- Get a blank checklist and fill out the administrative information.

Inspection Sequence: There are eight specific areas to be checked during the Quick Check inspection:

1. Overall appearance
2. Operator compartment
3. Exterior: operator's side
4. Exterior: front
5. Engine compartment
6. Exterior: passenger's side
7. Patient compartment
8. Exterior: rear

When the Full Check is discussed, the same eight areas will be used. More items will be covered and in greater detail during the Full Check.

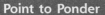

Point to Ponder

One organization might let a vehicle go on a run with a broken windshield wiper on a clear day; another organization might take the vehicle out of service. In either case, the problem should be documented and the repairs made as soon as possible. How would you handle this situation?

1. **Overall Appearance**
   - Check vehicle cleanliness.
     - The overall appearance to the public as a professional organization is enhanced by a clean, well-maintained vehicle.
     - Check general vehicle condition.
   - Is the vehicle sitting level?
     - Are there any puddles or other signs of visible fluid leaks?
     - Are there any signs of new, unreported body damage?
2. **Operator Compartment**
   - Check the vehicle log.
     - The most recently completed Full Check and Quick Check checklists should be in the log, along with blank copies of the run report and a complete inventory list of installed equipment.
   - Check for stowage of items.
   - Be sure switches for lights and communication equipment are in the "off" position.
   - Adjust the seat, seat belt, and side view mirrors.
   - Release the hood latch.
   - Turn the key to the ON position and check the fuel gauge.
   - Each organization has specific procedures for refueling.
   - An urban organization that makes several short runs each day may elect to refuel at the end of each day or when the quantity drops below half full. However, a rural organization that makes only a few runs each week may refuel after each run because runs of 40 to 100 miles are common and fuel may not be readily available.
     - Routine refueling should occur when the fuel level is between half and three-quarters empty. Follow the organization's procedures for refueling.
3. **Exterior Walk Around: Operator's Side**
   - Check left outside mirror bracket for general condition.
   - Check left side window for general condition.
   - Check left side of windshield and left wiper for general condition.
   - Check the left front wheel and tire for general condition.
   - Check the tire for a properly inflated appearance, but do not check tire pressure.
   - Check left front fender for general condition.
   - Check the pump panel and run the pump, if equipped.
4. **Exterior Walk Around: Front**
   - Inspect front of vehicle and grill for general condition.
     - Remove any obstructions to the grill, radiator, or lights.
   - Visually check condition of headlights and turn signals.
   - Visually check condition of emergency lights from the front.
5. **Engine Compartment**
   - Open hood and visually check engine for signs of leaks.
   - Visually check condition of belts.

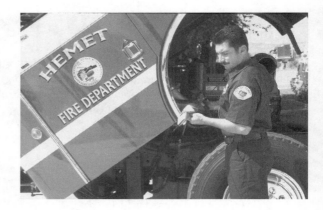

FIGURE 8.15 ◆ Regular maintenance needs to be conducted on the vehicle. (*Courtesy of Pearson Education/PH College*)

- Visually check condition of battery(ies).
- Check levels of engine oil (Figure 8.15), windshield washer fluid, and cooling system.
- Check coolant level at overflow reservoir; do not remove radiator cap to check.
- Replenish fluids according to local organization's requirements.
- Always replenish the engine oil when it is one quart low.
- Close the hood and ensure that it is latched.

6. **Exterior Walk Around: Passenger's Side**
   - Check right front fender for general condition.
   - Check the right front wheel and tire for general condition.
   - Check the tire for a properly inflated appearance, but do not check tire pressure.
   - Check right side of windshield, right wiper for general condition.
   - Check right side window for general condition.
   - Check right outside mirror bracket for general condition.
   - Check right rear fender for general condition.
   - Check the right rear wheel and tire for general condition.
   - Check the tire for a properly inflated appearance, but do not check tire pressure.

7. **Patient Compartment—Ambulances**
   - Open rear doors and visually check general condition of patient compartment.
   - Check that all equipment is properly secured.
     - Verify that no new equipment that may change vehicle weight has been added to patient compartment.
   - Close rear doors and ensure that they are properly latched.

8. **Exterior Walk Around: Rear**
   - Visually check the condition of emergency lights from the rear.
   - Visually check the condition of rear lights and turn signals.
   - Visually check the condition of external floodlights, if installed.
   - Check the left rear fender for general condition.
   - Check the left rear wheel and tire for general condition.
   - Check the tire for a properly inflated appearance, but do not check tire pressure.

This completes the items on the Quick Check. When this check is finished, the driver needs to decide whether to place the vehicle into service and sign and date the form. Place the completed checklist into the vehicle log.

NOTE: If the organization requires an operational check of the communications and emergency warning equipment, perform those checks after completing the visual inspection.

Point to Ponder

Conduct and record a Quick Check and Full Check on an emergency vehicle.

To conduct operational checks:

- Start the vehicle and drive it outdoors.
- Check the communications equipment, following local procedures.
- Operate and have the other crew member check the emergency lights.
- Check the siren, following local procedures.
- Secure the communications and emergency equipment and return the vehicle to its parking space.

Full Check. The Full Check includes additional items and should be adapted to meet the organization's requirements. Both checklists follow the same basic clockwise rotation around the vehicle to ensure a systematic inspection. Because this checklist is similar to the Quick Check checklist, we are not going to go over it item by item.

NEGLIGENCE RELATED TO INSPECTION

An operator might be judged to be negligent with regard to vehicle inspection for two main reasons:

- Failing to inspect a vehicle thoroughly according to the organization's requirements
- Knowingly operating a vehicle with a problem that should have caused it to be taken out of service

REFUSING TO DRIVE AN UNSAFE VEHICLE

The driver should never operate a vehicle that is not in safe operating condition. Although this seems pretty basic, faced with an emergency, some drivers might feel pressured to take an unsafe vehicle. A federal program, the Injury/Illness Prevention Program (IIP), supports an operator's right to refuse to drive an unsafe vehicle. Guidelines for this program are available from the Occupational Safety and Health Administration (OSHA).

◆ OPERATOR RESPONSIBILITY FOR VEHICLE MAINTENANCE

Vehicle maintenance is a critical part of an effective emergency response organization. If vehicles are not ready to respond to a service call, or if they break down during a run, the organization cannot mitigate the emergency effectively. Some general characteristics of a good maintenance program need to be discussed along with the operator's role in vehicle maintenance.

OPERATOR RESPONSIBILITIES FOR MAINTENANCE

The driver is an important part of the maintenance program. The primary responsibilities for maintenance follow:

- To document any needed maintenance you find
- To make sure needed maintenance has been completed before the vehicle is placed in service
- To perform any maintenance for which the organization makes the driver responsible

The driver will document needed maintenance on the inspection checklist or other form as required by the organization. Before the driver places the vehicle in service, it is important to make sure needed maintenance has been completed following the organization's procedures.

MAINTENANCE PROGRAMS

A comprehensive maintenance program anticipates the need for maintenance and completes it before a failure occurs and repairs are needed.

PREVENTIVE MAINTENANCE

There is a story that has been circulating among the emergency service community that talks about a huge fire raging out of control. A number of units are already on the scene making gallant efforts to extinguish the raging inferno. Over the crest of the hill a fire engine from a neighboring fire department comes speeding down the hill and into the fire. The firefighters jump off the vehicle and begin spraying water and before you know it the fire is extinguished. The owner of the property is elated with the fire department and offers a $10,000 reward for extinguishing the fire. The fire chief was interviewed and asked what the fire department would do with the money. Without hesitation the chief replied the first thing he would do is get new brakes put on the fire engine.

Humor is always a vital element in shedding light on troubling issues. However, vehicle maintenance is one of those issues that needs to be taken seriously and not left to chance. Vehicle maintenance is an ongoing process. It is every driver's responsibility to ensure that the vehicle in operation is functioning and safe to drive.

Preventive maintenance takes the form of three different classifications, which are typically referred to as **routine maintenance, scheduled maintenance,** and **crisis maintenance.** The last classification is not necessarily unavoidable, but efforts need to be made to reduce the potential of a maintenance crisis occurring.

Comprehensive Programs. A comprehensive program:

- Uses information from regular inspections to identify maintenance that may be needed
- Uses regular inspections, including those performed by the operator, that can provide an indication that maintenance is needed.
- Documents all inspections, work requests, and work completed
  - Remember: "If it's not in writing, it did not happen."
- Includes preventive maintenance

Preventive maintenance focuses on preventing the most likely vehicle malfunctions by replacing parts or making adjustments before a failure occurs. Preventive maintenance is maintenance performed according to the manufacturer's suggested schedule. It may include additional items identified by the organization.

Advantages of Preventive Maintenance. Preventive maintenance relies on fixing minor problems before they become major ones. It has several important advantages over repairing equipment when it breaks:

- It ensures safe, reliable vehicle operation.
- It reduces the total cost of repairs.
- It minimizes major equipment failure.

PERFORMING MAINTENANCE

Work Requests. A work request tells maintenance the work that is needed on a vehicle. When maintenance finishes the work, it records on the form the work performed, tests run, and the results of these efforts. This work request covers those problems that the driver finds during an inspection as well as routine preventive maintenance. An organization may or may not use a work request to track maintenance and repairs.

Vehicle Maintenance Logs. Information from the inspection checklists and work requests are written into a vehicle maintenance log. The vehicle maintenance log is a vehicle's central record:

- To list all maintenance needed and done, including routine maintenance and problems identified by inspections.
- To support the preventive maintenance program.
- To document that the vehicle has been properly maintained. Vehicle maintenance log pages are usually organized into binders and saved in an inspection file for use by a maintenance supervisor or manager.

Review. To determine whether the vehicle is in safe operating condition, the driver must know whether required maintenance has been performed. The driver must understand the organization's maintenance program in order to know the vehicle's maintenance status.

Operator Responsibilities for Vehicle Repairs. The driver's primary responsibilities for repairs are

- To document any needed repairs found during an inspection or during a run
- To make sure needed repairs have been completed before placing the vehicle in service
- To make any repairs for which the driver's organization makes him or her responsible

The driver will document needed repairs on the inspection checklist or other form as required by the organization. Before the driver places the vehicle in service, the driver will make sure needed repairs have been completed following the organization's procedures.

Making Repairs. In some organizations, drivers make a variety of repairs to the vehicles. In others, the driver is responsible for only minimal repairs. The driver should perform only those repairs for which he or she is trained and authorized.

Malfunctions During a Run. There may be a time when, in spite of all precautions, the vehicle breaks down during a run. When this happens, the driver should think the situation through carefully before taking action. The driver should also use communications to increase the options available. This decision aid will help the driver to focus on the most important information and make the correct decision about what action to take.

Decision Aid for Vehicle Malfunctions During a Run:

- Is the driver trained and authorized to make the repair?
  The driver should be both trained and authorized to make any repair. If the driver should not fix the problem, a call should be made for help.

- Is a backup readily available?

    The driver should use the communication system to inform dispatch of the situation and to find out if a backup is available. Develop a plan before starting any repair, in case the repair fails.

- If operating outside the normal service area, the driver may need to coordinate with an organization based in that service area.
- How quickly can the repair be made?
- Can the repair be made in less time than it takes for the backup to arrive?
- Can the vehicle's electrical system meet the demands made on it during the repair?

    If a long stay at the scene has depleted the system, the driver may need a backup vehicle even if the driver can make the repair.

- This decision aid applies for any vehicle problem during a run.
- The organization's policies and procedures may also discuss what to do when a malfunction occurs.

Point to Ponder

Find out some of the maintenance problems that would put an emergency vehicle out of service. Who decides that the emergency vehicle should be put out of service? Does everyone in the organization know how to contact the supervisors if they are not present? Does the standard operating procedure (SOP) cover maintenance procedures?

Repairs the Driver May Make on the Spot. A driver is generally expected or allowed to make only the most minor repairs during a run. For example:

- Change a flat tire.
- Use duct tape to make temporary repairs to a broken radiator hose (usually the upper radiator hose).

Problems That May Allow the Driver to Drive the Vehicle Safely. Drivers may find themselves in situations in which the vehicle has malfunctioned but is still drivable. For example, an ambulance with a power steering belt failure can be driven carefully with compensation for the lack of power steering. The driver's decision about whether to continue to drive the vehicle should be based on the organization's policies and procedures. The driver may be required to inform a supervisor of the situation instead of making the decision him- or herself.

◆ CASE STUDY RECAP

In this case study the operator did not follow established procedures to make sure that the vehicle was in safe operating condition. Additionally the organization may also be found at fault for not having an effective system to inform the operator of problems and for not making repairs promptly.

The driver is responsible for documenting any needed repairs found during an inspection or a run. Before the driver places a vehicle in service, make sure that needed repairs have been completed. The driver and his or her organization should have a strategy for dealing with vehicle malfunctions during a run.

Drivers should inspect their vehicles to determine whether they are in safe operating condition, and may be found negligent for driving vehicles that are not in compliance with their organization's maintenance program. Drivers are responsible for documenting any needed repairs they find during an inspection, or during a run. In addition, drivers are also responsible for confirming that needed repairs and scheduled maintenance have been completed prior to placing the vehicle back in service. It is critical for all drivers to understand their organization's maintenance program in order to know the maintenance status of each vehicle. Drivers and their organization should also establish a strategy for dealing with vehicle malfunction during a run.

Review Questions

1. What three things should drivers know before they decide that their vehicles are ready for service?
2. How do you decide whether a vehicle is in safe operating condition?
3. Describe the role of the EVT.
4. Describe the major components of a vehicle.
5. Describe the various types of braking systems.
6. Describe brake fade.
7. Describe the importance of tires being inflated to the proper pressure.
8. Diagram how to rotate tires.
9. Describe the three types of maintenance.
10. Describe the sequence for a vehicle inspection.
11. How does negligence play into vehicle maintenance?

Reference

Air brakes. Retrieved November 14, 2005, from http://auto.howstuffworks.com/ framed.htm?parent=drum-brake .htm&url=http://www.e-z.net/~ts/ts/ brakpg.htm

NFPA. 2000. *NFPA 1071, Standard for emergency vehicle technician professional qualifications.* Quincy, MA: National Fire Protection Association.

NFPA. 2000. *NFPA 1915, Standard for fire apparatus preventive maintenance program.* Quincy, MA: National Fire Protection Association.

Nice, K. 2005. *How antilock brakes work.* Retrieved November 14, 2004, from http://auto.howstuffworks.com/ anti-lockbrake.htm/printable

Pac brake. Retrieved November 14, 2005, from http://www.pacbrake.com/

Tires. Retrieved September 13, 2004, from http://www.nhtsa.dot.gov/cars/testing/ UTQG/

CHAPTER 9

Roadway Operations

Objectives

After completing this chapter, you should be able to:

- Explain the concept of roadway safety.
- List the core components of roadway/highway operations.
- Identify the ten best practices to ensure roadway safety.

Case Study

**Volunteer Fire Police Captain Dies from Injury-Related Complications
After Being Struck by Motor Vehicle While Directing Traffic—New Jersey**

According to NIOSH, on February 23, 2003, law enforcement and fire department units were dispatched to a motor vehicle incident (**MVI**) at a state highway/township road intersection. Emergency personnel (firefighters and fire police) were on the scene for approximately 30 minutes when a vehicle struck the victim while he was directing traffic in a heavy fog. On-scene personnel, trained as emergency medical technicians, came to the aid of the victim. He was then transported to the trauma center of a local hospital for further treatment. The victim was scheduled to be released from the hospital on March 1, 2003. But due to complications. The victim remained in the hospital until April 19, 2003, when he died as a result of complications from his injuries.

◆ INTRODUCTION

Emergency service organizations (ESOs) respond to a wide variety of incidents involving operations on or near a highway (Figure 9.1). These operations pose special risks to personnel performing fire, rescue, and EMS functions. Every year a significant number of emergency service personnel are killed or injured while operating on our highways. There may be a wide variety of reasons for these losses, but the point still remains, *they should never happen*! In many instances, an ESO responds to a *primary incident* on a highway, only to become the victim of a *secondary incident*—the nightmare in which a firefighter, EMS provider, or police officer is suddenly struck and killed by traffic. In a guest editorial for *Fire Rescue Magazine* (2006), noted expert

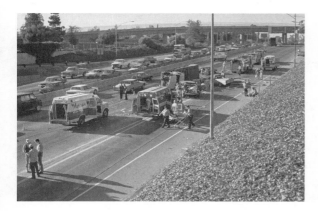

FIGURE 9.1 ◆ EMTs and firefighters work at accident scene on highway. (*Courtesy of PhotoEdit Inc.*)

Steve Kidd sums up the situation, "It's time to make traffic safety an integral part of any basic Fire or EMS training program."

The *Manual on Uniform Traffic Control Devices* (**MUTCD**) addresses virtually every component of highway safety. The MUTCD is published by the Federal Highway Administration (**FHWA**) under 23 **Code of Federal Regulations** (**CFR**), Part 655, Subpart F. The MUTCD is the national standard for all traffic control devices installed on any street, highway, or bicycle trail open to public travel. The MUTCD defines the purpose of traffic control devices, as well as the principles for their use, and is to promote highway safety and efficiency by providing for the orderly movement of all road users on streets and highways throughout the nation. Traffic control devices notify road users of regulations and provide warning and guidance needed for the reasonably safe, uniform, and efficient operation of all elements of the traffic stream.

Industry experts agree that to be effective, a traffic control device should meet five basic requirements:

1. Fulfill a need;
2. Command attention;
3. Convey a clear, simple meaning;
4. Command respect from road users; and
5. Give adequate time for proper response.

Design, placement, operation, maintenance, and uniformity are aspects that should be carefully considered in order to maximize the ability of a traffic control device to meet these five requirements. Vehicle speed should be carefully considered as an element that governs the design, operation, placement, and location of various traffic control devices. Personal protective equipment while working in these environments is also addressed.

Chapter 6 of the MUTCD specifically addresses temporary traffic control (**TTC**), which covers emergency scene operations. A TTC zone is an area of a highway where road user conditions are changed because of a work zone or an incident through the use of TTC devices, uniformed law enforcement officers, or other authorized personnel. An incident area is an area of a highway where temporary traffic controls are imposed by authorized officials in response to a traffic incident, natural disaster, or special event. It extends from the first warning device (such as a sign, light, or cone) to the last TTC device or to a point where road users return to the original lane alignment and are clear of the incident.

◆ TERMS

According to the USFA, the following terms shall be used during incident operations, postincident analysis, and training activities related to working in or near moving traffic.

1. **Advance warning.** Notification procedures that advise approaching motorists to transition from normal driving status to that required by the temporary emergency traffic control measures ahead of them.
2. **Block.** Positioning a fire department apparatus on an angle to the lanes of traffic, creating a physical barrier between upstream traffic and the work area. Includes "block to the right" and "block to the left."
3. **Buffer zone.** The distance or space between personnel and vehicles in the protected work zone and nearby moving traffic.
4. **Downstream.** The direction that traffic is moving as it travels away from the incident scene.
5. **Flagger.** A fire department member assigned to monitor approaching traffic and activate an emergency signal if the actions of a motorist do not conform to established traffic control measures in place at the highway scene.
6. **Shadow.** The protected work area at a vehicle-related roadway incident that is shielded by the block from apparatus and other emergency vehicles.
7. **Taper.** The action of merging several lanes of moving traffic into fewer moving lanes.
8. **Temporary work zone.** The physical area of a roadway within which emergency personnel perform their fire, EMS, and rescue tasks at a vehicle-related incident.
9. **Transition zone.** The lanes of a roadway within which approaching motorists change their speed and position to comply with the traffic control measures established at an incident scene.
10. **Upstream.** The direction that traffic is traveling from as the vehicles approach the incident scene.

◆ THE CHALLENGE

Understanding the factors that may cause these unfortunate events can lend itself to an intuitive awareness of surroundings. This raises the question of what has lead to the increased number of secondary highway incidents. Keep in mind that in most instances other drivers are more concerned about getting to their destinations with ill concern to happenings along the way. Perhaps it could be the inattentiveness of the emergency responders who are focused solely on the incident, lost in the potential crisis, sidetracked by other thoughts, or not thinking about the big picture. Maybe other drivers cannot even see you. The long and short of this is that the cause is most likely a combination of all of these issues.

Emergency responders must consider the provision of giving other vehicles on the roadway enough warning that an emergency lies ahead. In the environment of to-

---

Point to Ponder

As you read this chapter, ponder these issues as possible factors to consider toward confronting the challenge. The number of emergency incidents has increased; there may be more traffic; there are instances of inattentiveness of other drivers such as eating, drinking, smoking, reading, cell phone usage, radio or stereos blaring, applying makeup, and even using a computer.

day's highway safety awareness, providers should be attuned that two incidents often occur. The primary incident is the emergency to which you are responding to provide aid. A secondary incident is one in which you may become a victim.

The culture surrounding how emergency responders view their own respective safety at roadway incidents may be minimal at best. Getting providers to consciously acknowledge their own safety needs remains a challenge. To address the challenge, every ESO and specific provider should consider four key components applied to every emergency situation—planning, preparation, response, and recovery.

Safe positioning while operating in or near moving traffic is essential to responder safety. This procedure identifies parking practices for vehicles that will provide maximum protection and safety for personnel operating in or near moving vehicle traffic. It also identifies several approaches for individual practices to keep responders safe while exposed to the hazardous environment created by moving traffic.

It should be the policy of the ESO to position emergency and related vehicles at a vehicle-related incident on any street, road, highway, or expressway in a manner that best protects the incident scene and the work area. Such positioning shall afford protection to fire department personnel, law enforcement officers, tow service operators, and the motoring public from the hazards of working in or near moving traffic.

All personnel should understand and appreciate the high risk that personnel are exposed to when operating in or near moving vehicle traffic. Responders should always operate within a protected environment at any vehicle-related roadway incident.

Always consider moving vehicles as a threat to your safety. At every vehicle-related emergency scene, personnel are exposed to passing motorists of varying driving abilities. At any time, a motorist may be driving without a legal driver's license. Approaching vehicles may be driven at speeds from a creeping pace to well beyond the posted speed limit. Some of these vehicle operators may be vision impaired, be under the influence of alcohol and/or drugs, or have a medical condition that affects their judgment or abilities. In addition, motorists may be completely oblivious to your presence due to distractions caused by cell phone use, loud music, conversation, inclement weather, and terrain or building obstructions. Approaching motorists will often be looking at the scene and not the roadway in front of them. Assume that all approaching traffic is out to get you until proven otherwise.

Nighttime incidents requiring personnel to work in or near moving traffic are particularly hazardous. Visibility is reduced and driver reaction time to hazards in the roadway is slowed.

No solid data are available to support any of the progressive programs aimed at improving personnel safety related to vehicle and highway operations. There should be a national repository that collects data from all organizations. Because data are so fragmented and minimal, only anecdotal information is available to support the effectiveness of these safety practices or programs.

All emergency personnel are at great risk of injury or death while operating in or near moving traffic. Several specific tactical procedures should be taken to protect all crew members and emergency service personnel at the incident scene, including the following:

1. Never trust approaching traffic.
2. Avoid turning your back to approaching traffic.

3. Establish an initial "block" with the first-arriving emergency vehicle or fire apparatus.
4. Always wear Class III high-visibility reflective vests during daylight operations.
5. Always wear a structural firefighting helmet.
6. Wear full protective clothing plus the highway safety vest at all vehicle-related emergencies between the hours of dusk and dawn or whenever lighting levels are reduced due to inclement weather conditions.
7. Turn off all sources of vision impairment to approaching motorists at nighttime incidents including vehicle headlights and spotlights.
8. Use fire apparatus and police vehicles to redirect the flow of moving traffic initially.
9. Establish advance warning and adequate transition area traffic control measures upstream of incident to reduce travel speeds of approaching motorists.
10. Use traffic cones and/or cones illuminated by flares where appropriate for sustained highway incident traffic control and direction (Figure 9.2).
11. Establish a fire department member assigned to the **flagger** function to monitor approaching traffic and activate an emergency signal if the actions of a motorist do not conform to established traffic control measures in place at the highway scene

Listed here are benchmarks for safe parking of apparatus and emergency vehicles when operating in or near moving traffic.

1. Always position first-arriving apparatus to protect the scene, patients, and emergency personnel.
   a. Initial apparatus placement should provide a work area protected from traffic approaching in at least one direction.
   b. Angle apparatus on the roadway with a **block to the left** or a **block to the right** to create a physical barrier between the crash scene and approaching traffic.
   c. Allow apparatus placement to slow approaching motorists and redirect them around the scene.

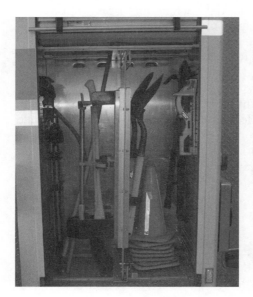

FIGURE 9.2A ◆ Traffic safety cones—inside compartment of fire engine.

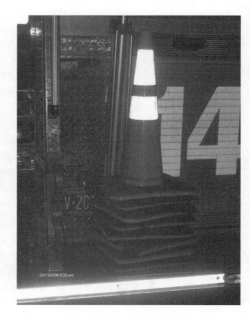

FIGURE 9.2B ◆ Traffic safety cones—mounted on rear bumper.

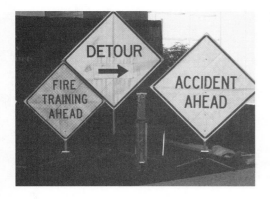

FIGURE 9.2c   ◆   Roadway safety signs.

    d. Use fire apparatus to block at least one additional traffic lane more than that already obstructed by the crashed vehicle(s).

    e. When practical, position apparatus in such a manner to protect the pump operator position from being exposed to approaching traffic.

2. Positioning of large apparatus must create a safe parking area for EMS units and other fire vehicles. Operating personnel, equipment, and patients should be kept within the "shadow" created by the blocking apparatus at all times.

3. When blocking with apparatus to protect the emergency scene, establish a sufficient size work zone that includes all damaged vehicles, roadway debris, the patient triage and treatment area, the extrication work area, the personnel and tool staging area, and the ambulance loading zone.

4. Ambulance should be positioned within the protected work area with its rear patient loading door area angled away from the nearest lanes of moving traffic.

5. Command shall stage unneeded emergency vehicles off the roadway or return these units to service whenever possible.

6. At all intersections, or where the incident may be near the middle lane of the roadway, two or more sides of the incident will need to be protected.

    a. Police vehicles must be strategically positioned to expand the initial safe work zone for traffic approaching from opposing directions. The goal is to effectively block all exposed sides of the work zone. The blocking of the work zone must be prioritized, from the most critical or highest traffic volume flow to the least critical traffic direction.

    b. For first-arriving engine or truck companies for which a charged hose line may be needed, block so that the pump panel is downstream, on the opposite side of oncoming traffic. This will protect the pump operator.

    c. At intersection incidents, consider requesting police response. Provide specific directions to the police officers as to exactly what your traffic control needs are. Ensure that police vehicles are parked in a position and location that provides additional protection of the scene.

7. Traffic cones shall be deployed from the rear of the blocking apparatus toward approaching traffic to increase the advance warning provided for approaching motorists. Cones identify and only suggest the transition and tapering actions that are required of approaching motorists.

8. Personnel shall place cones and flares and retrieve cones while facing oncoming traffic.

9. Traffic cones shall be deployed at 15-foot intervals upstream of the blocking apparatus with the farthest traffic cone approximately 75 feet upstream to allow adequate advance warning to drivers.

10. Additional traffic cones, when available, can be retrieved from police units to extend the advance warning area for approaching motorists.

◆ COMMAND AND CONTROL

The initial-arriving company officer and/or the incident commander must complete critical benchmarks to assure that a safe and protected work environment for emergency scene personnel is established and maintained, including the following:

1. Assure that the first-arriving apparatus establishes an initial block to create an initial safe work area.
2. Assign a parking location for all ambulances as well as later-arriving apparatus.
   - Lanes of traffic shall be identified numerically as Lane 1, Lane 2, and so on, beginning from the right to the left when right and left are considered from the approaching motorist's point of view. Typically, vehicles travel a lower speed in the lower number lanes.
   - Directions right and left shall be as identified as from the approaching motorist's point of view right or left.
   - Instruct the driver of the ambulance to block to the right or block to the left as it is parked at the scene to position the rear patient loading area away from the closest lane of moving traffic.
3. Assure that all ambulances on scene are placed within the protected work area (shadow) of the larger apparatus.
4. Assure that all patient loading into EMS units is done from within a protected work zone.
5. The initial company officer and/or incident commander must operate as the scene safety officer until this assignment is delegated.
6. Command shall assure that preemption strobe systems are turned OFF and that other emergency lighting remains ON.
7. At residential medical emergencies, command shall direct ambulances to park at the nearest curb to the residence for safe patient loading whenever possible.

◆ PERSONNEL FUNCTIONS

Listed here are benchmarks for safe actions of individual personnel when operating in or near moving vehicle traffic.

1. Always maintain an acute awareness of the high risk of working in or near moving traffic. They are out to get you!
2. Never trust moving traffic.
3. Always look before you move!
4. Always keep an eye on the moving traffic!
5. Avoid turning your back to moving traffic.
6. Personnel arriving in crew cabs of fire apparatus or patient compartment of ambulance should exit and enter the apparatus from the protected shadow side, away from moving traffic.
7. Officers, vehicle and apparatus operators, crew members in apparatus with individual jump seat configurations, and all ambulance personnel must exit and enter their units with extreme caution remaining alert to moving traffic at all times.
8. Protective clothing, **Class III safety vest**, and helmet must be donned prior to exiting the emergency vehicle.
   a. During normal daylight lighting conditions, don helmet and Class III safety vest or structural personal protective equipment (**PPE**) and Class III vest when operating in or near moving traffic.

b. During dusk-to-dawn operations or when ambient lighting is reduced due to inclement weather conditions, don helmet, full protective clothing, and Class III vest.

c. All staff personnel and assigned student trainee personnel arriving on an apparatus or emergency vehicle must don assigned helmet and Class III vest prior to exiting their vehicles.

9. Always look before opening doors and stepping out of apparatus or emergency vehicle into any moving traffic areas. When walking around fire apparatus or emergency vehicle, be alert to the individual proximity to moving traffic.

a. Stop at the corner of the unit, check for traffic, and then proceed along the unit remaining as close to the emergency vehicle as possible.

b. Maintain a reduced profile when moving through any area where a minimum buffer zone condition exists.

10. Police department personnel may place traffic cones or flares at the scene to direct traffic. This action builds on initial emergency vehicle (**EV**) cone deployment and can be expanded, if needed, as later-arriving police officers arrive. Always place and retrieve cones while facing oncoming traffic.

11. Placing flares, where safe to do so, adjacent to and in combination with traffic cones for nighttime operations greatly enhances scene safety. Where safe and appropriate to do so, place warning flares to slow and direct approaching traffic.

◆ LIMITED-ACCESS HIGHWAY OPERATIONS

Limited-access highways include the expressways, tollway, and multilane roadways within the ESO response area (Figure 9.3). The police department and department of transportation (DOT) have a desire to keep the traffic moving on these high-volume thoroughfares. When in the judgment of command it becomes essential for the safety of operating personnel and the patients involved, any or all lanes, shoulders, and entry/exit ramps of these limited-access highways can be completely shut down. This, however, should rarely occur and should be for as short a period of time as practical.

Unique safe parking procedures at expressway, tollway, and limited-access, high-volume multilane roadway incidents are as follows:

1. First-arriving vehicle or apparatus shall establish an initial block of the lane(s) occupied by the damaged vehicle plus one additional traffic lane.

2. In some departments, a ladder truck apparatus is automatically dispatched to all vehicle-related incidents on all limited-access, high-volume expressways, tollways, and highways.

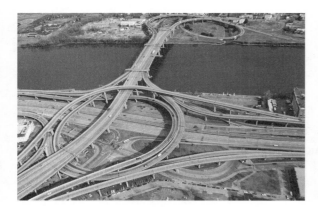

FIGURE 9.3 ◆ Limited access highways create unique challenges. (*Courtesy of Creative Eye/MIRA.com*)

3. As an example, one department uses the primary assignment of this truck company apparatus and crew to:
    a. Establish an upstream block occupying a minimum of two lanes plus the paved shoulder of the highway or blockage of three driving lanes of traffic upstream of the initial block provided by the first-due apparatus.
    b. The position of this apparatus shall take into consideration all factors that limit sight distance of the approaching traffic including ambient lighting conditions, weather-related conditions, road conditions, design curves, bridges, hills, and over- or underpasses.
    c. Traffic cones and/or cones illuminated by flares should be placed upstream of the ladder truck apparatus by the ladder truck crew at the direction of the company officer.
    d. Traffic cones on limited-access, high-volume roadways shall be placed farther apart, with the last cone approximately 150 feet upstream, to allow adequate warning to drivers. Personnel shall place cones and flares and retrieve cones while facing the traffic.
    e. Assign a flagger person to monitor the response of approaching motorists as they are directed to transition to a slower speed and taper into merged lanes of traffic.
    f. Notify command on the incident operating channel of any approaching traffic that is not responding to the speed changes, transition, tapering, and merging directions.
    g. Flagger shall activate a predetermined audible warning to operating personnel of a noncompliant motorist approaching.
    h. Driver/operator of ladder truck apparatus shall sound a series of long blasts on the apparatus air horn to audibly warn all operating personnel of the concern for the actions of an approaching motorist.
    i. Consider a separate communication channel for traffic control operations.
4. Police department vehicles can be used to provide additional blocking of additional traffic lanes as needed. EMS units should always be positioned within the safe work zone and allow for proper degrees.
5. Staging of additional companies off the highway may be required. Ambulances may be brought onto the highway scene one or two at a time. An adequate size multipatient loading area must be established.
6. Command should establish a liaison with the police department as soon as possible to coordinate a safe work zone jointly and to determine how most efficiently to resolve the incident and establish normal traffic flows.
7. The termination of the incident must be managed with the same aggressiveness as initial actions. Crews, apparatus, and equipment must be removed from the highway promptly, to reduce exposure to moving traffic and minimize traffic congestion.

◆ TEN CONES OF SAFETY

One emergency service insurance company has identified ten specific areas for emergency responders to pay particular attention to when operating on roadway/highway incidents (Figure 9.4).

In the planning stage management needs to consider agreements with all potential responding agencies. These include fire, emergency medical, rescue, and hazardous materials units; law enforcement; highway departments; wrecker/towing companies; public utility companies; media; medical examiners; toll road administrators; and mass transit agencies.

Planning should take place far in advance of a potential crisis. Planners must ensure that responders will be equipped with the proper tools and training (Cone 1) to perform

---

Ten Cones of Highway Incident Safety

🚧 There Is No Substitute for Training

🚧 Multi-Agency Coordination and Communications Are a Must – A
Unified Incident Command Is Essential

🚧 Limit Your Exposure … Limit Your Time

🚧 Give Traffic Plenty of Warning

🚧 Protect the Scene with Apparatus

🚧 Always Work Away from the Traffic

🚧 Be Prepared to Shut Down the Roadway

🚧 Be Seen and Not Hurt

🚧 Dress for the Occasion

🚧 Accountability Matters

FIGURE 9.4 ◆ Ten cones of highway incident safety. (*Courtesy of VFIS*)

required tasks. Most important to the planning process is for ESO management to establish a policy pertaining to highway safety and provide supporting standard operating procedures and guidelines (SOP/SOGs) for providers to use.

The ESO should coordinate efforts with other agencies to avoid confusion on the emergency scene. Responding agencies should meet on an annual basis to discuss and train with all possible agencies involved to ensure that everyone understands the overall process and specific tasks.

Critical to any response situation is being prepared. Highway incidents and operating alongside the roadway have inherent risks. This fact depicts the need for safety procedures and applications to not only be considered but also applied. Specific equipment needed to provide varying levels of protection includes vehicles, traffic cones, flares, signage, scene lighting, and personal protective equipment such as vests and hand lights.

Training is perhaps the most important component in the preparation phase.

Cone 1: There Is No Substitute for Training. Once the planning phase is complete and the applicable tools are purchased, every responder from every response agency should be trained. Training should include policy and SOP/SOG review, hands-on practice with the personal protective equipment, tabletop exercises (Figure 9.5), and actual field drills.

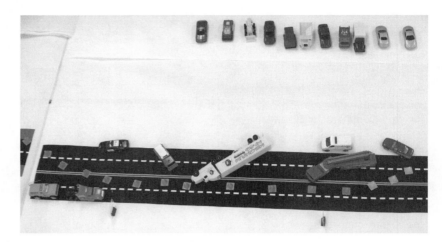

FIGURE 9.5 ◆ Highway/roadway safety tabletop training. (*Courtesy of R. Patrick*)

Cone 2: Multi-Agency Coordination and Communications Are a Must. Cone 2 also addresses the need for unified incident command. This is as essential to the planning section as it is to preparation. A unified incident command structure is imperative for agencies to function in a safe and cohesive environment. Interoperability of communications equipment is critical and will permit responding agencies to function better within a unified command structure. Be prepared by cross training with multiagency responders. Such training will further identify and address coordination and communication issues critical to the overall safety of the operation.

On-Scene Operations: First-arriving crews need to take the whole scene into account (Figure 9.6). Crews need to know how they are safely going to operate at the incident scene and then have safe incident termination including proper egress. Do your crews have the right training and equipment to properly ensure safe operations? Management cannot make the decision for you; however, it needs to provide the support for

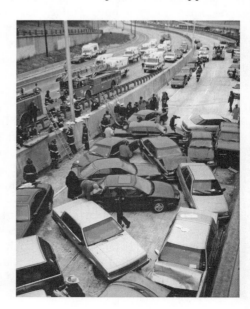

FIGURE 9.6 ◆ Multiple agency response to MVC. (*Courtesy of AP Wide World Photos*)

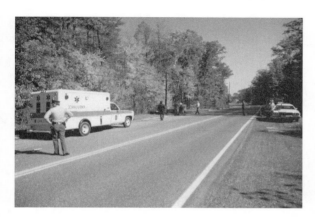

FIGURE 9.7 ◆ First-arriving ambulance blocks to the right. (*Courtesy of Pearson Education/ PH College*)

you to make the best judgment for the situation. This is accomplished with supporting SOP/SOGs.

Cone 3: Limit Your Exposure . . . Limit Your Time. Determine what needs to be done to mitigate the incident and complete the task as quickly and safely as possible. The MUTCD divides the TTC work zone into four areas: the advance warning area, the transition area, the activity area, and the transition area.

Cone 4: Give Traffic Plenty of Warning. Placing vehicles, signs, cones, and flares (when appropriate) as pre-incident warning creates a buffer zone for all responders and public on the roadway. This buffer zone provides notice that an emergency incident lies ahead and should direct motorists to merge, yield, detour, or even stop as indicated.

Cone 5: Protect the Scene with Apparatus. Positioning response vehicles strategically permits a safer operating tactic in the initial 10 to 15 minutes of scene arrival. The first-arriving vehicle should position itself in a block left or block right position. The purpose of blocking is to angle vehicles in a strategic way to protect the scene. If a blocking emergency vehicle is struck, the emergency vehicle can absorb the impact and be pushed in a direction away from the active scene. Blocking left or right is depicted in the Figure 9.7. A second vehicle's blocking position should be at least 150 feet (depending on road conditions) to the rear of the first vehicle.

Cone 6: Always Work Away from the Traffic. Responders should make every attempt to stay away from traffic (Figure 9.8). This stresses the importance of assuring a

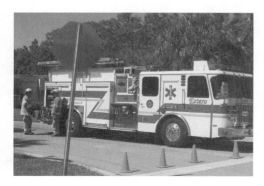

FIGURE 9.8 ◆ Emergency responders working away from traffic.

FIGURE 9.9 ◆ Blocked roadway.

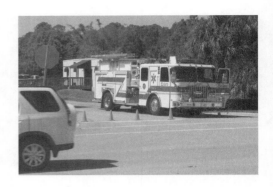

safe working zone. Although no zone may be 100 percent safe, consciously alert responders, safe positioning of vehicles, and cone and sign use, can enhance a safe working environment.

Cone 7: Be Prepared to Shut Down the Roadway. Although blocking the entire roadway is not always a popular decision, it must be kept as an option (Figure 9.9). This should be an ongoing consideration of the incident commander. Cones, signs, and vehicles should be used to direct detours. Direction should be continued until traffic is redirected back onto the designated route.

Cone 8: Be Seen and Not Hurt. The use of warning signs, message boards, cones, flares, and personnel directing traffic is of vital importance (Figure 9.10). We cannot expect someone who is traveling in the fast lane at 70 miles per hour to anticipate a stopped emergency vehicle in the lane of travel. The same argument can be made for any motorist traveling in any lane, on any roadway, at any time of day. It is not reasonable to think that the general public would be anticipating a roadway being

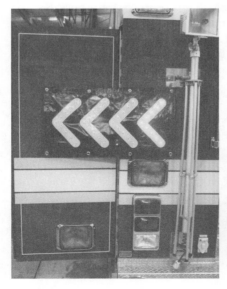

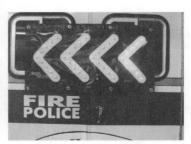

FIGURE 9.10 ◆ Warning signs on emergency vehicles. (*Courtesy of R. Patrick*)

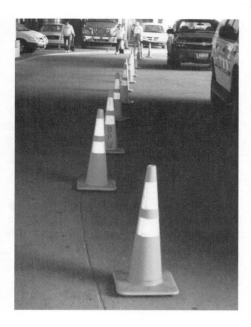

FIGURE 9.11 ◆ Cones set up on roadway. (*Courtesy of R. Patrick*)

obstructed for any reason without warning. Prior notification to the traveling public is essential. Depending on the situation, advanced warning may need to be placed as much as 2,500 feet (depending on road conditions) prior to the incident.

Cones shall be predominantly orange and shall be made of a material that can be struck without causing damage to the impacting vehicle (Figure 9.11). The MUTCD provides outlines of cone applications and details. For daytime and low-speed road-ways, cones shall be not less than 18 inches (450 mm) in height. When cones are used on freeways and other high-speed highways or at night on all highways, or when more conspicuous guidance is needed, cones shall be a minimum of 28 inches (700 mm) in height. For nighttime use, cones shall be **retroreflectorized** or equipped with lighting devices for maximum visibility. Retroreflectorization of 28 inches (700 mm) or larger cones shall be provided by a white band 6 inches (150 mm) wide located 3 to 4 inches (75 to 100 mm) from the top of the cone and an additional 4-inch (100 mm) wide white band approximately 2 inches (50 mm) below the 6-inch (150 mm) band. Cone tapering is also referenced by the MUTCD. One lane taper should have a 100-foot **taper** with cones placed at 10 to 20 feet apart. Downstream tapers should have 100 feet per lane with cones placed at 10 to 20 feet apart.

MUTCD states that traffic cones may be used to channelize road users, divide op-posing motor vehicle traffic lanes, divide lanes when two or more lanes are kept open in the same direction, and delineate short duration maintenance and utility work (Figure 9.12).

According to the MUTCD, an advanced warning sign should be placed 4 to 8 times the speed limit in miles per hour (**MPH**), expressways and freeways at one-half mile, and 8 to 12 times the speed limit in MPH in rural areas. The second advanced warning sign should be placed at 100 feet in low-speed urban areas, 350 feet in high-speed urban areas, 1,500 feet on expressways and freeways, and 500 feet in rural areas. (See Table 9.1.)

Buffer areas should consist of 30 MPH—625 feet; 40 MPH—825 feet; 50 MPH—1,000 feet; 60 MPH—1,300 feet; and 70 MPH—1,450 feet.

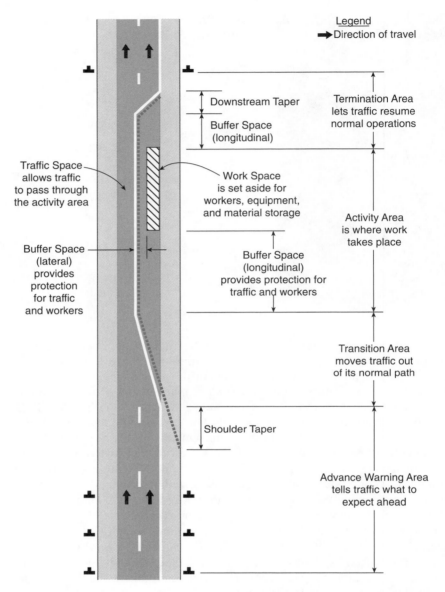

FIGURE 9.12 ◆ Component Parts of Temporary Traffic Control Zone. (*MUTCD, 2003*)

Cone 9: Dress for the Occasion. Responders who place warning devices and assist with directing traffic need to be properly trained (Cone 1) and equipped (Cones 8 and 9). Be seen at the scene. All responders must don Class III reflective vests or other protective clothing suitable to the conditions in which they are operating (Figure 9.13). Traditional bunker gear worn by emergency service responders does not provide sufficient visibility. Any responders who are not participating in the actual directing of traffic need to stay within the protected work area.

Properly donned apparel is essential for provider safety. The MUTCD identifies specific reflective vest requirements, which represent the most visible attributes.

TABLE 9.1 ◆ Suggested Advance Warning Sign Spacing

| Road Type | Distance Between Signs** | | |
	A	B	C
Urban (low speed)*	30 (100)	30 (100)	30 (100)
Urban (high speed)*	100 (350)	100 (350)	100 (350)
Rural	150 (500)	150 (500)	150 (500)
Expressway / Freeway	300 (1,000)	450 (1,500)	800 (2,640)

* Speed category to be determined by highway agency
** Distances are shown in meters (feet). The A dimension is the distance from the transition or point of restriction to the first sign. The B dimension is the distance between the first and second signs. The C dimension is the distance between the second and third signs. (The third sign is the first one in a three-sign series encountered by a driver approaching a TTC zone.)
Source: MUTCD, Chapter 6C.

Personnel visibility is critical during highway operations, especially at night. Being struck by a vehicle is a constant danger. Dawn, dusk, and inclement weather compromise visibility and increase the risk of being struck. It is imperative that workers be visible as a person among the flashing lights and other apparatus marking. **ANSI/ISEA** Standard 107-1999 specifies the minimum amount of fabric and reflective materials to be placed onto safety garments that are worn by workers near vehicular traffic. This standard is now the most commonly used standard associated with safety vests.

Reflective vests should be used to increase worker visibility, regardless of the use of turnout gear. The reflective vests used by emergency workers should have both retroreflective and fluorescent properties. Retroreflective material returns the majority of light from the light source back to the observer. Fluorescent material absorbs **UV** light of a certain wavelength and regenerates it into visual energy (see Figure 9.14). The apparel

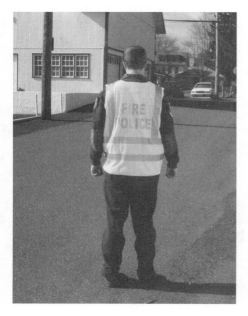

FIGURE 9.13 ◆ Safety vest. (*Courtesy of R. Patrick*)

FIGURE 9.14 ◆ Safety vest. (*Courtesy of R. Patrick*)

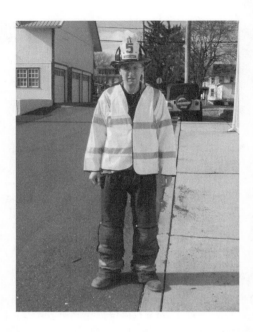

background (outer) material shall be either fluorescent orange-red or fluorescent yellow-green, as defined in the standard. The retroreflective material color shall be either orange, yellow, white, silver, yellow-green, or a fluorescent version of these colors, and shall be visible at a minimum distance of 1,000 feet (300 m). The retroreflective safety apparel shall be designed to identify the wearer clearly as a person.

Scene lighting (Figures 9.15a, 9.15b, and 9.15c) lends itself as well to Cone 8: Be Seen and Not Hurt. Scene lighting currently used by emergency responders may actually do more harm than good. According to the **FEMA**-USFA *Emergency Vehicle Safety Initiative* (2004), emergency vehicle lighting, although important, provides warning only and provides no effective traffic control. It is often confusing to road users, especially at night. Road users approaching the traffic incident from the opposite direction on a divided highway are often distracted by emergency vehicle lighting and slow their vehicles to look at the traffic incident, posing a hazard to themselves and others traveling in their direction.

Scene lighting should be directed at illuminating the functioning portion of the incident. Ideally, high-level lighting directed down on the operations is best. When traffic around the scene is considered secure, forward facing headlights should be turned off, and limiting the number of flashing red lights is also recommended.

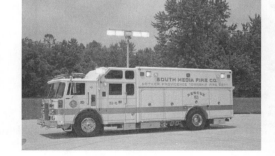

FIGURE 9.15A ◆ Scene lighting. (*Courtesy of Pearson Education/PH College*)

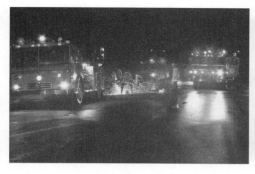

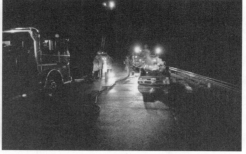

FIGURE 9.15B ◆ Nighttime scene lighting using headlamps. (*Courtesy of Pearson Education/PH College*)

FIGURE 9.15C ◆ Nighttime lighting. (*Courtesy of Pearson Education/PH College*)

Cone 10: Accountability Matters. Everyone is personally accountable and should be accounted for. The incident commander needs to establish a command post quickly, appoint a safety officer, and designate an accountability officer to oversee safe operations. Even though best practices suggest a designated safety officer, every emergency responder in essence is a safety officer and thus should be consciously aware of the surroundings.

Safety practices during roadway operations are numerous. Here are several other considerations for all emergency responders. Do not congest the work area with un-needed equipment. Consider vehicle staging off-site until needed. When you increase the number of vehicles and personnel on the scene, it increases exposures and the chance of a secondary incident involving the emergency responders. Summon additional vehicles as needed and instruct them where to position their units (Figure 9.16).

If EMS are needed and are not already on scene, place those personnel and vehicles within the protected area so they can triage, treat, and prepare for transport of patients safely (Figure 9.17). All emergency personnel should be trained to exit the vehicles on the downstream side, away from moving traffic, if possible. The reduction of emergency lighting can be helpful, as strobes and red flashing lights can blind, attract, or confuse the general public. The use of amber lights, arrow boards, arrow sticks, message boards, and police vehicles are generally effective in slowing traffic. The use of overhead lighting to illuminate the scene is preferable when visibility is limited.

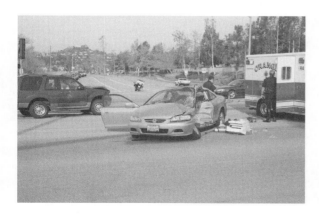

FIGURE 9.16 ◆ Ambulance arriving first on scene of MVC. (*Courtesy of PhotoEdit Inc.*)

FIGURE 9.17 ◆ EMTs should work within the protected area at the emergency scene. (*Courtesy of Pearson Education/ PH College*)

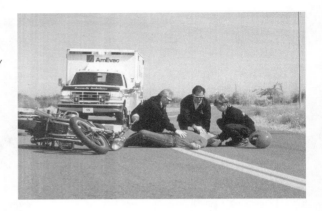

Always expect the unexpected. When the incident is mitigated, the incident commander needs to limit time on scene. Incident termination can be as dangerous as any component of the operation. Limiting scene time reduces exposure. Emergency responders should be accounted for and then placed in available status as soon as possible. Cones and signage should be removed in the reverse order of how they were set up. Start at the incident scene and work in reverse until the last warning device is secured. This is a very dangerous task, and traffic must remain under control until the last cone is picked up and all emergency responders have left the scene.

◆ OFFICER'S SAFE PARKING "CUE CARD"

Block with first-arriving apparatus to protect the scene, patients, and emergency personnel.

- Block at least one additional lane.
- Block so pump panel is downstream.
- Block most critical or highest traffic volume direction first.
- Consider requesting additional PD assistance.

Crews wear proper PPE with helmet.

- Class III vests at all times
- Helmet at all times
- Full PPE plus Class III vest between dusk and dawn or inclement weather

Establish more than adequate advance warning.

- Place traffic cones at 15-foot intervals.
- Deploy minimum five cones upstream.
- Cones only "suggest"; they don't block!
- Expand initial safe work zone.

For the direct placement of ambulances:

- Assure ambulances park within shadow of larger apparatus as directed.
- Lane 1 is farthest right lane, next is Lane 2, then Lane 3, and so on, from approaching motorist's point of view.
- Direct ambulance to block to the right or block to the left to protect loading doors.
  - Place ambulance patient loading area facing away from closest lane of moving traffic.
- All patient loading into med units is done from within a protected work zone.

You are the scene safety officer.

- Consider assigning a responder as an upstream spotter as necessary for approaching traffic.

At night or in reduced light conditions:

- Turn OFF vehicle headlights.
- Turn OFF preemption devices.
- Provide overall scene lighting.
- Have all personnel in PPE with helmets.
- Illuminate cones with flares.
- Consider additional vehicle(s) for additional upstream block.

In limited-access, high-volume highway incidents:

- Establish initial block: minimum two lanes.
- Consider ladder truck to establish upstream block.
  - Two lanes plus paved shoulder, or
  - Three driving lanes
- Place cones and/or cones illuminated by flares upstream of first apparatus.
  - Last cone approximately 150 feet upstream of apparatus
- Establish flagger position.
  - Monitor approaching traffic.
  - Sound emergency signal as necessary.
- Driver/operator of first apparatus.
  - Sound a series of long blasts on apparatus air horn as necessary.
- Use other EV and police department vehicles for additional blocking.
- Stage additional companies off highway.
- Establish liaison with police department.
- Terminate incident aggressively.

Unlike other workplaces, the roadway is not a closed environment. Preventing work-related roadway crashes requires strategies that combine traffic safety principles and sound safety management practices. Although employers cannot control roadway conditions, they can promote safe driving behavior by providing safety information to workers and by setting and enforcing driver safety policies. Crashes are not an unavoidable part of doing business. Employers can take steps to protect their employees and their companies.

◆ THE PUBLIC YIELDING TO EMERGENCY VEHICLES

Our society is mobile. Every year the volume of traffic increases and interstate systems become more complex. We spend hours traveling to and from work in urban areas. In response, automobile manufacturers make vehicles as comfortable as possible. They control noise and provide a variety of entertainment, including radios, CDs, and screens for watching videos.

We also are a society in a hurry. Because we must spend more time on the roadways, we conduct many activities while traveling from point *A* to point *B*. Studies have shown that these activities include eating, putting on makeup, combing hair, reading the paper, and the ever-present talking on the cell phone. All these activities decrease focus on driving and traffic flow.

FIGURE 9.18 ◆ Traffic passing an emergency scene.

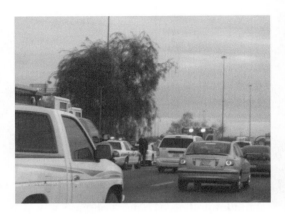

We are curious when seeing emergency lights along the roadside (Figure 9.18). Drivers routinely try to see what is going on, often missing an altered traffic pattern. Any impairment from fatigue, alcohol, or drugs increases the potential for poor judgment and a mishap.

Highway operations should be handled in the same manner as other types of operations. Departments must preplan highway emergency incidents with an emphasis on tactical considerations and personnel safety. This section will review practices that provide a safer environment and improve the protection of emergency responders involved in highway operations.

The privately owned vehicle (**POV**) operator is not without responsibility. **Move-over-laws** that exist in many states depict the responsibility of the lay public to yield the right-of-way to emergency response vehicles (Figure 9.19). Emergency vehicle operators must remember that they do not have, should not take, and cannot take the right-of-way. They must be yielded the right-of-way.

The Georgia Move-Over-Law states:

a. The operator of a motor vehicle approaching a stationary authorized emergency vehicle that is displaying flashing yellow, amber, white, red, or blue lights shall approach the authorized emergency vehicle with due caution and shall, absent any other direction by a peace officer, proceed as follows:

  1. Make a lane change into a lane not adjacent to the authorized emergency vehicle if possible in the existing safety and traffic conditions; or

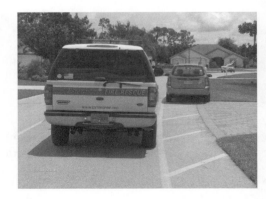

FIGURE 9.19 ◆ Private vehicle yielding to right.

2. If a lane change under paragraph (1) of this subsection would be impossible, prohibited by law, or unsafe, reduce the speed of the motor vehicle to a reasonable and proper speed for the existing road and traffic conditions, which speed shall be less than the posted speed limit, and be prepared to stop.

b. The operator of a motor vehicle approaching a stationary towing or recovery vehicle or a stationary highway maintenance vehicle that is displaying flashing yellow, amber, or red lights shall approach the vehicle with due caution and shall, absent any other direction by a peace officer, proceed as follows:

1. Make a lane change into a lane not adjacent to the towing, recovery, or highway maintenance vehicle if possible in the existing safety and traffic conditions; or

2. If a lane change under paragraph (1) of this subsection would be impossible, prohibited by law, or unsafe, reduce the speed of the motor vehicle to a reasonable and proper speed for the existing road and traffic conditions, which speed shall be less than the posted speed limit, and be prepared to stop.

c. Violation of subsection (a) or (b) of this Code section shall be punished by a fine of $500.00.

See Figure 9.20 for another example of a move-over law.

State: Michigan	**Citation:** MCLS § 257.653a (2002)

Move-Over-Law: § 257.653a. Stationary emergency vehicle giving visual signal; duty of approaching vehicle to exhibit due care and caution; violation; penalty.

Sec. 653a. (1) Upon approaching and passing a stationary authorized emergency vehicle that is giving a visual signal by means of flashing, rotating, or oscillating red, blue, or white lights as permitted by section 698, the driver of an approaching vehicle shall exhibit due care and caution, as required under the following:

(a) On any public roadway with at least 2 adjacent lanes proceeding in the same direction of the stationary authorized emergency vehicle, the driver of the approaching vehicle shall proceed with caution and yield the right-of-way by moving into a lane at least 1 moving lane or 2 vehicle widths apart from the stationary authorized emergency vehicle, unless directed otherwise by a police officer. If movement to an adjacent lane or 2 vehicle widths apart is not possible due to weather, road conditions, or the immediate presence of vehicular or pedestrian traffic in parallel moving lanes, the driver of the approaching vehicle shall proceed as required in subdivision (b).

(b) On any public roadway that does not have at least 2 adjacent lanes proceeding in the same direction as the stationary authorized emergency vehicle, or if the movement by the driver of the vehicle into an adjacent lane or 2 vehicle widths apart is not possible as described in subdivision (a), the approaching vehicle shall reduce and maintain a safe speed for weather, road conditions, and vehicular or pedestrian traffic and proceed with due care and caution, or as directed by a police officer.

(2) Except as provided in subsections (3) and (4), a person who violates this section is guilty of a misdemeanor punishable by a fine of not more than $500.00 or imprisonment for not more than 90 days, or both.

(3) A person who violates this section and causes injury to a police officer, firefighter, or other emergency response personnel in the immediate area of the stationary authorized emergency vehicle is guilty of a felony punishable by a fine of not more than $1,000.00 or imprisonment for not more than 2 years, or both.

(4) A person who violates this section and causes death to a police officer, firefighter, or other emergency response personnel in the immediate area of the stationary authorized emergency vehicle is guilty of a felony punishable by a fine of not more than $7,500.00 or by imprisonment for not more than 15 years, or both.

FIGURE 9.20 ◆ Example of move-over law.

The number of firefighters struck and killed by motor vehicles has dramatically increased within recent years. During the 5-year period between 1995 and 1999, 17 firefighters were struck and killed by motorists. This represents an 89 percent increase in the number of line-of-duty deaths over the previous 5-year period (between 1990 and 1994), when 9 firefighters were struck and killed by motor vehicles (NFPA, 2000). Under the Fire Fighter Fatality Investigation and Prevention Program, NIOSH investigated two separate incidents involving firefighters who were struck and killed while providing emergency services along roadways during 1999 (NIOSH, 1999, 2000). These incidents and data demonstrate that hazards to the fire service are not limited to structural or wildland fires. Motorists accustomed to a clear, unobstructed roadway may not recognize and avoid closed lanes or emergency workers on or near the roadway. In some cases, conditions can reduce a motorist's ability to see and avoid firefighters and apparatus. Some examples include weather, time of day, scene lighting (i.e., area lighting and optical warning devices), traffic speed and volume, and road configuration (i.e., hills, curves, and other obstructions that limit visibility). These hazards are not limited to the fire service alone. Other emergency service providers such as law enforcement officers, paramedics, and vehicle recovery personnel are also exposed to these hazards.

◆ CASE STUDY

On August 5, 1999, one firefighter died, and a second firefighter and another person were severely injured when they were struck by a motor vehicle that lost control on a wet and busy interstate highway (NIOSH, 1999). A heavy-rescue squad and a ladder truck had been dispatched to a single motor vehicle crash on an interstate highway. Approximately two minutes after they arrived on the scene and took a position to the rear of the rescue squad (protecting the initial vehicle crash scene), another car collided with the back of the ladder truck. While attending to the injuries of the driver who struck the ladder truck, two firefighters and the injured driver were struck by a third car, causing one firefighter to be fatally injured and the second firefighter and the driver (who had collided with the back of the ladder truck) to be severely injured. On September 27, 1999, a firefighter died after being struck by a tractor-trailer truck while directing traffic along a four-lane highway (NIOSH, 2000). The victim was standing in front of an apparatus that was parked (facing north) in the outer emergency lane for the southbound traffic. The emergency lights of the apparatus were on and functioning properly at the time of the incident. He was called out to provide assistance for a neighboring fire department that had responded to a tractor-trailer crash. The initial tractor-trailer crash and subsequent firefighter fatality occurred during a heavy rainstorm along a one-mile stretch of a four-lane highway. Thirty-nine collisions have occurred on this one-mile stretch of road since 1994.

◆ APPARATUS PLACEMENT

The Phoenix, Arizona, Fire Department made major revisions to its positioning SOP after the loss of a firefighter in 1994. The firefighter/paramedic was struck by a drunk driver while loading a patient into the back of an ambulance. Prior to this fatality, the use of an emergency vehicle as a barrier to protect on-street incidents was well established. The SOP was used for highway and freeway emergencies, but not for incidents in residential areas. The positioning SOP was changed to place emphasis on the dangers in residential areas as well as on highways. Personnel interviewed for this report stated that the level of awareness of apparatus positioning is significantly higher than before the 1994 fatality (FEMA, USFA, 2004).

A line-of-duty fatality that occurred in Midwest City, Oklahoma, prompted the Plano, Texas, Fire Department to institute an apparatus-positioning policy. On August 5, 1999, two career firefighters were struck by a motor vehicle on a wet and busy interstate. One firefighter was killed and one was seriously injured. The NIOSH report of this incident is available online at http://www.cdc.gov/niosh/summ9927.html

At the time, there was no consistency for securing a highway incident scene in Plano. Although the department had not suffered a catastrophic loss, it realized the potential and the need to develop a highway safety operations policy. As in other growing urban/suburban areas, increases in traffic volume and speed also contributed to the need for improved safety on the roadways. The Plano policy mirrors the policy developed by the Phoenix Fire Department.

Fairfax County, Virginia, Fire and Rescue developed a manual to outline appropriate highway operations. This manual, *Operating Procedures for Highway Incidents,* is now used in place of an SOP. The manual was developed in response to an increase in the incidence of near misses while operating on the highway. It is based on information from federal DOT publications and was developed in consultation with VDOT. The SOPs of all three departments provide graphic examples of vehicle placement.

When the apparatus-positioning SOP was changed in Phoenix, much of the training was done using videos that were aired on the cable television Phoenix Fire Network (PFN). PFN, a 24-hour-a-day operation, schedules programs based on input from operations personnel and the safety officer. Practical training was done at the district level, using demonstrations of how to position, how to set up work zones, and some simulated scenes for hands-on practice.

The Plano training included classroom presentation of the Midwest City incident. Videos, pictures, and other information regarding that incident served as the basis for the safety discussion. A tabletop exercise planned the placement of apparatus at various intersections and locations on various roadways. This was followed by a roadway exercise with apparatus to emphasize the points of the classroom and tabletop exercise. Personnel consistently remarked that the concept was discussed so often in advance of the policy and training, it seemed like second nature when it went into effect.

Fairfax County recruits receive the highway operations manual while at the academy. Other personnel are given the manual when they go through driver training. Policy change is communicated via an intranet. The change may be in the form of a general order, a training or safety bulletin, or a manual change. This is usually followed by an instation discussion and/or training or may involve quarterly training at the academy.

◆ SCENE LIGHTING AND MARKING

Lighting specifications for new apparatus for all departments interviewed are based on NFPA 1901. Fairfax County Fire and Rescue personnel cite an increased use of amber lighting in conjunction with emergency lighting, but amber lights are not used in isolation. The current policy is to leave all emergency lights on at the scene. Headlights are turned off when facing oncoming traffic.

Several ESOs use directional arrows on the rear light bar of apparatus and then turn off headlights and leave rotators and flashing beacons on while operating at highway incidents. When floodlights are used, they are raised to a height that allows light to be directed down on the scene. Personnel believe this provides the optimum working conditions at night, improves vision, and reduces the trip hazard. "The more lights, the safer the providers" is the consensus among Plano line personnel. The Plano Police Department also has a support pickup truck with cones that can be called to help divert traffic from an incident scene.

The Virginia Beach Fire and Rescue SOP for highway markings was developed as the result of proactively reviewing safety aspects of highway operations and an increasing number of responses for highway incidents. Line personnel also identified the number of near misses they experienced and injuries in the neighboring Norfolk Fire Department as factors that prompted the desire for the SOP at their level.

Virginia Beach used a team approach to develop the SOP, which is based on the Fairfax County and Phoenix departments' policies, NFPA standards, state regulations, and what Fort Collins, Colorado, was doing related to lighting issues. The department also consulted public safety, law enforcement, VDOT, and the private EMS provider to identify their needs and recommendations.

The policy for highway marking distances for a working incident zone (300 feet when light, 500 feet when dark) was based on vision and distance changes at night. The policy also identifies the minimum requirements for the work zone. The incident commander can adjust these distances, request additional units for protection, and block the entire road as dictated by existing conditions. The state police are responsible for traffic control outside the fire department's established work zone.

The "best" light color(s) and lighting pattern for highway operations are still being debated. Research by the National Institute of Standards and Technology has shown that as the number of flashing lights increases, the ability of drivers to quickly respond to the emergency message decreases. A 1988 study conducted by Boff and Lincoln at Wright-Patterson AFB showed an emergency flashing light is noticed quickly if there are no other flashing lights in the field of view.

Dr. Stephen Solomon, an ophthalmologist who has studied emergency vehicle colors and lighting, notes that the fire service philosophy has been to attract as much attention as possible through a combination of lights and light colors with varying degrees of reflection and flashes. Strong stimuli hold central gaze and drivers tend to steer in the direction of gaze. If fatigue, alcohol, or drugs impair the driver, the potential and degree of drift increases. He suggests this practice actually makes the fire apparatus a "visual, magnetic target." He recommends reducing the time span of looking toward a complex flashing light display by reducing the number, brightness, and array of color, revolving strobe, and reflecting lights during emergency travel; and using either filament bulbs in one or two amber flashers (mounted on the upper level of the vehicle on each corner) blinking in tandem or revolving beacons when the vehicle is parked along the road or at a curb and clear of all active traffic lanes.

The use of emergency vehicle lighting (Figure 9.21) is also addressed in the *Manual on Uniform Traffic Control Devices* (MUTCD). The manual revision had a target finalization date of October 2003. The manual addresses the use of emergency lighting as follows.

Support. The use of emergency vehicle lighting is essential, especially in the initial stages of a traffic incident, for the safety of emergency responders and persons involved in the traffic incident as well as road users approaching the traffic incident. Emergency vehicle lighting, however, provides warning only and provides no effective traffic control. It is often confusing to road users, especially at night. Road users

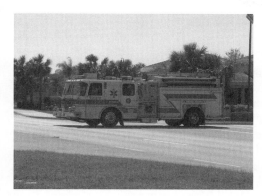

FIGURE 9.21 ◆ Emergency vehicle lighting.

approaching the traffic incident from the opposite direction on a divided facility are often distracted by emergency vehicle lighting and slow their vehicles to look at the traffic incident, posing a hazard to themselves and others traveling in their direction.

The use of emergency vehicle lighting can be reduced if good traffic control has been established at a traffic incident scene. This is especially true for major traffic incidents that might involve a number of emergency vehicles. If good traffic control is established through placement of advanced warning signs and traffic control devices to divert or detour traffic, then public safety agencies can perform their tasks on scene with minimal emergency vehicle lighting.

Guidance. Public safety agencies should examine their policies on the use of emergency vehicle lighting, especially after a traffic incident scene is secured, with the aim of reducing the use of this lighting as much as possible while not endangering those at the scene. Special consideration should be given to reducing or extinguishing forward-facing emergency vehicle lighting, especially on divided roadways, to reduce distractions to oncoming road users.

◆ REFLECTIVE VESTS

Reflective vests should be used to increase worker visibility, regardless of the use of turnout gear. The reflective vests used by emergency workers should have both retroreflective and fluorescent properties. Retroreflective material returns the majority of light from the light source back to the observer. Fluorescent material absorbs UV light of a certain wavelength and regenerates it into visual energy. Plano Fire Department requires all personnel involved in highway operations to wear a Class II vest with a lime-green background and orange/gray stripes.

◆ STANDARD OPERATING PROCEDURES

Seven fire departments in northern Virginia have formed a regional committee to review highway safety policies and recommend changes to them when necessary. The committee is made up of the following departments:

◆ Fairfax County Fire and Rescue Department
◆ Arlington County Fire Department

- Fort Belvoir Fire Department
- Fairfax City Fire Department
- Reagan National Airport Fire Department
- Dulles Airport Fire Department
- Alexandria County Fire Department

Any member of any of the participating fire departments can submit a proposed change. The proposed change is passed through the chain of command to the committee for review. In Fairfax County, the safety officer and an operations chief review the proposed change before it is advanced to the committee. Committee recommendations go to all department chiefs, who ultimately decide whether the recommendation will be implemented in the individual department. The regional committee does not mandate changes to individual departments. It serves primarily as an information sharing forum to improve interoperability among participating departments.

The Virginia Beach Fire and Rescue SOP, Operations of Fire Department Vehicles, was in the process of revision at the time of this writing. Any member of the department can submit suggested policy changes. Suggestions go first to a specific committee, such as the safety committee or apparatus committee, for review. If the suggestion has merit, it is forwarded to the SOP committee. The SOP committee forwards its final recommendation to the chief for a decision on implementation. It is not unusual for changes to go back and forth between the chief and the SOP committee several times until consensus is reached. After approval, the SOP is implemented as an interim policy for 90 days for evaluation and any necessary modification before it becomes final.

EFFECT ON HIGHWAY OPERATIONS

The design and insulation of new passenger and commercial vehicles, combined with operating radio/CD and air conditioning, can significantly hinder a driver's ability to hear emergency vehicle audible warning devices and realize emergency vehicles are approaching. Departments must engrain safety into all activities; and personnel must view safety as their job, both individually and collectively.

According to the *Emergency Vehicle Safety Initiative, no* department interviewed had any specific data to support current apparatus placement or lighting patterns. However, personnel had several subjective comments regarding the effects. All Phoenix Fire Department field personnel, including chiefs, believed that crew communication and apparatus positioning were the primary methods of providing a safe operational environment.

Plano Fire Department personnel also unanimously agreed that apparatus placement is the most effective of all methods used on scene to improve safety of providers. They believed the department's placement policy had definitely improved safety and decreased near misses. Blocking a lane with apparatus slows traffic speed and impedes traffic flow. The blocking policy increases the feeling of safety for both fire and law enforcement personnel, but all remain vigilant. Even when proper blocking is used, personnel have witnessed drivers going over curbs, cones, and even between blocking apparatus. Vehicles have struck blocking apparatus. Had the apparatus not been there, the vehicle could have breached the work zone and injured personnel.

All the departments placed less importance on lighting patterns versus apparatus placement. Phoenix fire personnel considered lighting secondary and, in many cases, unreliable. Some believed that any lighting pattern was useless at night when extensive floodlights were used. Some Fairfax County personnel believed that directional signaling (light sticks, arrows, etc.) seemed to help traffic flow, but identified pulling all the information together and discipline as the keys to successful highway operations, and rapid mitigation as the key to improving and restoring traffic flow.

LIMITATIONS

Plano Fire Department personnel identified forgetting to shut off apparatus headlights and civilian motorists paying more attention to what is going on at the scene than to traffic flow as their biggest problems during highway operations. Another challenge is dealing with neighboring districts that do not use similar apparatus placement practices, which can result in confusion and policy issues when responding with mutual aid. In an effort to reduce this problem, Plano shared its policies with neighboring departments. It must be remembered that SOPs and operating manuals serve as a basis for safe practice. Actual practices depend on the existing conditions identified by the company officer or incident commander.

◆ RECOMMENDATIONS FOR SAFE ROADWAY/HIGHWAY OPERATIONS

The USFA *Emergency Vehicle Safety Initiative* identified the following basic best practices when operating on a roadway/highway regardless of the incident nature.

- During roadway/highway operations, position the vehicle at a 45-degree angle to the lanes.
- Fire engines should attempt to position the pump panel toward the incident and the front wheels rotated away from the incident.
- Rescue vehicles should attempt to position the vehicle with the primary extrication equipment accessible to the incident scene.
- Ambulances should be positioned with patient compartment access facing away from traffic flow and preferably upstream from the incident. Do not allow the ambulance to get blocked in by other response vehicles.
- Turn off forward-facing emergency vehicle lighting, especially on divided roadways.
- Reduce the use of lighting as much as possible at the scene.
- Require crew members to wear highly reflective material when conducting roadway/highway operations.
- Remain vigilant during all phases of roadway/highway operations.
- Work with neighboring ESOs to develop similar roadway/highway operation policies.
- Allow all members to submit suggestions for policy enhancements.

POLICIES

- Assign a key member of the management team responsibility and authority to set and enforce comprehensive driver safety policy.
- Enforce mandatory seat belt use.
- Do not require workers to drive irregular hours or far beyond their normal working hours.
- Do not require workers to conduct business on a cell phone while driving.
- Develop work schedules that allow employees to obey speed limits and to follow applicable hours-of-service regulations.

FLEET MANAGEMENT

+ Adopt a structured vehicle maintenance program.
+ Provide company vehicles that offer the highest possible levels of occupant protection.

SAFETY PROGRAMS

+ Teach workers strategies for recognizing and managing driver fatigue and in-vehicle distractions.
+ Provide training to workers operating specialized motor vehicles or equipment.
+ Emphasize to workers the need to follow safe driving practices on and off the job.

DRIVER PERFORMANCE

+ Ensure that workers assigned to drive on the job have a valid driver's license and one that is appropriate for the type of vehicle to be driven.
+ Check driving records of prospective employees, and perform periodic rechecks after hiring.
+ Maintain complete and accurate records of workers' driving performance.

For more information on crash prevention and vehicle safety programs, see *Prevention Strategies for Employers* (NIOSH DHHS Publication No. 2004-136, March 2004).

VEHICLE PLACEMENT

Placement of Vehicles at Emergency Incidents. Every emergency service organization should have standard operating guidelines (SOGs) for placing emergency vehicles at emergency incidents. These guidelines should address, at a minimum, the following issues:

+ Placement of vehicles at emergencies located on streets and highways
+ Positioning of emergency vehicles at incidents so as to minimize the blinding effect of the warning lights on approaching and passing vehicles
+ Identification of potential hazards affecting placement of vehicles at emergency scenes
+ Identification of appropriate safe distances from certain types of emergencies (such as vehicle fires) for the placement of emergency vehicles
+ Consideration for the ease of leaving the scene because of changing conditions at the emergency incident; or, a directive to leave the scene to respond to another incident or to be available for any potential issues

PERSONNEL AWARENESS

Any responder working along any type of roadway runs the risk of being struck by a motorist. Even though the following information references NIOSH fire service investigation and reporting, similar practices should be exercised by all ESOs and responders.

To prevent such incidents, NIOSH recommends that fire departments and firefighters take the following actions.

Fire Departments

+ Develop, implement, and enforce standard operating procedures (SOPs) regarding emergency operations for roadway incidents.
+ Implement an incident management system to manage all emergency incidents.

- Establish a unified command for incidents that occur where multiple agencies have jurisdiction.
- Ensure that a separate incident safety officer (independent of the incident commander) is appointed.
- Develop pre-incident plans for areas that have a high rate of motor vehicle crashes.
- Establish pre-incident agreements with law enforcement and other agencies such as the highway department.
- Ensure that firefighters are trained in safe procedures for operating in or near moving traffic.
- Ensure that firefighters wear suitable high-visibility apparel, such as a strong yellow-green or orange reflecting flagger vest, when operating at an emergency scene.

Firefighters

- Ensure that the fire apparatus is positioned to take advantage of topography and weather conditions (uphill and upwind) and to protect firefighters from traffic.
- Park or stage unneeded vehicles off the roadway whenever possible.
- If police have not yet arrived at a scene involving a highway incident or fire, first control the oncoming vehicles before safely turning your attention to the emergency.
- Position yourself and any victim(s) in a secure area that maximizes your visibility to motorists when it is impossible to protect the incident scene from immediate danger.
- Use a traffic control device that maximizes your visibility to motorists when controlling traffic.

VEHICLE MARKINGS

Striping with Diamond Grade fluorescent material in a herringbone pattern improves driver recognition while the apparatus is on the roadways. Vehicles should have high visibility. Contrasting colors can add to this effect. These factors are not highly dependent on driver behavior. For example, the Plano Fire Department uses additional lighting of a contrasting color to the vehicles.

The installation of contrasting color restraints and a rearview mirror above the officer's seat will lend a hand to ensuring compliance accountability. NFPA 1901 states, "If available from the chassis manufacturer, the seatbelt webbing shall be bright red in color." The committee suggested that "international orange" is not the best color because it shows dirt. A rearview mirror above the officer's seat allows him or her to assure that all personnel are wearing restraints without the distraction of having to turn around. These practices make it easier to ensure that all personnel are restrained before the apparatus moves.

Backing and Preemption.   Even though cameras and other devices that assist with backing the apparatus do provide some measure of safety, there is no substitute for having at least one, preferably two, spotters to guide the driver while the apparatus is being operated in reverse. NFPA 1500 requires spotters for backing, regardless of whether the apparatus is equipped with cameras or other backing safety equipment. One spotter should be equipped with a portable radio in the event that he or she needs to contact the driver during the backing operation.

Consider optical traffic preemption systems to improve emergency vehicle movement through controlled intersections. With activation at half a mile, optical traffic preemption usually clears the intersection before the unit arrives, allowing continued travel without the need to stop. However, drivers must not assume they will have a clear path when they arrive at the intersection; they must verify visually that all traffic has stopped.

Always bring units to a complete stop at red lights, stop signs, and activated or unguarded rail crossings before proceeding.

Even though optical preemption devices can provide a clear path for emergency units through traffic signals, drivers must not anticipate a change so far ahead that they cannot stop the apparatus safely or avoid striking another vehicle. Pursue a working relationship with your state department of transportation and local law enforcement to identify criteria for responses that would incorporate the DOT resources to aid in traffic control and improve safety for responders involved in roadway operations.

An intelligent transportation system, a traffic operations center, and Department of Transportation (DOT) freeway motorist assist patrollers, if available, can provide considerable assistance to emergency response departments for traffic control at a highway operations scene.

Point to Ponder

- Drivers should extinguish forward-facing EV lighting (Figure 9.22). This is very important on divided roadways. This will help reduce distractions and glare to oncoming drivers. The headlights on the EV can temporarily blind approaching drivers, resulting in the problem of glare recovery. It takes at least six seconds, going from light to dark, and three seconds from dark to light for vision to recover.
- Responders should consider the reduction of lighting as much as possible at the scene. Establish good traffic control, including placement of advance warning signs and traffic control devices to divert or detour traffic. This will allow responders to reduce emergency vehicle lighting. This is especially true for major traffic incidents that might involve a number of emergency vehicles.
- ESOs should require members to wear highly reflective material when conducting highway operations. Personnel visibility is critical during highway operations. In addition to PPE, high-visibility vests should meet the ANSI III Standard. ANSI III provides the highest level of both retroreflective and fluorescent properties. It makes workers conspicuous through a full range of body movements at 1,280 feet.

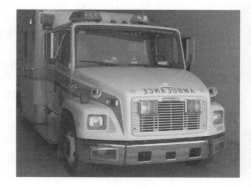

FIGURE 9.22 ◆ Emergency vehicle with lights turned off.

REMAIN VIGILANT

Even with all safety precautions in place, personnel are at risk from drivers who may violate safety zones, thereby blocking apparatus, cones, curbs, and so on. Use law enforcement personnel to help secure and protect the scene. If necessary, appoint a safety officer to monitor traffic. ESOs should work with neighboring ESOs to develop similar roadway safety policies. Mutual aid departments using the same apparatus positioning and marking policies will improve the overall safety of all members at the incident, through understanding of and familiarity with operating procedures. Responders who work at highway operations on a daily basis can provide a critical review of existing policy and valuable information to improve safety based on experience.

Assess code responses using a risk management matrix. Identify the low-frequency, low-severity incidents. Use preset dispatch questions and respond in a nonemergency mode.

Multiple EMS studies have shown, with the exception of a few conditions, that there is no statistically significant difference in patient outcomes with emergency driving on ambulances versus nonemergency driving. It is logical to assume that in many situations the results related to incident outcome would be duplicated with fire apparatus. St. Louis Fire Department found responding without lights and sirens reduced its crash rate. There are commercial dispatch programs available for priority dispatching, as discussed in Chapter 10.

Training. Organizations that deliver driver training should ensure that their instructors meet local and state certification requirements for emergency service instructors. These instructors should also have specialized training and experience in safe and proper operation of emergency vehicles.

Students should be provided with the theory and concepts associated with the safe operation of emergency vehicles and highway emergency scene safety. If driving simulators are available, they should be used to familiarize driver candidates with principles of vehicle operation. Tabletop scenarios also can be used for simulations. Practical driving exercises should be conducted on a controlled driving course and over public thoroughfares.

A driving simulator is an effective tool to familiarize driver candidates with vehicle operations. It can also be used to place experienced drivers in special situations that cannot be reproduced practically or safely using actual vehicles. It is most appropriate for high-risk situations, such as intersections and conflict management. It also allows remedial training to be tailored to a specific problem. However, a simulator cannot replace practical driver training exercises using actual emergency vehicles. All driver training programs must include the operation of actual vehicles in order to ensure candidates are capable of operating the real thing.

The ESO's in-service training program must stress continuous maintenance and improvement of driver skills. In order to ensure that emergency vehicle drivers maintain their skills at an acceptable level, they should be required to prove their proficiency by recertifying at least every three years, coupled with continuing education on an annual basis.

Responders who are going to drive and operate EVs must be familiar with all the different types of EVs operated by the ESO. One method of developing this familiarity is to require personnel to complete a task book before taking the driver's examination. This practice ensures that the responders are familiar with all of the different models of EVs that they may encounter and any driving course specifications. The tasks should be minimum requirements and provide a foundation for future learning.

Sharing incident information, the surrounding circumstances, and the findings of the investigation in a timely manner can be a valuable training tool. If the investigation is prolonged, release a preliminary findings report. This is exceptionally beneficial in near-miss investigations.

◆ SAMPLE SOP/SOGs

The following samples are from the USFA EV driving initiative:

Part 1: Fairfax County Fire and Rescue Operating Procedures for Highway Incidents
Part 2: Phoenix Fire Department Safe Parking While Operating in or near Vehicle Traffic

FAIRFAX COUNTY FIRE AND RESCUE OPERATING PROCEDURES FOR HIGHWAY INCIDENTS PREFACE

The primary objectives for any operation at the scene of a highway incident are preserving life, preventing injury to emergency workers, protecting property, and restoring traffic flow.

Managing a highway incident and other related problems is a team effort. Each responding agency has a role to play in an effective incident operation. The police, the Virginia Department of Transportation, and the Fire and Rescue Department all play important roles in the management of highway incidents. It is not a question of "Who is in charge?" but "Who is in charge of what?"

Care of the injured, protection of the public, safety of the emergency responders, and clearance of the traffic lanes should all be priority concerns of the incident manager operating at the scene of a highway accident. It is extremely important that all activities that block traffic lanes be concluded as quickly as possible and the flow of traffic be allowed to resume promptly. When traffic flow is heavy, a small savings in accident scene clearance time can greatly reduce traffic backups and reduce the probability of a secondary incident. Restoring the roadway to normal or to as near normal as soon as possible creates a safer environment for the motorist and emergency responders. Additionally, it improves the public's perception of the agencies involved and reduces the time and dollar loss resulting from the incident.

Purpose. The purpose of this manual is to provide the incident officers and members of the Fire and Rescue Department with a uniform guide for safe operations at incidents occurring on the highway system. It is intended to serve as a guideline for decision making and can be modified by the incident officers as necessary to address existing incident conditions. The most common occurrence and the one that has possibly the greatest potential for an unfavorable outcome to department personnel is emergency operations at the scene of a vehicle accident. Each year many significant incidents occur on roadways within Fairfax County. Whether it is on the interstate highway or on a secondary road, the potential for injury or death to a member of the department is overwhelming.

Response. Fire and Rescue Department personnel shall operate safely and make every effort to minimize the risk of injury to themselves and those who use the highway system. Personnel shall wear appropriate gear and be seated with restraint straps on prior to their vehicle responding to all incidents.

Apparatus operating in the emergency mode shall operate warning devices and follow the guidelines outlined in Department SOP 1.8.03.

Warning Lights:	Emergency warning lights shall remain operational while responding and, when necessary, while working at incidents.
Headlights:	Apparatus headlights shall be operational during all responses and incidents regardless of the time of the day. Caution should be used to avoid blinding oncoming traffic while on the scene.
Siren and Air Horn:	When operating as an emergency vehicle, siren and air horn will be utilized.

Emergency response to incidents on limited-access highways should include at least one unit traveling each direction on the highway. When units respond together in the same direction, they should remain in single file in relatively close proximity to one another. This reduces confusion to the motorists on the highway as to how to appropriately yield the right-of-way to emergency apparatus.

The preferable lane of response should be the left travel lane. When the shoulder must be utilized, apparatus operators must use extreme caution. Be aware of road signs, debris, guardrails, oversized vehicles, and stopped vehicles. Fire and Rescue Department vehicle operators must reduce speed of their vehicle when using the shoulder of the road to access the incident.

Response on access ramps shall be in the normal direction of travel, unless an officer on the scene can confirm that oncoming traffic has been stopped and no civilian vehicles will be encountered on the ramp.

Median strip crossovers marked "Authorized Vehicles Only" shall be used only for turning around and crossing to the other travel lanes, when apparatus can complete the turn without obstructing the flow of traffic in either travel direction or all traffic movement has stopped. Under no circumstances shall crossovers be utilized for routine changes in travel direction.

Utilization of U-turn access points in "Jersey" barriers on limited access highways is extremely hazardous and shall be utilized only when the situation is necessary for immediate lifesaving measures.

On-Scene Actions. The proper spotting and placement of apparatus is the joint responsibility of the driver and officer. The proper positioning of apparatus at the scene of an incident assures other responding resources of easy access, a safe working area, and helps to contribute to an effective overall operation.

The unit officer is responsible for the safety of the unit and his or her crew from the time the apparatus leaves quarters until its return. Safety of the crew is foremost while they are operating, in both emergency and nonemergency situations.

Arrival. Standard practice shall be to position apparatus in such a manner as to ensure a safe work area at least one lane wider than the width of the incident. This may be difficult to accomplish at incidents on secondary and one-lane roads. Position the apparatus in such a manner as to provide the safest work area possible. A work zone shall be established allowing EMS units and the rescue squad to position in close proximity of the incident.

The engine placement should be back some distance from the incident, utilizing it as a safety shield blocking only those travel lanes necessary. The engine shall be placed at an angle to the lanes, with the pump panel toward the incident and the front wheels rotated away from the incident.

In the event that a motorist strikes the engine, the engine will act as a barrier and in the unlikely event the engine is moved on impact, it will travel away from the work zone. The pump panel should face the incident to provide protection for the operator while monitoring apparatus functions.

Before exiting apparatus at an incident, personnel shall check to ensure that traffic has stopped to avoid the possibility of being struck by a passing vehicle. Personnel should remember to look down to ensure that debris on the roadway will not become an obstacle, resulting in a personal injury. All crew members shall be in full protective clothing or traffic vests as the situation indicates.

As soon as possible, the engine operator should place out flares and traffic cones. Traffic cones assist in channeling traffic away from the incident. Cones shall be used whenever department vehicles are parked on or about any road surface.

Placement of cones and/or flares shall begin closest to the incident, working toward oncoming traffic. Cones and/or flares shall be placed diagonally across the roadway and around the incident. This assists in establishing a safe work zone. When placing cones or flares, care should be exercised to avoid being struck by oncoming traffic.

The speed of traffic must be considered when establishing a safe work area. Utilize Figure 9.23 to determine how far to place the first cone or flare away from the incident scene.

When channeling traffic around the incident, cones shall also be used in front of the incident with the same diagonal placement to direct traffic safely around the work zone (Figure 9.24).

It is possible to channel traffic around a curve, hill, or ramp provided the first cone is placed such that the oncoming driver is made aware of imminent danger. The first cone should be placed well before the curve, hill, or ramp. The rest of the cones shall be placed diagonally across the lanes around the work zone.

A four point system will be used whenever vehicles are parked in an area that does not require the channeling of traffic. One cone will be placed at each corner of the vehicle approximately four feet from each corner. This will assist the motorist and incoming units to identify the established work zone. When utilizing this system around aerial apparatus and rescue squads, additional cones should be placed to identify extended outriggers, booms, and heavy equipment.

Parking of Response Vehicles. Providing a safe work area for emergency responders is a priority at every emergency incident. However, consideration must be given to keeping as many traffic lanes as possible open. Except for those vehicles needed in the operation and those used, as a shield for the work area, other response vehicles should be parked together in a designated area. Parking should be on the shoulder or median area, if one exists. Parking response vehicles completely

Posted Speed Limit	Distance
35 MPH	100 ft
45 MPH	150 ft
55 MPH	200 ft
>55 MPH	250 ft plus ...

FIGURE 9.23 ◆ Spacing cones or flares at incident scene.

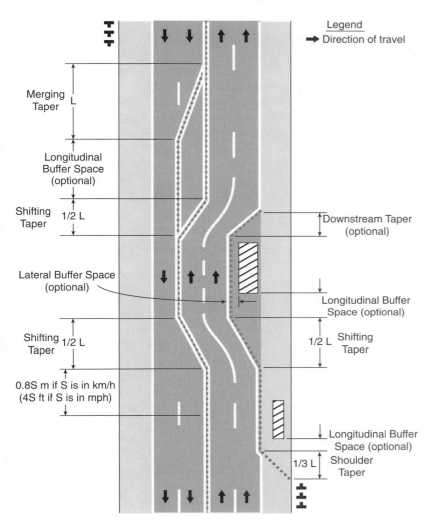

Legend
→ Direction of travel

Merging Taper — L

Longitudinal Buffer Space (optional)

Shifting Taper — 1/2 L

Lateral Buffer Space (optional)

Shifting Taper — 1/2 L

0.8S m if S is in km/h
(4S ft if S is in mph)

Downstream Taper (optional)

Longitudinal Buffer Space (optional)

1/2 L Shifting Taper

Longitudinal Buffer Space (optional)

1/3 L Shoulder Taper

FIGURE 9.24 ◆ Types of Tapers and Buffer Spaces. (*MUTCD, 2003*)

out of available travel lanes greatly assists in the movement of traffic. If not needed to illuminate the scene, drivers should remember to turn vehicle headlights off when parked at incidents.

Apparatus Visibility at Night. As the human eye becomes adapted to the dark, the first color to leave the spectrum is red. This is important due to the fact that our warning lights are red. The color red tends to blend in to the nighttime surroundings. Glare vision and recovery is the amount of time required to recover from the effects of glare once a light source is passed through the eye. This takes at least six seconds, going from light to dark and three seconds from dark to light for vision to recover.

At 50 miles per hour, the distance traveled during a second is approximately 75 feet. Thus, in six seconds, the vehicle has traveled 450 feet before the driver has fully regained night vision. This is extremely important when operating on roadways at night.

The headlights on the apparatus can temporarily blind drivers that are approaching fire and rescue apparatus. Drivers of oncoming vehicles will experience the problem of glare recovery. This essentially means individuals are driving by the emergency scene blind. The wearing of protective clothing and/or traffic vests will not help the blinded driver see department members standing in the roadway.

Studies conducted show that at two-and-a-half car lengths away from a vehicle with its headlights on, the opposing driver is completely blinded. The best combination of lights to provide maximum visibility is as follows:

+ Red warning lights on
+ Headlights off
+ Fog lights off
+ Pump panel lights on
+ Spotlights on rear (and front if equipped) on and directed on to a traffic cone
+ Traffic directional boards operating
+ Low-beam headlights utilized to light the emergency scene, using care as to light only the immediate scene

Clearing Traffic Lanes. When outside of a vehicle on a major roadway, both civilian and emergency responders are in a very unsafe environment. Therefore, it is imperative to take every precaution to protect ourselves as well as civilians at incident scenes (Figure 9.25). Positioning apparatus to serve as a shield for work areas is a prudent practice on any incident on a major roadway. But, we must remember that reducing and/or shutting down traffic lanes creates other problems and safety concerns. Therefore, it is critical when operational phases (extrications, medical care, and suppression) are completed, that apparatus be repositioned to allow traffic to flow on as many lanes as possible.

Remember that unnecessarily closing or keeping traffic lanes closed greatly increases the risk of a secondary incident occurring in the resulting traffic backup. One minute of stopped traffic causes an additional four-minute delay in traffic.

Clearing the Scene. Management of incidents on the interstate system and local roadways requires the expertise and resources of the Fire and Rescue Department, police department, Virginia State Police, local police departments, and the Virginia Department of Transportation working in concert. Although the safety of emergency services personnel is the paramount concern for the officer in charge, the flow of traffic must be kept in consideration at all times. The closing of roadways disrupts traffic throughout the area as well as having a significant impact on businesses throughout the region.

Keeping the safety of all personnel in mind and coordinating the needs with the other emergency services, the officer in charge should begin to open closed lanes utilized for extrication and place units in service as soon as practical.

PHOENIX FIRE DEPARTMENT SAFE PARKING WHILE OPERATING IN OR NEAR VEHICLE TRAFFIC

(Sample policy continued)

+ Overview
+ Safety Benchmarks
+ Freeway Operations

Overview. This procedure identifies parking practices for fire department apparatus that will provide maximum protection and safety for personnel operating in or near moving vehicle traffic. It also identifies several approaches for individual practices to keep firefighters safe while exposed to vehicle traffic.

It shall be the policy of the Phoenix Fire Department to position apparatus at the scene of emergencies in a manner that best protects the work area and personnel from vehicle traffic and other hazards.

Traffic Control Safety Checklist/Worksheet   ❋VFIS.

Location: _____   Date: _____   Incident #: _____

Incident Commander: _____   Safety Officer: _____

Vehicles on Scene: _____

Type of Incident: _____

Estimated Time On Scene: ☐ Less than 20 minutes   ☐ 20 – 60 minutes   ☐ More than 60 Minutes

Time of Day: _____   Type of Roadway: _____   Posted Speed Limit: _____

Weather Conditions: _____   Light Conditions: _____

Traffic Conditions: ☐ Low   ☐ Moderate   ☐ Heavy

Initial Traffic Control (Less than 60 minutes)   √**Completed**

Work area evaluated for hazards	☐
Emergency vehicle positioned properly	☐
Safety vests WORN	☐
Advanced warning sign (1) placed (100' – 1000')	☐
Traffic cones placed for taper (max of 20' intervals) (100' length)	☐
Traffic cones placed along work area (max of 40' intervals)	☐
Emergency warning lights reduced	☐
Law enforcement notified	☐
Staging area established	☐
Incident terminated - cones/signs removed	☐

Set-Up (Initial) **Equipment Needed:** Traffic cones (12), Emergency scene sign (1), Class 2 safety vest (2), Road flares (10)

Advanced Warning Area:	Distance _____	# of Signs _____
Transition Area (taper):	Distance _____	# of Cones _____
Work Area:	Distance _____	# of Cones _____

Temporary Traffic Control (More than 60 minutes)   √**Completed**

Work area evaluated for hazards	☐
Emergency vehicle positioned properly	☐
Safety vests WORN	☐
Advanced warning signs (2) placed (100' - 1500')	☐
Transition area (taper) established (Cones – max of 20' intervals) (max 100' length)	☐
Buffer space established	☐
Work area established	☐
Termination area established (Downstream taper) (max of 100' per lane)	☐
Flaggers with equipment positioned properly	☐
Emergency air siren cans issued	☐
Portable radios issued	☐
Emergency warning lights reduced	☐
Law enforcement traffic control points established	☐
Local department of transportation on scene with advanced warning signs in place	☐
Staging area established	☐
Incident terminated - cones/signs removed	☐

Set-Up (Temp.) **Equipment Needed:** Traffic cones (25-50), Emergency scene sign (2), Flagger signs (2), Stop/slow paddles (2), Emergency air siren cans (3), Portable radios (3), Class 2 safety vest (4), Road flares (1 case)

Advanced Warning Area:	Distance _____	# of Signs _____	# of Flaggers _____
Transition Area (taper):	Distance _____	# of Cones	
Buffer Area:	Distance _____	# of Cones	
Work Area:	Distance _____	# of Cones	
Termination Area:	Distance _____	# of Cones	

FIGURE 9.25 ◆ Traffic Control Safety Checklist. (*Courtesy of VFIS*)

Drawing

Miscellaneous Information

1. One advanced warning sign – Urban (Low speed) – 100', Urban (High speed) – 350', Rural – 500', Expressways/Freeways – 1000'

2. Second advanced warning sign – Urban (Low speed) – 100', Urban (High speed) – 350', Rural – 500', Expressways/Freeways – 1500'

3. Buffer area – 30 MPH – 625', 40 MPH – 825', 50 MPH – 1000', 60 MPH – 1300', 70 MPH – 1450'

4. One lane taper – 100' max. – cone placement 10' – 20'

5. Downstream taper – 100' per lane – cone placement – 10' – 20'

6. The equipment listed is the minimum required.   Additional safety vests may be required based on the number of personnel on the scene

For additional information check with your State Department of Transportation and the Federal Highway Administration's *Manual on Uniform Traffic Control Devices, Millennium Edition,* http//mutcd.fhwa.dot.gov.

C10:213 (Rev. 4/03)

FIGURE 9.25 ◆ (*continued*)

All personnel should understand and appreciate the high risk that firefighters are exposed to when operating in or near moving vehicle traffic. We should always operate from a defensive posture. Always consider moving vehicles as a threat to your safety. Each day, emergency personnel are exposed to motorists of varying abilities, with or without licenses, with or without legal restrictions, and driving at speeds from creeping to well beyond the speed limit. Some of these motorists are the vision impaired and the alcohol and/or drug impaired. On top of everything else, motorists will often be looking at the scene and not the road.

Nighttime operations are particularly hazardous. Visibility is reduced and the flashing of emergency lights tends to confuse motorists. Studies have shown that multiple headlights of emergency apparatus (coming from different angles at the scene) tend to blind civilian drivers as they approach.

Safety Benchmarks. Emergency personnel are at great risk while operating in or around moving traffic. There are approaches that can be taken to protect yourself and all crew members:

1. Never trust the traffic.
2. Engage in proper protective parking.
3. Wear orange, high-visibility reflective vests.
4. Reduce motorist vision impairment.
5. Use traffic cones and flares.

Listed here are benchmarks for safe performance when operating in or near moving vehicle traffic.

1. Always maintain an acute awareness of the high risk of working in or around moving traffic. Never trust moving traffic. Always look before you step! Always keep an eye on the traffic!
2. Always position apparatus to protect the scene, patients, emergency personnel, and provide a protected work area. Where possible, angle apparatus at 45 degrees away from curbside. This will direct motorists around the scene.
   a. Apparatus positioning must also allow for adequate parking space for other fire apparatus (if needed), and a safe work area for emergency personnel. Allow enough distance to prevent a moving vehicle from knocking fire apparatus into the work areas.
3. At intersections, or where the incident may be near the middle of the street, two or more sides of the incident may need to be protected. Block all exposed sides. Where apparatus is in limited numbers, prioritize the blocking from the most critical to the least critical.
4. For first-arriving engine companies where a charged hose line may be needed, angle the engine so that the pump panel is downstream, on the opposite side of oncoming traffic. This will protect the pump operator.
5. The initial company officer (or command) must assess the parking needs of later-arriving fire apparatus and specifically direct the parking and placement of these vehicles as they arrive to provide protective blocking of the scene. This officer must operate as an initial safety officer.
6. During daytime operations, leave all emergency lights on to provide warning to drivers.
7. For NIGHTTIME operations, turn OFF fire apparatus headlights. This will help reduce the blinding effect to approaching vehicle traffic. Other emergency lighting should be reduced to yellow lights and emergency flashers where possible.
8. Crews should exit the curbside on the nontraffic side of the vehicle whenever possible.

9. Always look before stepping out of apparatus or into any traffic areas. When walking around fire apparatus parked adjacent to moving traffic, keep an eye on traffic and walk as close to fire apparatus as possible.

10. Wear the orange safety vest any time you are operating in or near vehicle traffic.

11. When parking apparatus to protect the scene, be sure to protect the work area also. The area must be protected so that patients can be extricated, treated, moved about the scene, and loaded into Rescues safely.

12. Once enough fire apparatus have "blocked" the scene, park or stage unneeded vehicles off the street whenever possible. Bring in Rescue companies one or two at a time and park them in safe locations at the scene. This may be downstream from other parked apparatus, or the Rescue may be backed at an angle into a protected loading area to prevent working in or near passing traffic. At residential medical emergencies, park Rescues in driveways for safe loading where possible. If driveways are inaccessible, park Rescues to best protect patient loading areas.

13. Place traffic cones at the scene to direct traffic. This should be initiated by the first company arriving on the scene and expanded, if needed, as later arriving companies arrive on the scene. Always place and retrieve cones while facing oncoming traffic.

14. Placing flares, where safe to do so, adjacent to and in combination with traffic cones for nighttime operations greatly enhances scene safety. Place flares to direct traffic where safe and appropriate to do so.

15. At major intersections a call for police response may be necessary. Provide specific direction to the police officer as to exactly what your traffic control needs are. Ensure the police are parking to protect themselves and the scene. Position Rescues to protect patient loading areas.

Freeway Operations. Freeway emergencies pose a particular high risk to emergency personnel. Speeds are higher, traffic volume is significant, and civilian motorists have little opportunity to slow, stop, or change lanes.

The Department of Public Safety will also have a desire to keep the freeway flowing. Where need be, the freeway can be completely shut down. This, however, rarely occurs.

For freeway emergencies, we will continue to block the scene with the first apparatus on the scene to provide a safe work area. Other companies may be used to provide additional blocking if needed.

The initial company officer, or command, must thoroughly assess the need for apparatus on the freeway and their specific positions. Companies should be directed to specific parking locations to protect the work area, patients, and emergency personnel.

Other apparatus should be parked downstream when possible. This provides a safe parking area.

Staging of Rescue companies off the freeway may be required. Rescues should be brought into the scene one or two at a time. A safe loading area must be established.

Traffic cones should be placed farther apart, with the last cone approximately 150 feet upstream, to allow adequate warning to drivers. Place and retrieve cones while facing the traffic.

Command should establish a liaison with the Department of Public Safety as soon as possible to jointly provide a safe parking and work area and to quickly resolve the incident.

The termination of the incident must be managed with the same aggressiveness as initial actions. Crews, apparatus, and equipment must be removed from the freeway promptly to reduce exposure to moving traffic.

RECOMMENDATION #1

Fire departments should ensure that the placement of various types of warning devices (portable signs, orange traffic cones, flares, and/or portable changeable message signs) informs drivers of what to expect when approaching an incident scene.[1–4]

Discussion. Part 6 of the November 2003 edition of the *Manual on Uniform Traffic Control Devices (MUTCD)* includes Chapter 6I—"Control of Traffic Through Traffic Incident Management Areas." Chapter 6I defines a traffic incident management area as "an area of highway where temporary traffic controls are imposed by authorized officials in response to a road user incident, natural disaster, or special event. It extends from the first warning sign or emergency warning lights on a vehicle to the last temporary traffic control device or to a point where vehicles return to the original lane alignment and are clear of the traffic incident."

Warning devices are a means by which emergency personnel can convey information to motorists approaching an incident scene, referred to as the "advance warning area." The advance warning area may vary from a single sign or high-intensity rotating, flashing, oscillating, or strobe lights on a vehicle to a series of signs in advance of the incident scene. NFPA 1500, section 8.4.27 requires that department of transportation (DOT) approved warning devices such as traffic cones, retroreflective signs stating "Emergency Scene," and illuminated warning devices such as highway flares and/or other appropriate warning devices be used to warn oncoming traffic of the emergency operations. These warning devices can be used independently or in tandem based on the volume and speed of traffic, weather and road conditions, and visibility of the incident scene by approaching motorists. For rural highways, the effective placement of the first warning device should range from 8 to 12 times the posted speed limit in mph (e.g., 50 mph speed limit multiplied by 8 would equal 400 feet from the incident site to the placement of the first warning device). Weather conditions, curves, and hills that limit visibility of the incident scene require that the advance warning devices be placed at an even greater distance. An incident occurring in an intersection requires advance warning signs, devices, and markings to be used on all cross streets, as appropriate.

Portable signs can be transported on an emergency vehicle to the incident scene where they can be placed in a location that allows maximum visibility to oncoming traffic. The *Manual on Uniform Traffic Control Devices* (MUTCD) states, "where special emphasis is needed, signs may be placed on both the left and right sides of the roadway. Signs mounted on portable supports may be placed within the roadway itself. Signs may also be mounted on or above barricades."

Flares and orange traffic cones may be used individually or together to provide advance warning. To enhance the visibility of the orange traffic cones, flares may be placed next to them, where the glow from the burning flare would reflect off of and illuminate the cone.

Portable changeable message signs can be used as temporary traffic control devices. The flexibility to display various messages allows the signs to be used in a wide variety of applications (e.g., at a crash or for emergency incident management). The primary purpose of portable changeable message signs is to advise the road user of unexpected situations. Some typical applications may include where the speed of vehicular traffic is expected to drop substantially, where crash or incident management is needed, or where changes in road user pattern occur.

At this incident, flares and traffic cones were used. The flares were placed down the center of the highway for 220 feet in both directions, and traffic cones were placed in the vicinity of the personnel directing traffic. The driver of the vehicle that had struck the victim reported to law enforcement that he had seen the emergency flares but thought they were red traffic reflectors. No other traffic control devices such as signs were used.

RECOMMENDATION #2

Fire departments should consider positioning flaggers on or near the shoulder of the roadway upstream (approaching traffic) from the incident scene.[1,5]

Discussion. When establishing traffic control, flaggers should be positioned on or near the shoulder of the roadway while remaining within clear view of approaching motorists. Flaggers should take into consideration possible escape routes from their operating position in the event that an approaching motorist loses control of his or her vehicle. The flagger's position will be upstream at a distance (based on the posted speed limit) that provides ample warning to approaching motorists of the incident scene.

Recommended Minimum Distance of Flagger Upstream of Incident Scene
35 mph posted speed limit 250 feet
40 mph posted speed limit 305 feet
55 mph posted speed limit 495 feet
65 mph posted speed limit 645 feet

Source: U.S. Department of Transportation http[1]

Additionally,

RECOMMENDATION #3

Incident management agencies (e.g., department of transportation) should consider disseminating traffic control and road condition information to motorists utilizing local commercial and public radio and television broadcasts.[6]

Discussion. Traffic reports on radio and television stations have been a traditional means by which motorists receive traffic information, including incident-related warnings. Radio and television stations receive the traffic information they use in their reports from a variety of sources that may include public transportation agencies or by simply monitoring emergency (police and fire) radio frequencies. Public agencies, radio, and television stations can communicate important incident-related information to motorists, who will be more prepared and perhaps able to avoid the incident scene.

Niosh references

1. U.S. Department of Transportation, Federal Highway Administration. 2003. Part 6—Temporary traffic control of the *Manual on Uniform Traffic Control Devices* (MUTCD) 2003 edition. Fredericksburg, VA: American Traffic Safety Services Association.

2. NIOSH. 2001. *NIOSH Hazard ID: Traffic Hazards to Fire Fighters While Working Along Roadways.* Cincinnati, OH: U.S. Department of Health and Human Services, Public Health Service, Centers for Disease Control and Prevention, National Institute for Occupational Safety and Health, DHHS (NIOSH) Publication No. 2001-143.

3. Moore, R. 2003. *Vehicle rescue safety.* Respondersafety.com. [http://www.respondersafety.com/news/2004/0623_VRSI.html]. Date accessed: June 29, 2004.

4. NFPA. 2002. *NFPA 1500: Standard on fire department occupational safety and health program.* Quincy, MA: National Fire Protection Association.

5. Moore, R. 2004. *Safe parking—part 4: Personal survival skills.* Respondersafety.com. [http://www.respondersafety.com/news/2004/0623_UESP.html]. Date accessed: June 29, 2004.

6. U.S. Department of Transportation, Federal Highway Administration. 2000. *Traffic incident management handbook.* Prepared by PB Farradyne. [http://www.itsdocs.fhwa.dot.gov/jpodocs/rept_mis/@9201!.pdf]. Date accessed: June 29, 2004.

◆ **CASE STUDY RECAP**

Functioning at incidents on or near roadways requires a heightened sense of safety by every emergency responder. The case study referenced a traffic control responder who was struck and later died. In this particular incident, NIOSH investigators concluded that, to minimize the risk of similar occurrences, fire departments (all ESOs) should:

- Ensure that the placement of various types of warning devices (portable signs, orange traffic cones, flares, and/or portable changeable message signs) informs drivers of what to expect when approaching an incident scene.
- Consider positioning flaggers on or near the shoulder of the roadway upstream (approaching traffic) from the incident scene.

Additionally,

- Incident management agencies (e.g., department of transportation) should consider disseminating traffic control and road condition information to motorists utilizing local commercial and public radio and television broadcasts.

◆ **SUMMARY**

Emergency service organizations respond to a wide variety of incidents involving operations on or near a highway. These operations pose special risks to personnel performing fire, rescue, EMS and various other functions. Preventing injury to responders must be at the forefront during any emergency situation. Basic responder awareness during response and on scene can dramatically reduce the potential of a secondary incident. Strategically positioning vehicles, wearing personal protective and reflective apparel, placing appropriate signage/coneage, and reducing exposure time can enhance scene safety for all responders.

Review Questions

1. How does the concept of highway/roadway safety best practices enhance scene safety?
2. What are the core components of roadway/highway operations?
3. Identify the ten best practices to enhance highway/roadway safety.
4. What does blocking mean in the context of highway/roadway scene safety?
5. What does the tapering of cones mean?
6. A safe transition of traffic flow to normal conditions should occur after the incident scene. What provisions should the responders take to assure this safe transition?
7. What is the significance of the MUTCD as it pertains to emergency service responders?
8. How far apart should warning signs be placed on an expressway? Low-speed roadway?
9. What is the best reflective color for warning signs?
10. Explain how signs and cones should be retrieved when the emergency scene is terminated.

References

Boff, K. R., and Lincoln, J. E. 1988. Wright-Patterson Air Force Base, *Emergency finishing light study.*

Colorado firefighter struck, killed at accident scene. Retrieved February 4, 2004, from http://www.Firehous.com.

Davis, C. C. 1982. *Accidents involving stopped vehicles on freeway shoulders*. Automobile Club of Southern California.

FEMA. (USFA). 1994–2001. *Fire fighter fatality in the United States.*

FEMA. (USFA). August 2004. *Emergency vehicle safety initiative*, FA-272.

Gurba, R. M. 2004. *Highway safety for emergency service personnel.* York, PA: VFIS.

Hall, R., and Adams, B., eds. 1998. *Essentials of fire fighting*, 4th ed. Stillwater, OK: Board of Regents, Oklahoma State University.

Kahn, C. A., Pirrallo, R. G., and Kuhn, E. M. (2001). "Characteristics of fatal ambulance crashes in the United States: An 11-year retrospective analysis." *Prehospital Emergency Care*, 5, 261–269.

Kipp, J. D., and Loflin, M. E. 1996. *Emergency incident risk management: A safety and health perspective.* New York: Van Nostrand Reinhold.

Kidd, S. 2006 *Fire Rescue Magazine.*

Manual on Uniform Traffic Control Devices, millenium edition. DOT-FHWA.

Manual on Uniform Traffic Control Devices (MUTCD), 3rd ed. Fredericksburg, VA: American Traffic Safety Services Association, Chap. 6.

Mitterer, D. M. 2000. *Risk management for EMS and ambulance transportation industry.* York, PA: VFIS.

National Safety Council. 1998. *Defensive driving course*, 7th ed.

NFPA. 1995. *NFPA 1561, standard on fire department incident management system.* Quincy, MA: National Fire Protection Association.

NFPA. 1999. *NFPA 1500: Standard on fire department occupational safety and health program.* Quincy, MA: National Fire Protection Association.

NFPA. 2000. *U.S. fire fighters struck by vehicles, 1977–1999.* Quincy, MA: National Fire Protection Association. Unpublished.

NFPA. 2005. *NFPA 1901: Standard for automotive fire apparatus.* Quincy, MA: National Fire Protection Association.

NIOSH. 1999. *One fire fighter died and a second fire fighter was severely injured after being struck by a motor vehicle on an interstate highway—OK.* Cincinnati, OH: U.S. Department of Health and Human Services, Public Health Service, Centers for Disease Control and Prevention, National Institute for Occupational Safety and

Health, DHHS (NIOSH) Publication No. 99F-27.

NIOSH. 2000. *Volunteer fire fighter died after being struck by an eighteen-wheel tractor trailer truck—SC.* Cincinnati, OH: U.S. Department of Health and Human Services, Public Health Service, Centers for Disease Control and Prevention, National Institute for Occupational Safety and Health, DHHS (NIOSH) Publication No. 99F-38.

NIOSH. March 2004. *Prevention strategies for employees.* NIOSH DHHS Publication No. 2004-16.

NIOSH. December 2005. *Hazard notification sheet niosh traffic hazards to fire fighters while working along roadways description of hazard.* http://www.cdc.gov/niosh/hid12.html

OSHA and National Highway Traffic Safety Administration (NHTSA). 2004. *Traveling on federal business?* 428 KB PDF.

Patricks R.W. May 2005. "Follow the cones—Highway scenes and your protection." *Journal of Emergency Medical Services.*

U.S. Department of Health and Human Services, Centers for Disease Control and Prevention. February 28, 2003 "Ambulance crash-related injuries among emergency medical services workers—United States, 1991–2002." *Morbidity Mortality Weekly Report, 52*(8), 154–156.

U.S. Department of Health and Human Services, National Institute for Occupational Safety and Health. 2001. *26-year-old emergency medical technician dies in multiple fatality ambulance crash—Kentucky.* Pub. No. FACE-2001-11.

U.S. Department of Transportation, Federal Highway Administration. 1998. "Standards and guides for traffic controls for street and highway construction, maintenance, utility, and incident management operations." Part VI of the *Manual on Uniform Traffic Control Devices.* http://www.fhwa.dot.gov/reports/tswstudy/vehiclsaf.htm

Van Natter, C., Steffens, J., and Lindsey, J. 2003. *Dynamics of emergency vehicle response.* York, PA: VFIS.

VFIS. November 2005. *Privately owned vehicle operations, answering the call safely.*

CHAPTER 10

Special Operations

Objectives

After completing this chapter, you should be able to:

- Identify critical subject areas that present the need for special hazard awareness for the emergency and related vehicle operator.
- Describe the considerations needed for safe operation in each subject area.
- Discuss the importance of each specialty topic as it applies to emergency vehicle operations.

◆ INTRODUCTION

Operating any vehicle for the purpose of emergency services could present special conditions or considerations that should be understood by everyone in the ESO. Specifically, the driver and passengers of these vehicles must be familiar with these conditions, applicable considerations, and safe operating practices. The knowledge and special training required must be understood in order for the vehicle to be operated safely in the various situations. Key subjects include preparing to drive, off-road driving, rollover, private vehicle use, vehicle security, emergency dispatch, collision and near-miss investigation, and training program safety.

◆ PREPARING TO DRIVE

OBJECTIVES

- Identify the components of driver readiness.
- Explain the concept and purpose of route planning.

CASE STUDY

You are dispatched to a report of a structure fire. Knowing the location, you take the most familiar route. Committed en route you come on a working road crew with the route of travel blocked and impassable and traffic building behind your units. You find yourself blocked in. Multiple **911** reports depict a working fire with injuries. Additional units have to be sent in place of your units. An occupant of the involved building has severe injuries and later dies. The structure is a total loss.

TOPIC REVIEW

Route planning is essential to the overall response. Safety considerations should be taken in order to allow the driver to focus on driving tasks, thus avoiding hazards and minimizing the potential for collisions. Route planning can also affect response times based on the most logical route during specific times of day, weather, and traffic conditions.

Effective Start-up Procedures. Driver readiness also plays a role. Fatigue, health issues, and personal problems can affect the safety of everyone. Being mentally prepared and physically capable of doing the job is an ongoing obligation of the responder. The driver should conduct a circle of safety inspection prior to any response. *The driver should always circle the emergency vehicle prior to starting and moving it for any reason.* The driver has sufficient time to undertake this activity while other crew members are donning their gear or obtaining additional incident information.

Adjustment of cab features including the seat, mirrors, and related in-cab controls should be made prior to vehicle movement. Wearing of occupant restraint systems should be ensured, and a signal from the right front seat officer should be received before vehicle motion is engaged.

Volunteer departments typically conduct weekly and monthly vehicle checks. Based on time commitments and use of vehicles, this is generally considered acceptable. Regardless, the EV driver must understand that these vehicle checks do not replace the need to conduct primary safety inspections and basic vehicle operational functions. Every response is a new and different one that may present variables that could result in an unsafe vehicle or response.

CASE STUDY RECAP

Preparing to Drive. The case study depicts an incident that resulted in the EV response being delayed due to road construction. Preparing to drive requires many components, and in this situation prior knowledge of the road construction could have provided the needed information to allow a response via another route. This daily and sometimes dynamic knowledge can avert such tragic situations as depicted in the case study, loss of life and property.

SUMMARY

Planning and preparation are critical to the emergency response. Drivers and crew are mutually responsible for assuring the vehicle and equipment are capable to respond at a moment's notice. In addition, knowing various routes to get to the same destination is essential. Because responders cannot predict all possible response obstacles, preplanning of alternate routes and escape options should be considered. Daily reports from roadway/highway departments can aid in this process. Assuring the vehicle and crew are prepared for the response is also a responsibility of the driver. Cursory checks of exterior cabinet doors for closure, crew status, and restraint mechanisms in place are important components the driver should acknowledge before going en route.

In the case study, if the responding crew would have been aware of the construction site activity, they may have been able to take an alternate route of travel. In essence, the injured person may have had less serious injuries and the structure may not have been lost.

REVIEW QUESTIONS

1. List three key components of driver readiness.
2. What is the purpose of route planning?
3. What hazards exist that could interfere with the response?

◆ OFF-ROAD DRIVING

OBJECTIVES

- Identify two critical components needed for off-road driving.
- List the best practices for off-road driving.

CASE STUDY

On August 8, 2002, a 28-year-old male volunteer firefighter (the victim) was fatally injured when he was run over by the left front tire of a brush truck. The victim was attacking a grass fire with a charged hose line from a work platform on the front of a moving brush truck. The brush truck was making a U-turn on the roadway through heavy smoke when a vehicle skidded into it. The victim was ejected from the left side of the work platform and run over by the brush truck. The victim was pronounced dead at the scene.

TOPIC REVIEW

Various types of emergency-related vehicles are operated on off-road terrain. The terrain is often unknown or unfamiliar to the vehicle driver. Caution should be exercised in all cases when a vehicle leaves a designated roadway. Vision and speed are critical components to the safe operation and handling of the vehicle. Ensure that you can see and know what you are traveling on. Drive slowly because speed will increase the possibility of something going wrong. Specialized off-road vehicles have unusual handling characteristics. These characteristics must be understood by the driver to prevent circumstances such as rollover.

Industry experts recommend the following best practices:

1. If equipped, place the vehicle into all-wheel drive prior to proceeding off road.
2. Always proceed slowly and ensure that the vehicle is under control at all times.
3. Do not "cut" a new road unless there is no other way to traverse the area.
4. Have someone on foot scout an unknown route or one with dense underbrush in order to identify hidden hazards.
5. Go straight up the hill; do not angle across the face of a steep hill.
6. If the vehicle starts to slide, steer going downhill but do not steer going uphill.
7. Set the emergency brake if the vehicle stalls on a hill.
8. Never coast down a hill; always proceed slowly in low gear.
9. When crossing a ditch or gully, advance slowly and proceed at an angle to avoid "bottoming out" the vehicle.

NIOSH RECOMMENDATIONS/DISCUSSIONS

Recommendation #1. *Fire departments should ensure that firefighters attack a brush fire from a safe place on the apparatus or walk alongside the moving apparatus.*[1-4]

Discussion: In this case, the victim was holding a charged hose line and attacking the fire from the front-bumper-mounted working platform on the brush truck. There was a 39-inch metal guardrail open-sided at both ends. The platform was mounted on the front bumper, which is where the victim was working while the brush truck was moving. According to the International Fire Service Training Association (IFSTA), there are two proper methods for making a moving fire attack: "The first method is to have firefighters use a short section of hose and walk alongside the apparatus and extinguish the fire as they go." NFPA 1500, *Standard for Fire Department Occupational Safety and Health Program,* concurs with this recommendation. Further, this standard strongly recommends that "two firefighters, each with a hose line, walk ahead and beside of the vehicle's path, both firefighters on the same side of the uninvolved terrain. This allows the firefighters to operate in an unhurried manner, with a clear view of fire conditions and the success of the extinguishment."

The second IFSTA recommendation is to use nozzles that are remotely controlled from the inside of the cab. The practice of firefighters riding on the outside of vehicles and fighting wildland fires from unprotected positions is not recommended by NFPA Standards.

Recommendation #2. *Fire departments should ensure that adequate traffic control is in place before turning their attention to the emergency.*[4,6,7]

Discussion: The incident commander sized up the grass fire area and called for traffic control for both the east and west entrances to the rural road. The deputy sheriff was blocking the west entrance, and traffic control was en route to the east entrance when the incident occurred. According to Dunn, "When a fire company arrives on the scene of a roadway emergency and there are no police at hand to control traffic, firefighters themselves should first control the oncoming vehicles before safely turning their attention to the emergency. It is recommended that warning signal devices such as flares, flags, road blocks, or road signs be placed at a minimum of 350 feet from the incident scene (farther distance may be required taking into account line of sight, visibility, road and weather conditions) and positioned so they are visible to oncoming traffic for at least 350 feet beyond that. This placement allows the driver a minimum of 700 feet in which to stop a vehicle.

Recommendation #3. *Fire departments should enforce standard operating procedures that require operators of fire apparatus to wear seat belts (restraints) whenever operating the vehicle.*[1,2,5]

Discussion: Firefighters make many life and death decisions during a tour of duty, and one of the most important is snapping on a seat belt after climbing aboard an emergency apparatus that is called to respond. As stated in NFPA 1500, "All persons riding in or on fire service vehicles should be seated in approved riding positions and should be secured to the vehicle by seat belts whenever the vehicle is in motion. Riding on tail steps, running boards, side steps, or in any other exposed position should be prohibited." The fire department in this incident did have a written safety policy on the use of seat belts at the time of the incident; however, no enforcement policy was utilized. The department also has an SOP that specifies that members obey all traffic laws while responding to any call. Texas has a mandatory seat belt law.

Niosh references

1. NFPA. 1997. *NFPA 1451, Standard for a fire service vehicle operations training program.* Quincy, MA: National Fire Protection Association.
2. NFPA. 2000. *NFPA 1500, Standard for fire department occupational safety and health program.* Quincy, MA: National Fire Protection Association.
3. International Fire Service Training Association. 1999. *Pumping apparatus driver/operator handbook,* 1st ed. Stillwater, OK: Oklahoma State University, Fire Protection Publications, p. 12.
4. Dunn, V. 1992. *Safety and survival on the fireground.* Saddle Brook, NJ: Fire Engineering Books and Videos.
5. Texas Transportation Code, http://www.Capitol.state.tx.us/statutes/tntoc.html. Date accessed: November 27, 2002.
6. Hall, R., and Adams, B., eds. 1998. *Essentials of fire fighting,* 4th ed. Stillwater, OK: Oklahoma State University.
7. Federal Highway Administration. 1998. "Standards and guides for traffic control for street and highway construction, maintenance, utility and incident management operations." Part IV of the *Manual on Uniform Traffic Control Devices* (MUTCD), 3rd ed.

Even though the case study and the NIOSH report reference a fire department, all emergency responders should heed the advice and recommendations of NIOSH. The firefighter killed in the case study might still be alive today if the ESO had had policy and compliance mechanisms in place. In addition, driver and firefighter attentiveness for their surroundings in this tragic situation could have lead to avoidance.

CASE STUDY RECAP

Off-Road Driving. Drive slowly. NIOSH investigators in the case study concluded that, to minimize the risk of similar occurrences, fire departments should

- Ensure that firefighters attack a brush fire from a safe place on the apparatus or walk alongside the moving apparatus.
- Ensure that adequate traffic control is in place before turning attention to the emergency.
- Enforce standard operating procedures that require operators of fire apparatus to wear seat belts (restraints) whenever operating the vehicle.

SUMMARY

Driving off road is unlike normal roadway driving. Use caution, know your vehicle, ensure you know and can see where you are driving, know the terrain you are driving over, and make sure that there are no persons in harm's way. Take the time to familiarize yourself with the geography and topography in your response area. Conduct regular off road driving exercises to enhance personnel skills.

REVIEW QUESTIONS

1. Identify the two critical components needed for off-road driving.
2. List five best practices for off-road driving.
3. How could the fatality in the case study have been prevented?

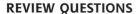

◆ ROLLOVER

OBJECTIVES

- ◆ Identify the recommended best practices to maintaining vehicle control.
- ◆ List the five primary components needed to be understood to avoid a rollover crash.

CASE STUDIES

Under the Fire Fighter Fatality Investigation and Prevention Program, NIOSH investigated two separate incidents involving firefighters who were killed in tanker truck rollovers during 1999 and 2000 (NIOSH, 2000a, 2000b). Both incidents involved volunteer fire departments providing mutual aid with water tanker trucks.

Case 1. On October 28, 1999, a captain and a firefighter (the driver) responded to a mutual aid call in a full, elliptical-shaped, 1,800-gallon water tanker truck equipped with baffles (NIOSH, 2000a). The tanker was traveling west, and as it approached a curve, the driver lost control. The vehicle drifted toward the shoulder of the road as the driver tried to correct the direction of travel. Just past the curve, the tanker veered off the road into a cornfield. The tanker rolled onto the passenger side and continued to roll over several times. The driver was ejected from the tanker. The captain was trapped in the crushed upside-down cab and had to be extricated. He was taken to a local hospital and died 7 days later. The driver was taken to a local hospital, then flown by helicopter to a trauma center. He died 86 days after the incident.

Case 2. On January 17, 2000, a fire chief died after responding to a mutual aid call in a full T-shaped, 641-gallon, handmade water tanker truck that was not equipped with baffles and was attached to a converted pickup truck (NIOSH, 2000b). The tanker was traveling west when the chief lost control of the tanker as he approached a slight curve in the road. As the tanker began to skid, the right tires left the pavement and entered the shoulder. The tanker continued on the shoulder until it entered a ditch and became airborne. Next the tanker crossed a lane on a side street, struck a center median, and crossed a second lane on the side street. The tanker then struck a guardrail and flipped end-over-end until it landed in a concrete culvert. The chief was killed instantly.

TOPIC REVIEW

The number of emergency service vehicle rollovers has escalated over the past few years. ESOs need to know that the majority of rollover crashes, like most crashes, can be prevented. A large number of the crashes that have occurred are single vehicle related. According to investigative reports from NIOSH and the USFA's white paper report on vehicle rollovers, the leading contributing factor is driver error. In addition to driver error, many other factors can contribute to vehicle rollovers. These factors include wet roads, poor visibility, and distractions from both inside and outside the cab. Although more common in fire apparatus, ambulances too can and do roll over. Proper driver training, responder attentiveness, and an understanding of the causes of vehicle rollovers can help prevent these tragic incidents.

The FEMA report titled *Safe Operation of Tankers* (2004) states that in order to implement a program to reduce the frequency and severity of crashes involving fire department tankers, it is necessary to review and understand the factors that have influenced such incidents in the past. When reviewing the various reports and case histories of tanker crashes that have occurred in the past ten years or so, numerous common factors or trends begin to emerge. With this information in hand, fire department officers and training personnel are able to develop standard operating procedures, policies, and training programs that address this issue effectively.

Remember: Laws of Physics + Mechanics of Vehicle Operation + Driver Error = LOSS OF VEHICLE CONTROL

In its manual titled *Pumping Apparatus Driver/Operator Handbook* (2002), the International Fire Service Training Association (**IFSTA**) suggests that the causes of all fire apparatus crashes can be grouped into one of five categories:

1. **Improper Backing of the Apparatus.** Backing crashes are among the most frequent of all types of fire apparatus crashes. Although they are seldom serious in terms of injury or death, they do account for a significant portion of overall damage costs.
2. **Reckless Driving by the Public.** This category includes a variety of reckless actions, including failure to obey traffic signals, excessive speed, failure to yield to emergency vehicles, and other common civilian driving behaviors.
3. **Excessive Speed by the Fire Apparatus Driver.** Excessive speed may result in the driver losing control of the vehicle or being unable to stop the vehicle before hitting another vehicle or object.
4. **Lack of Driving Skill and Experience by the Fire Apparatus Driver.** This may be due to insufficient training of the driver or unfamiliarity with the exact vehicle being driven.
5. **Poor Apparatus Design or Maintenance.** Although this can be the case with custom-built fire apparatus, it is a more significant problem in departments that use retrofitted or home-built apparatus.

The same FEMA report claims that five subfactors were identified within the referenced categories. They include

1. Human factors
2. Apparatus design factors
3. Driving surface factors
4. Emergency scene factors
5. Other factors

According to VFIS (2005), the components of a rollover crash include

- The driver
  - Training
  - Experience
  - Physical conditioning
  - State of mind

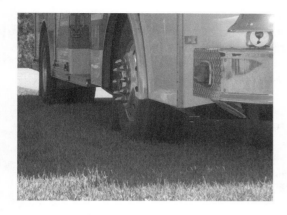

FIGURE 10.1 ◆ Emergency vehicle running on soft shoulder of roadway.

- The vehicle
  - Height, weight, width
  - Suspension
- Common rollover circumstances
  - Excessive relative speed
  - Soft shoulder drop-off (Figure 10.1)
  - Uneven surface drop-off and improper recovery
- Physical dynamics of vehicle operations (discussed in Chapter 5)
  - Inertia
  - Momentum
  - Center of gravity
  - Friction
  - Centrifugal force
- Mechanics of vehicle operations
  - Relative speed
  - Specific road conditions
  - Effects of **body roll**, center of gravity, and tire sidewall flexibility
  - Effects of weight transfer, understeering, braking, and uneven surfaces
  - Steering angle and tire friction
  - **Liquid slosh effect**

Mobile water supply vehicles, known as tankers or tenders, are widely used to transport water to areas beyond a water supply system or where the water supply is inadequate (Figure 10.2). Incidents involving motor vehicles account for approximately

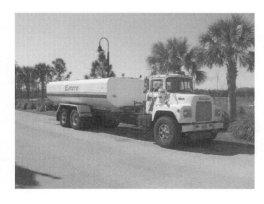

FIGURE 10.2 ◆ Water tanker truck.

25 percent of U.S. firefighter deaths each year; cases involving tankers are the most prevalent of these motor vehicle incidents. During 1977–1999, 73 deaths occurred in 63 crashes involving tankers. Of those deaths, 54 occurred in 49 crashes in which tankers rolled over (no collision), and 8 occurred in 6 crashes in which the tankers left the road (no collision). The other cases involved collision with another vehicle (10 deaths in 7 crashes) and collision with stationary object(s) (1 death) (NFPA, 2000d).

Tanker drivers may not be fully aware that tanker trucks are more difficult to control than passenger vehicles. A tanker truck requires a much greater distance to stop. Tankers weigh substantially more, and their air brake systems take more time to activate than the hydraulic/mechanical brake systems on smaller passenger cars. The effect is influenced by the amount of water the tanker is hauling and whether the tanker is baffled.

To reduce the risk of tanker truck rollovers, NIOSH recommends that fire departments take the following precautions:

- Develop, implement, and enforce standard operating procedures (SOPs) for emergency vehicles—particularly with regard to the use of seat belts.
- Ensure that drivers have necessary driving skills and experience, and provide them with periodic refresher training.
- Consider terrain, weather, and bridge and road conditions when purchasing a mobile water supply vehicle.
- Adhere to the requirements of NFPA 1915 for keeping a vehicle on a maintenance schedule and documenting the performance of the maintenance (NFPA, 2001).
- Inspect the complete vehicle at least once per year to comply with federal and state motor vehicle regulations.
- Adhere to the requirements of NFPA 1901 for an approved mobile water supply vehicle (NFPA, 2001).
- Equip all vehicles with seat belts.
- Ensure that water tank capacity is adequate and has proper tank mounting and sufficient front and rear weight distribution.
- Ensure that the weight of the fully loaded vehicle does not exceed the gross axle weight rating of any axle and the gross vehicle weight rating of the chassis.
- Ensure that the center of gravity of the vehicle does not exceed the chassis manufacturer's specified center of gravity.
- Provide proper baffles to control water movement for all vehicles equipped with water tanks.
- Verify that vehicles are of proper design and have adequate suspension, steering, and braking ability.
- Ambulances also fall within these parameters.

The best practices for maintaining vehicle control follow:

- Always wear your seat belt.
- Do not panic.
- Get control of your speed.
- Maintain control of the steering wheel.
- Steer straight ahead and slow down.
- Take your foot off the accelerator, but do not brake.
- Allow the vehicle to slow down on its own.
- When you reach a slow, safe speed, turn the steering wheel to the left and gently steer the vehicle back onto the highway.
- Do not jerk your steering wheel.

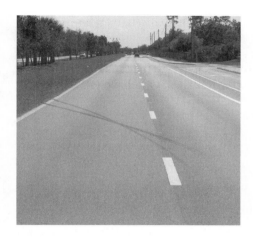

FIGURE 10.3 ◆ Photo depicts "yew."

Drivers of any emergency or related vehicle should do the following:

- Recognize that they are responsible for the safe and prudent operation of the vehicle under all conditions.
- Wear a seat belt when operating a vehicle.
- Take training to meet the job performance requirements stated in NFPA 1002 before driving and operating the vehicle (NFPA 2001).
- Take refresher driver training at least twice per year.
- Understand the vehicle characteristics, capabilities, and limitations.
- Be aware of the potential for unpredictable driving by the public (excessive speed, failure to yield to emergency vehicles, inattentiveness, etc.).

CASE STUDY RECAP

Rollover. The two case studies referenced in this section carry common themes. Understanding a vehicle's center of gravity and the relating dynamic forces are essential to prevent such incidents. Low-force defensive driving will keep the vehicle on the roadway. In the unfortunate instance when a vehicle leaves the road surface, knowledge on how to control the vehicle to avoid a rollover situation is priceless. This occurs through proper education and training.

SUMMARY

Most situations resulting in a rollover could have been prevented. Several subject areas and contributing factors must be taken into account. Excessive relative speed is common in most rollover crashes. Relative speed is determined in relation to your environment, road conditions, and your vehicle. Drivers must always maintain a slow, steady, and safe speed. Specific road conditions that affect rollovers include a high center crown, reverse or negative camber, S curves, and restrictions of lane widths.

The effects of body roll, center of gravity, and tire sidewall flexibility must also be considered. The body of a vehicle pivots around the center of gravity side to side. Drivers must keep body roll to a minimum. Radial tires are designed to flex;

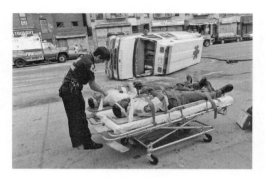

FIGURE 10.4 ◆ Ambulance rollover. (*Courtesy of David Handschuh, Photographer*)

uncontrollable conditions can cause the tires to flex too much and contribute to vehicle rollover(Figure 10.3).

Drivers must also consider moving loads in an ambulance, such as the movement of medics in the back of the vehicle (Figure 10.4). Speed is a major contributor to weight shifting back and forth and control of the vehicle. Effects of weight transfer, understeering, braking, and uneven surfaces must be understood. Know how your vehicle handles under emergency and nonemergency conditions. Braking and deceleration have an effect on weight transfer. Overcompensation and oversteering can cause the vehicle to go out of control. The steering angle and subsequent tire friction are important. Six patches of rubber are the only things holding you to the road. Do not oversteer if your vehicle drops off the road surface.

The slosh effect from liquid is a frequent contributor to rollover incidents. Solid loads tend to be steady, more controllable, and hold in place. Liquid loads slosh side to side and front to rear. Baffling is used to minimize the slosh effect in tankers, but it still occurs. Ideally the apparatus should be totally full or totally empty.

Adjust speed when driving on wet or icy roads, in darkness or fog, or under any other conditions that make emergency vehicle operation especially hazardous.

Applied basic defensive driving concepts could have avoided the results in both of the case studies. Policies with enforcement and low-force driving practice simulations can build the knowledge base of drivers in order to prevent or avoid such instances from occurring.

REVIEW QUESTIONS

1. List three of the recommended best practices to maintaining vehicle control.
2. List the five primary components needed to be understood to avoid a rollover crash.
3. Explain the concept of center of gravity.
4. How does crew movement in the patient compartment or crew cab affect rollover potential?

◆ PRIVATE VEHICLE USE

OBJECTIVES

- Understand basic privately owned vehicle (**POV**) use during ESO operations.
- Review applicable state laws.
- Identify areas that can get POV operators into trouble.

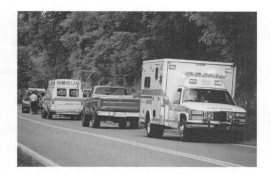

FIGURE 10.5 ◆ Emergency responder's privately owned vehicle sitting between ambulances at incident scene. (*Courtesy of The Stock Connection*)

CASE STUDY

A fire lieutenant was responding to a call for a structure fire. His lights and siren were activated at the time. It is his personal vehicle, but it is registered and authorized to be used by the fire department, which provided the emergency lights and siren equipment. At an intersection, he hits another car broadside. The 23-year-old female driver dies two days later, but never regained consciousness prior to her death. The lieutenant receives several broken bones and other moderate trauma, but survives. The call he was responding to had been downgraded to a nonemergency response of "unattended cooking" just after this crash occurred. The family of the female driver sues the volunteer lieutenant, the department, the town, and the town's board of commissioners. Their insurance companies' share of court settlement is for slightly over $1 million. The fire lieutenant is sentenced to 12 to 23 months in the county jail, gets a $185 fine, and has to pay $5,000 in funeral costs for his victim. He also loses his personal driver's license for one year, and his insurance rates will be adversely affected.

TOPIC REVIEW

Having the use of a private vehicle can be crucial to your ability to respond to emergencies in a timely manner (Figure 10.5). The more than 43,000 annual roadway deaths in the United States should paint a permanent picture for the need to instill basic driving practices in the minds of all responders. From a different perspective, 43,000 deaths means there are approximately 118 deaths per day or approximately 5 per hour. When an emergency responder drives rapidly to the ESO or emergency scene, such driving exacerbates the potential of a POV collision.

Most volunteer emergency service agencies rely heavily on their members' ability to respond to emergency calls, to either the scene or the station, in their private vehicles (Figure 10.6). Yours may be one. Although this practice is essential if your organization is to react quickly to emergencies, there are inherent risks associated with it.

The most significant risk—which all too often results in collisions—is that members tend to operate their private vehicles as if they are emergency vehicles. While motor vehicle laws vary from state to state, all address the use of private vehicles by volunteers. Their common theme: Although licensed emergency vehicles may be permitted prudently to exceed the posted speed limit, move against traffic flow, and proceed through a negative intersection control device, private vehicles are not

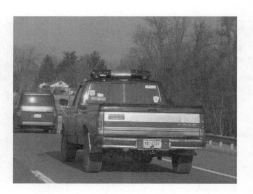

FIGURE 10.6 ◆ Privately owned vehicle responding to an incident. (*Photo by R. Patrick*)

emergency vehicles and therefore are not permitted the same, if any, exemptions from state motor vehicle laws.*

There may also be a reference in these laws regarding the use of blue or red "courtesy lights" (Figure 10.7). Basically, these lights are a request for other drivers to be courteous enough to let you pass them. They are not a grant of, nor legitimate demand for, right-of-way. Neither do they permit you to illegally pass or speed up to overtake another vehicle.

While everyone recognizes that quick response to an emergency is important, all drivers must understand one critical fact—privately owned vehicles (POV) in most states are not emergency vehicles and therefore cannot claim any exemptions or special privileges under the law. That means any drivers caught breaking traffic laws or operating private vehicles in an aggressive or unsafe manner are subject to disciplinary action including suspension or loss of driving privileges and withdrawal of their courtesy light permit.

It is common practice for members of volunteer fire and EMS departments to respond to the station (and, in some instances, to an incident location) using their private vehicles (Figure 10.8). Many states allow volunteer members to equip their POV with emergency lights. Acceptable color for those lights varies from state to state. Some states allow only red lights, some allow only blue lights, some allow green, and some allow a combination. In addition, departments may specify the color based on the rank held by the individual (e.g., red is used only by chief officers). Regardless of color, a review of the data in the USFA *Fire Fighter Fatality in the United States* reports from 1990 to 2000 showed that 25 percent of firefighters who died in motor vehicle crashes were killed in privately owned vehicles.

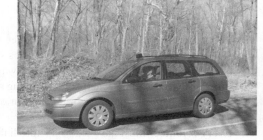

FIGURE 10.7 ◆ Privately owned vehicle with blue light. (*Photo by R. Patrick*)

*In some states, a firefighter's privately owned vehicle can be considered an emergency vehicle with the chief's approval. Nevertheless, the driver must still adhere to all applicable motor vehicle laws.

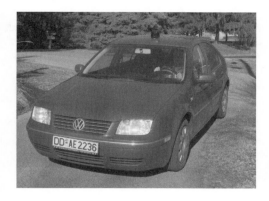

FIGURE 10.8 ◆ Privately owned vehicle at incident scene. (*Photo by R. Patrick*)

Although volunteers in Utah can legally run with warning lights on a POV, the state requires them to have authorization from local law enforcement and a rider on their personal auto insurance policy. Therefore, volunteers in the Salt Lake Valley do not run with warning lights on POVs. There have been no issues related to response times because they travel with normal traffic when responding to the station.

Point to Ponder

What should your organization do to reduce the risks associated with private vehicles? Your volunteers must understand that, first and foremost, they have to arrive at the emergency scene or the station safely in order to be of any help to the public.

Essential to the understanding and acceptance is the development and enforcement of standard operating procedures and guidelines (SOP/SOGs) that include, but are not limited to, the following:

1. Limit POV use in emergency situations.
2. Train personnel on proper SOP/SOGs pertaining to safe driving practices.
3. Assess and prioritize responses using an approved risk management protocol.
4. Respond to low-severity incidents in a nonemergency mode.
5. Volunteers responding in personal vehicles should obey their state motor vehicle code with respect to courtesy light and siren privileges.
6. Courtesy lights should not be used by volunteers as a license to operate their personal vehicle as if it were an emergency vehicle. All courtesy lights should be approved by the chief and a written permit be issued. The permit should include the "rules of the road" applying to the expected usage.
7. Volunteers responding in personal vehicles should never exceed the posted speed limit.
8. Volunteers responding in personal vehicles should *always* stop at every stop sign and red traffic signal and wait for normal right-of-way before proceeding.
9. Procedures for at-the-scene parking/staging should be included in the SOPs.
10. Train dispatchers in the use of preset questions to determine emergency versus nonemergency response.
11. Every volunteer must have personal auto liability insurance with appropriate liability limits that protect not only the volunteer but also your organization. This should be verified in each instance.

Two sample SOGs are shown at the end of this chapter (Figures 10.21a and 10.21b).

CASE STUDY RECAP

Private Vehicle Use. Private vehicle use for emergency response is a common practice in emergency services. The case study depicts the use of lights and siren on a private vehicle. Although state laws vary on the use of L&S devices on private vehicles, few states provide special privileges unless the vehicle is classified as an emergency vehicle. All responders should be educated on their respective state laws and ESO policy related to private vehicle use. Basic driving practices should be followed in all circumstances. This tragic incident might have been avoided had the lieutenant simply stopped at the intersection.

SUMMARY

The use of POVs for response in the emergency service arena is essential to many ESOs. Responders must think about their response attitude and mode from the moment the alert tones activate. Acknowledging the adrenaline rush can allow the responder to act responsibly and drive sensibly. The associated inherent risks must be addressed by the ESO management and sound doable policy established. All responders should be trained annually on best practices and on the applicable policies. These basic management processes coupled with appropriate training and enforcement can avoid situations and the potential consequences as depicted in the case study.

REVIEW QUESTIONS

1. Does your personal automobile insurance policy cover you if you are involved in an private emergency vehicle response collision?
2. Does the insurance company that insures your fire department or ambulance service have a policy that extends its coverage to cover you if you have insufficient policy limits to cover your exposure to this type of a collision?
3. Does your department have sufficient liability limits in the case of a POV collision?
4. Do you have safe operating policy with SOP/SOGs that identify what drivers can and cannot do when responding in their personal vehicles as well as in your department or service vehicles?
5. Do these SOP/SOGs comply with your state's emergency vehicle code?

◆ VEHICLE SECURITY

OBJECTIVES

- Describe the importance of maintaining vehicle security.
- Identify the key components of vehicle security.
- Discuss the purpose for ESO policy pertaining to vehicle security.

CASE STUDY

An EMS crew responded to a medical emergency, business as usual. The crew arrived on scene, positioned their vehicle along the street, grabbed their equipment, and entered the residence. While attending to the patient, an unknown suspect entered the vehicle, with engine running, and then drove off. The ambulance was found

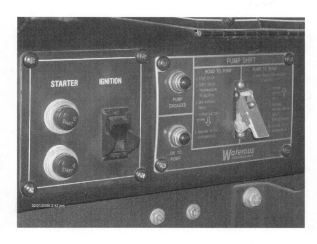

FIGURE 10.9 ◆ Vehicle ignition system. Turn battery on and push to start. (*Photo by R. Patrick*)

abandoned two hours later in a field. The vehicle received moderate damage and a medication kit was missing. The suspect was nowhere to be found.

TOPIC REVIEW

The security of all vehicles, inside and outside the station, should be an everyday practice for emergency responders. The accountability of all vehicles—marked and unmarked—is a modern-day necessity. Such accountability includes tracking vehicles that are in service, out of service, on reserve status, in the maintenance garage, and even those that are for sale or going for salvage. Unattended emergency and related vehicles should not be left running or with the keys left in the ignition (Figure 10.9).

The tracking of vehicle use and access should be conducted. Such tracking should include to ensure that vehicles in the station are secured in such a manner that significantly increases the difficulty of unauthorized access and use (Figure 10.10). Assignment and inventory of vehicle keys should be conducted. Routine and random vehicle audits are encouraged along with review of vehicle and station key access logs.

Ensure that all vehicles that are off the premises are accounted for, especially when not in direct possession of the ESO (Figure 10.11). This includes, in addition to government-based repair facilities, contracted vendor services that require the vehicle to be shipped off-site such as radio repair firms, mechanical and biomedical repair, and warranty service.

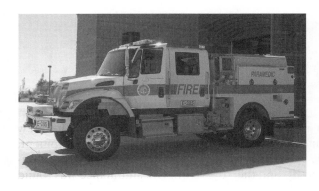

FIGURE 10.10 ◆ Unattended fire engine with door open. (*Photo by R. Patrick*)

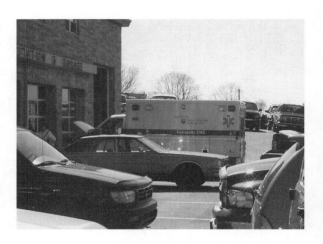

FIGURE 10.11 ◆ Unattended ambulance at repair shop. (*Photo by R. Patrick*)

ESOs are strongly encouraged to discuss security measures with repair facilities and vendors to confirm that they understand the requirements to secure the vehicle and the ESO compliance expectations. Such requirements may include the following.

- Secure the vehicle indoors overnight when facility is closed.
- Do not leave the engine running or lock the vehicle when on scene.
- Do not leave the keys in the vehicle.
- Do not allow the vehicle to be taken off vendor premises for any reason other than directly related to the repair and return of the unit to the ESO.
- Report to the ESO and law enforcement officials any unusual interest in the vehicle while in their possession.
- Educate crews regarding the importance of stations' security through meetings, tail board chats, information postings in station, and/or supervisory shift briefings. Do so on a periodic basis.
- Consider key controls for all vehicles when in station.
- Keep the station locked, especially when the nation is on heightened alert (code orange, code red).
- Account for ALL department vehicles regardless of location (in service, out of service, maintenance locations, etc.).
- Keep your vehicle bay doors closed unless the bays are physically occupied by a department member. When leaving the station, *ensure,* after exiting the bay, that the bay door is closed (Figure 10.12).

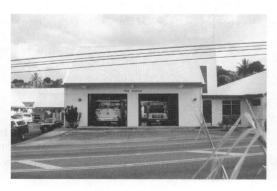

FIGURE 10.12 ◆ Station with bay doors open equals open invitation. (*Courtesy of Dorling Kindersley Media Library*)

- Inform maintenance facilities of security procedures including parking vehicles out of sight or locking them inside overnight, securing keys when not in use, and making sure who is/is not permitted to pick up vehicles.
- Make sure vehicles are attended to at all times on the scene of an incident or when conducting routine business.
- Unattended vehicles should not be left running or with the keys in the ignition.
- Change combinations on keypads frequently.
- Limit access to the station. Require visitors to sign in and leave identification. Visitors should be escorted. Confirm the identity of reporters, and know your vendors.

Decommissioned vehicles slated for resale, but not to another bona fide emergency response organization, or vehicles scheduled for salvage should be stripped of ESO identifying markings by complete removal or destruction by grinding. Uninstalling of emergency warning devices and any other emergency service–related markings is strongly encouraged.

CASE STUDY RECAP

Vehicle Security. In the case study, the emergency vehicle was left running and unattended. Although, this is considered a common practice in the emergency services, ESOs should identify best practices and implement SOP/SOGs to thwart such situations. If the providers in the case study had locked the vehicle prior to entering the scene, the perpetrator would not have had such easy access to the vehicle. Another approach may be to turn off the vehicle's engine when functioning out of sight of the vehicle.

SUMMARY

Vehicle security, inside and outside the station, should be an everyday practice for emergency responders. The accountability of all vehicles—marked and unmarked—is a modern-day necessity. Such accountability includes tracking vehicles that are in service, out of service, on reserve status, in the maintenance garage, and even those that are for sale or going for salvage. Unattended emergency and related vehicles should not be left running or with the keys left in the ignition. If the ESO had a policy addressing the security of vehicles during on-scene operations, and the policy were adhered to, the suspect from the case study would have had to have worked harder to gain access to the ambulance or the attempt would have been thwarted.

REVIEW QUESTIONS

1. What controls can be established to maintain vehicle security?
2. List five key components of vehicle security measures.
3. How do SOP/SOGs come into play when dealing with vehicle security?

◆ **EMERGENCY DISPATCH**

OBJECTIVES

- Describe the concept of emergency dispatch protocols.
- Identify the vehicle risk control–related feature of emergency dispatch protocols.
- Discuss practical applications of emergency dispatch protocol use pertaining to vehicle response.

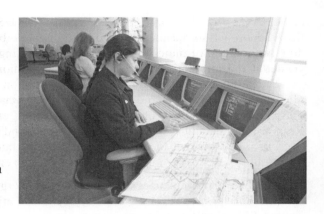

FIGURE 10.13 ◆ "911" dispatch center. (*Courtesy of Photo Researchers, Inc.*)

CASE STUDY

Associated Fire-Rescue was dispatched to an automatic fire alarm. En route to the scene the second responding engine, running hot, passed through a controlled intersection against a red signal. The engine broadsided a minivan resulting in multiple injuries and severe damage. Department policy is that the first-out engine responds hot and all other vehicles respond cold unless upgraded by the public safety answering point (**PSAP**), incident command, or first-arriving unit. The automatic fire alarm was a malfunction.

TOPIC REVIEW

EV operators and emergency dispatchers are faced with many stressful circumstances (Figure 10.13). From dispatch to incident termination, we must control many unnatural actions. Unfortunately, many of these unnatural actions result in tragedy. Don't let the emergency vehicle operator commit **sirencide**. Start the call out right! Sirencide is a term used to describe the emotional reaction of emergency vehicle operators when they begin to feel a sense of power and urgency that blocks out reason and prudence drivers begin to go faster and faster. It leads to the reckless operation of the emergency vehicle and increases as siren use increases.

As one of our colleagues has referenced, Dr. Jeff Clawson's book (1998) addresses this topic; however, for effective and efficient benefit, it has to result in a system-wide change that begins at the PSAP. Using emergency dispatching criteria as a risk control tool can have profound rewards. Simply put, it can send the right equipment/personnel to the right emergency under the right response mode . . . essentially setting the tone of the call right from the beginning of emergency services involvement. Your state's motor vehicle code addresses some of the use issues surrounding this topic. Use them as guidance and have a risk control expert and your solicitor provide recommendations.

A policy on light and siren (**L&S**) use would best encompass responsible best practices. Implementing emergency dispatch (**ED**) protocols may be the best practice, but in light of politics and the pending time commitment, using existing sample SOPs to frame your policy is suggested. Then educate your staff on the policy and supporting procedures. You may find that involving the staff with the development of the SOPs will result in a stricter policy (which you may have to water down), but, most importantly, buy-in and compliance from the staff. L&S issues should not necessarily be about whether responders should have L&S or not, but about responsible use of the devices. When utilized appropriately/responsibly, L&S use should provide enough notice of approach so reasonable action can be taken by the public at large. In no case do responders have the right-of-way; they are asking for the right-of-way, and when yielded it, it is imperative to proceed with due caution.

The position paper of the National Association of Emergency Medical Service Physicians (**NAEMSP**), and the National Association of State EMS Directors (**NASEMSD**), titled "Use of Warning Lights and Siren in Emergency Medical Vehicle Response and Patient Transport," identified issues and needed policy relating to the safe operation of emergency medical vehicles. Position statement three from this document specifically addresses the implementation and use of emergency dispatch protocols.

- **EMS dispatch agencies should utilize an emergency medical dispatch priority reference system that has been developed in conjunction with and approved by the EMS medical director to determine which requests for prehospital medical care require the use of warning lights and siren.**

Sound dispatch prioritization systems establish a patient's level of severity, which then allows the determination of the type of vehicle(s) that should respond and the urgency of that response. Emergency medical dispatch centers should implement the protocols and monitor adherence to them (Figure 10.14).

Responses that are true emergencies (both fire and EMS) are limited. Yet, tradition dictates that vehicles and apparatus respond using lights and siren to all calls received through a PSAP. Responding in the emergency mode increases the risk for vehicular crashes resulting in damage to property, and injuries and fatalities to both emergency responders and civilians.

The use of warning lights and sirens on fire and EMS emergency vehicles is a basic component of emergency response and patient transport in this country. Over the past several years, the effectiveness of this long-standing tradition in affecting patient outcome or decreasing property or financial loss has come into question. What is known is that the majority of emergency vehicle crashes occur when warning lights and siren are in use. Multiple studies have been conducted comparing ambulance response times with and without the use of lights and sirens. Separate studies conducted by Addario et al. (2000) and Kupas, Dula, and Pino (1994) have demonstrated that, although response times are faster with lights and siren, the time saved had no significant impact on patient outcome, except in cardiac arrest and obstructed airway.

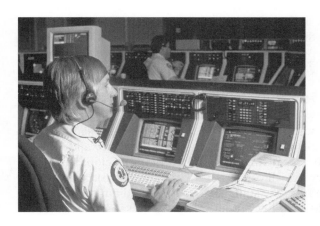

FIGURE 10.14 ◆ Dispatcher utilizing dispatch protocols. (*Courtesy of Pearson Education/PH College*)

A dispatcher receiving accurate and complete information from the caller should be able to determine whether the condition warrants a lights and siren response from this information. Sound priority dispatching relies on trained dispatchers and preset, algorithmic questions. There are commercial programs with preset questions available for both fire and EMS conditions. Many ESOs have also developed their own preset questions.

According to the USFA EV Driver Safety initiative, Salt Lake County and Phoenix Fire have addressed Emergency Medical Dispatch (**EMD**). Responses within Salt Lake County, with the exception of Salt Lake City, are automatic and cross jurisdictional boundaries. All calls are dispatched based on the closest station rather than the jurisdiction of the incident location. Testing of Automatic Vehicle Locator (AVL) dispatching began in May 2003. All fire apparatus have Global Positioning Satellite (GPS) locators installed. During the testing phase, units are dispatched using both the closest unit (AVL) and the closest station. Data are being collected to compare and ensure the closest unit is actually being dispatched. Response times will also be compared between the two systems. A plan is in place to dispatch a second unit to ensure the first AVL unit dispatched does not remain out of its jurisdiction on consecutive calls.

Priority dispatch for both fire and EMS has been part of the Salt Lake County system for all departments for 25 years. Priority dispatch began with Dr. Jeff Clawson's (EMD), which he developed while medical director for Salt Lake City Fire Department (1998). Over time, the concept was extended to fire calls. Currently Salt Lake City uses Clawson's system, which must be purchased. The nine departments that provide services for the rest of Salt Lake County organized a committee of representatives, including chiefs, who developed the priority questions that are used by the Valley Emergency Communications Center (**VECC**) to determine priority dispatch codes.

Phoenix fire apparatus is initially dispatched to respond with lights and siren on the majority of calls. If the first-arriving unit finds nothing, the remaining responding units are downgraded to continue without lights and siren. Virginia Beach Fire and Rescue uses the same approach on multiunit emergency responses. If an emergency situation does not exist, the first-arriving unit transmits a radio downgrade to all responding units. This downgrade transmission includes a brief description of findings. All other responding units continue to the scene in nonemergency mode, until cleared by command.

Certain conditions are dispatched nonemergency (no lights and siren.) In Phoenix, all company officers have the authority to change the level of response and are encouraged to err on the side of caution and firefighter safety. If the code is changed, it is recorded in the dispatch center records by the Mobile Data Terminal (**MDT**) transmission.

As all issues are within the Phoenix Fire Department, a labor–management committee, with input from the medical director, determined the nonemergency response EMS conditions. The EMS dispatch codes were developed about 1998 and, as of this writing, had not undergone a review. Units dispatched in the nonemergency mode can be preempted and redirected to an emergency response.

The average response time for a Phoenix nonemergency dispatch is seven minutes and just under five minutes for an emergency dispatch. The dispatch supervisor believed that most increases in response times are a result of annexation and larger coverage areas. If a response time exceeds ten minutes, dispatch receives an electronic notice and follows up by contacting the unit to determine the cause.

Response Matrix. With the exception of Salt Lake City, all the fire departments in the Salt Lake Valley belong to a user alliance, which meets on a monthly basis. The

CODE	BDALE	COUNTY	MIDVALE	MURRAY	SANDY	SJORDAN	SOSL	WJORDAN	WVALLEY
ALARM	1E	1E	1E	1E	1E	1E,1A	1E	1E	1E
ALRMCO	1E	1E	1E	1E	1E	1E	1E	1E	1E
ALRMR	1E	1E	1E, CS	1E	1E	1E, 1A	1E	1E	1E
ALRMW	1E, 1T	1E, 1T	1E, 1T	1E, 1T	1E, 1T	1E, 1T, 1A	1E, 1T	1E, 1T	1E, 1T

ADMINISTRATIONS: 840-4100 / FAX: 840-4040		DISPATCH: 840-4000 / FAX: 840-4039
Date Received:	VECC CAD#:	Date Assigned:
Date Completed:	VECC Case#:	VECC Supervisors Initials:

FIGURE 10.15 ◆ Example of Salt Lake Valley Fire Response Matrix. (*Source: USFA, Emergency Vehicle, Safety Initiative*)

departments developed a recommended response matrix for each incident type, which was sent to each department's chief for approval. Each department chief had the option to disapprove or modify the response matrix. An example from the matrix is found in Figure 10.15.

The Virginia Beach department's response matrix includes two engines responding from opposing directions to all collisions on the interstate. Members cannot jump or navigate jersey barriers dividing the highway in order to reach a collision scene from the opposite lane. Apparatus proceeds in a manner that allows it to position in the lane and direction of travel where the incident occurred. Responding engines that are not on the incident side of the highway contact the officer of the apparatus that is to find out if the unit will be needed, should stage until further evaluation is completed, or should clear. If the unit is needed, it continues to the next exit and reenters the highway system to assist from the same lane and direction. If the unit is asked to stage, it proceeds to the next exit and stages at an appropriate location until cleared.

CASE STUDY RECAP

Emergency Dispatch. Compliance with the ESO policy of first unit responds hot and all others respond no L&S would most likely have averted the situation in the case study. Emergency dispatch protocols have been shown to reduce the number of response-related collisions with minimal time delays in the actual response. Because this ESO had a response policy in place, enforcement for compliance becomes the predominating factor. All responders onboard the vehicle should be knowledgeable of safe response procedures and held accountable for safe operations.

SUMMARY

Safe operation on any vehicle rests with the driver and crew. The use of ED protocols lends itself as a risk reduction tool for the response process. Regardless of fire or emergency medical response, sending the right equipment to the right emergency situation in the right response mode equates a safer response and positive outcome for all involved. Front line decisions can make the difference when deciding emergency vehicle response levels. Dispatchers are the eyes and ears of the emergency responder during the response phase. If they start it right, the system will get the credit. If they start it wrong, the customer pays . . . dearly!

REVIEW QUESTIONS

1. Describe the concept of emergency dispatch protocols.
2. Identify the vehicle risk control–related feature of emergency dispatch protocols.
3. What are practical applications of emergency dispatch protocol use pertaining to vehicle response?

◆ COLLISION AND NEAR-MISS INVESTIGATION

OBJECTIVES

- Identify the procedures for reporting unsafe conditions.
- Identify the procedures for crash investigations.
- Describe the process for remediation of investigation findings.
- Define the concept of a near miss.

CASE STUDY

An ambulance arrives at the local hospital's emergency department. While backing into the off-loading entrance, the EV driver collides with an ambulance parked at the emergency department. Minor damage resulted to both vehicles. The unrestrained **EMT** in the patient compartment of the backing ambulance is thrown against the side wall of the ambulance and injures her neck. A care provider restocking equipment in the parked ambulance is also jolted from the collision but offers no complaints.

TOPIC REVIEW

Reducing collisions, injuries, and preventing reoccurrence should be the goal of any collision investigation program. The ESO should complete an analysis of any vehicle collision, loss, or near miss. The root cause(s) of the loss or near miss should be determined and corrective action(s) taken by your organization to try to prevent any future losses.

Every collision, including a minor injury collision and a near-miss collision, offers a potential lesson to be learned (Figure 10.16). The unreported collision is automatically a lesson that has gone unlearned. When injury collisions are not reported, their causes usually go uncorrected. Thus the collision can recur, perhaps causing a serious injury or fatality. All collisions must be investigated to determine the cause of the collisions and to ensure that actions to prevent recurrence are implemented.

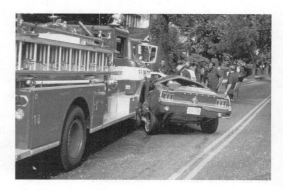

FIGURE 10.16 ◆ Fire engine collides with car. (*Courtesy of Pearson Education/PH College*)

The purpose of a collision investigation is to determine facts and prevent recurrence, not to find fault or assess blame. The investigator collects information on how and why the collision occurred, analyzes the information to determine the cause(s) of the collision, and develops recommendations to prevent the situation from recurring. The ESO should investigate collisions not to determine individual fault, but to understand the consequences of the incident. According to VFIS (2000), the failure to keep the collision investigator's investigation and the ESO investigation separate may

◆ Cause personnel to view the ESO's safety effort as a punitive program.
◆ Cause the safety manager (or collision investigator) to be seen as someone who sides with management against individual employees.
◆ Create a climate of fear among personnel.
◆ Diminish the ability to prevent recurrence by reducing the quality of information and evidence collected following a mishap.

A formal collision investigation is conducted for all fatalities, serious or potentially serious injuries, and significant equipment damage collisions. The Serious Incident Investigation Review is conducted when a collision results in a fatality or potential fatality. The following guidelines describe the types of collisions that should be formally investigated:

◆ A collision/mishap resulting in personal injury or death to any party.
◆ Any collision/mishap that may involve violation of a company policy, procedure, or regulation.
◆ Any collision or mishap involving the care or handling of a patient.
◆ Any collision or mishap that involves a vehicle not owned by the company and has the potential for a serious claim. Serious claims can result from any injury.

Collision investigations are designed to ensure a safe workplace is maintained. The objectives of collision investigations are to

◆ Provide a safe and healthful work environment for all personnel.
◆ Identify all collision causes and develop corrective actions to eliminate those causes.
◆ Implement all recommendations in a timely manner to prevent collision recurrence.
◆ Develop safety awareness so that potential unsafe acts and conditions are identified and actions taken to prevent a collision.

Specific procedures can be implemented for reporting unsafe conditions. Examples include written SOP/SOGs addressing

◆ Comprehensive apparatus maintenance program
◆ Who is authorized to perform maintenance functions
◆ How problems are corrected and reported when detected
◆ How the process is documented
  ◆ Date and time problem or risk was discovered
  ◆ Description of complaint
  ◆ All actions taken
  ◆ Personnel that discrepancy was reported to
  ◆ Date and time corrective action was taken

Procedures for collision investigations should first identify what incidents require investigation. Management should be responsible for developing and implementing a crash investigation procedure. The following incidents should trigger an investigation: a vehicular collision, a severe loss collision, a collision in which there has been a loss of life, or a near-miss situation.

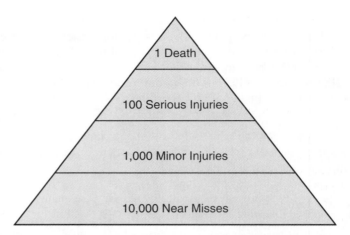

FIGURE 10.17 ◆ The chart references near-miss consequences. (*Source: Firefighter Near Miss Reporting. www.firefighternearmiss.com*)

All crashes, injuries, fatalities along with all violations of rules, regulations, laws, and orders involving emergency service vehicles should be investigated. The root causes shall be determined and full documentation provided. The ESO should take whatever corrective action is necessary to avoid repetitive occurrences of all collisions and/or violations regardless of injury or fatality results. The driver training program shall include a review and critique of crash scenarios, both local and national, to serve as an objective learning experience.

Near Misses. According to Dennis Mitterer (2005), risk and safety consultant for the emergency services industry, the concept and understanding of a near miss is as varied as the number of personalities who work in emergency services. As drivers, we should be evaluated on the close calls or near misses. It is in this evaluation process that an organization can determine how close "statistically" it is to having a serious or fatal crash. The theory depicted in Figure 10.17 illustrates this point, but a bit of an explanation is necessary. Looking at the pyramid, you see the top number is 1. This represents a death or major property loss. For every 1 death that occurs, there are roughly 100 serious injuries or significant property losses. For every 1 death that occurs, there are roughly 1,000 treatable injuries or minor property losses. For every 1 death, there are roughly 10,000 near misses.

Mitterer states that most organizations wait until a death or serious injury occurs and then decide to look at their program to avoid that specific event from ever occurring. Fact is, THIS event will probably never occur again, but the circumstances that caused the event will. Organizations need to be proactive and look at the near misses or close calls. By reducing the number of near misses, the statistical chance of having a serious or fatal event decreases. Why? Because by looking at the near misses, you begin to see the reasons for both the near misses and potentially fatal incidents. ATTITUDE and education can begin to change these behaviors. It is in this change of behavior that drivers will begin to value their role and understand that it is completely within their grasp to arrive safely.

Data Collection and Record Keeping. A safety committee should be appointed to investigate all collisions, injuries, and fatalities. In addition, the ESO should establish a data collection system and maintain permanent records of all on-duty crashes and injuries involving emergency service vehicles. Data collection systems shall maintain individual employee records of all on-duty crashes and injuries involving motor vehicles, service vehicles, and fire apparatus (Figure 10.18).

Records shall include but shall not be limited to

- Annual motor vehicle record checks
- On-duty motor vehicle crash history
- Preventable versus nonpreventable collision determination
- Remedial training recommended and/or provided as a result of previous crashes
- Safety review committee recommendations
- All investigative/review committee reports of crashes

Permanent records should be maintained on all crash and injury prevention recommendations and corrective actions taken to correct unsafe acts, conditions, or practices involving ESO vehicles or apparatus.

The NIOSH Firefighter Fatality Investigation and Prevention Program conducts investigations of both fire ground and non–fire ground fatal firefighter injuries resulting from a variety of circumstances, including motor vehicle incidents. NIOSH staff also conducts investigations of selected nonfatal injuries. Each investigation results in a report summarizing the incident and includes recommendations for preventing future similar events. Congress began funding the independent NIOSH investigations in 1998 in response to the need for further efforts to address the continuing national problem of occupational firefighter fatalities. More information and specific investigation results and recommendations are available on the NIOSH Web site at http://www.cdc.gov/niosh/firehome.html

NIOSH also publishes Hazard ID fact sheets and Alerts related to all aspects of firefighter safety. The NIOSH Hazard ID, Traffic Hazards to Firefighters While Working Along Roadways, can be found in Appendix H. Other Hazard IDs and Alerts can be accessed online at http://www.cdc.gov/niosh/othpubs.html

The following sample policy statements are from the Pennsylvania Department of Health Bureau of EMS guidelines for ambulance services. Any ESO can adapt these basic concepts to existing or enhancement of SOP/SOGs.

Should any company vehicle be involved in an collision, the vehicle operator, if able to do so, will immediately bring the vehicle to stop in a safe location and contact the appropriate supervisor immediately.

In the case of a minor collision the crew should ascertain if any injuries have occurred to staff, the occupant(s) of any other vehicle(s), and the patient if a patient is onboard.

If a patient is onboard, is in stable condition, and the providers are able to contact additional units or local communications center an additional transporting unit should be contacted to respond and transport the patient.

If a patient is onboard, is in unstable condition, and the ambulance is able to be operated safely, the crew will determine if additional unit(s) are to be contacted for patient transport or if transport should continue by present crew.

Once above conditions are met, immediately begin to document the collision. All aspects of the collision should be documented. Information included should be time of day, weather conditions, traffic conditions, response mode, and so forth.

Do NOT discuss the collision with anyone except for the police.

Gather any witness information available.

Do NOT admit fault or any type reparation.

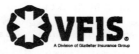

Vehicle Accident/Loss Investigation Report

(This is not a claim form)

Fire Department _____ Date _____

Address _____

Name of Driver_____ Vehicle ID/Unit Number _____

Type of Vehicle _____

Date Driver Last Certified On Above Vehicle _____

Date of Accident_____ Time_____ Date Reported _____

Location of Accident _____

Roadway

- ☐ Straight _____
- ☐ Curve _____
- ☐ On Grade _____
- ☐ Level _____
- ☐ Hillcrest_____
- ☐ Dry _____
- ☐ Wet _____
- ☐ Muddy_____
- ☐ Snowy_____
- ☐ Icy_____
- ☐ Oily _____

- ☐ 2-lane
- ☐ 3-lane
- ☐ 4-lane
- ☐ Divided
- ☐ Rural
- ☐ Other_____
- ☐ Lanes marked
- ☐ Lanes unmarked
- ☐ No road detects
- ☐ Holes, ruts, etc.
- ☐ Loose material
- ☐ Other

Accident Occurred:

- ☐ At station
- ☐ Responding to emergency
- ☐ At emergency scene
- ☐ Returning from emergency
- ☐ Training
- ☐ Convention or parade
- ☐ Other _____
- ☐ Sleet

Type of Loss

- ☐ Personal injury
- ☐ Property damage
- ☐ Vehicle damage

Weather

- ☐ Clear
- ☐ Rain
- ☐ Snow

- ☐ Fog
- ☐ Other _____

Description Of Accident _____

_____

_____

_____

_____

_____

Motor Vehicle Diagram

Complete the following diagram showing direction and positions of automobiles involved, designating clearly point of contact.

Indicate North ↑

Instructions:
1. Show vehicles and direction of travel
2. Use solid line to show path of each vehicle before accident

Give Street Names and Directions
Your Vehicle
dotted line after accident...
Other Vehicle 1 2

-over-

FIGURE 10.18 ◆ Sample of an accident investigation form. (*Courtesy of VFIS*)

CASE STUDY RECAP

Collision and Near-Miss Investigation. Investigating and determining the underlying causes of vehicle-related incidents is paramount to keeping a similar incident from re-occurring. Near-miss situations are the crash that could have been. In the case study, the occupant in the rear of the moving vehicle should have been restrained, thus reducing the potential severity of the incident. If a crew member would have been used as a spotter for backing, the incident would most likely not have occurred. Proper investigation

Safety Analysis

What acts, failures to act and/or conditions contributed most directly to this accident? (Immediate Cause)

_____
_____
_____
_____
_____

What are the basic or fundamental reasons for the existence of these acts and/or conditions? (Fundamental Cause)

_____
_____
_____
_____
_____

What action has or will be taken to prevent recurrence? Place "X" by items completed.

_____
_____
_____
_____
_____

Safety Supervisor's Comments _____

_____
_____
_____
_____
_____
_____

Driver's Signature _____   Date _____

Supervisor's Signature _____   Date _____

Safety Supervisor's Signature _____   Date _____

WP\WINWORD\VFIS\SAFETYKITFORMS\vehaccidentloss.doc   C10:004 Rev. 7/02

FIGURE 10.18 ◆ (*continued*)

technique supported by the ESO's SOP/SOG for such incidents can determine root cause issues and allow the ESO to hone policy in an effort to avert future incidents.

SUMMARY

Collision and near-miss investigation is critical to the safety of any ESO. The reduction of collisions, injuries, and preventing reoccurrence should be the goal of any collision/near-miss investigation program. Every collision, including a minor injury collision and a near-miss collision, offers a potential lesson to be learned. The unreported collision is automatically a lesson that has gone unlearned.

The case study demonstrates that even if policy were in place, it might not have been followed. This would be a basic discovery in the investigation process. Investigations look for the root cause(s) but often focus on the result of the collision, the energy transfer, and the driver. Often, the major root cause(s) are with management dysfunction or, simply put, no policy, no training, no compliance, and no remediation.

REVIEW QUESTIONS

1. What are the basic procedures for reporting unsafe conditions?
2. List the procedures for crash investigations.
3. Describe the process for remediation of investigation findings.
4. Define the concept of a near miss.

◆ TRAINING PROGRAM SAFETY

OBJECTIVES

- Understand the importance of training safety.
- Discuss safety measures that could avoid injury in the training environment.
- Identify key areas that place safety as the highest priority.

CASE STUDY

Volunteer Training/Safety Officer Dies from Injuries Received in Fall from Pickup Truck Following Training Exercise—Tennessee. On May 18, 2003, a 28-year-old male volunteer training/safety officer (the victim) was seriously injured when he fell from a moving pickup truck. He had completed a three-day training course and at the time of the incident was being transported within the training grounds. The victim was riding on the lowered tailgate of a pickup truck when he fell onto the road. He suffered severe head trauma and was treated at the scene by fellow firefighter/emergency medical technicians (EMTs) and on-site emergency medical services. The victim was transported by medical helicopter to a local trauma center where he died from his injuries on May 24, 2003.

TOPIC REVIEW

The topic of safety is often referenced in every function of the emergency services arena. Safety takes on various meanings and applications by all levels of personnel. But what does *safety* really mean? According to *Webster's Dictionary*, safety is defined as "freedom from danger." Safety is a culture that must be instilled in every aspect of the work environment and beyond. Abraham Maslow's hierarchy of basic human needs addresses personal safety expectations as one of five basic needs that must be satisfied prior to higher-level needs. The topic of safety is so broad based that it can be discussed and virtually applied to every conceivable human activity.

Through attitude and behavior, organization leaders must reflect the importance of safety in all aspects dealing with vehicles. This attitude must be infused in

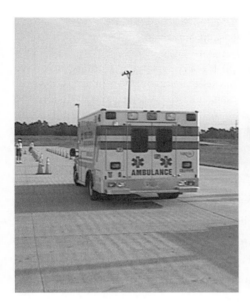

FIGURE 10.19A ◆ Ambulance vehicle on competency course. (*Photo by R. Patrick*)

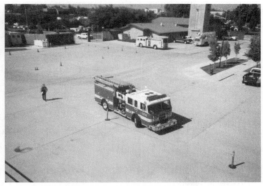

FIGURE 10.19B ◆ Fire vehicle on competency course. (*Photo by R. Patrick*)

all organizational policies and training. Department commitment to driver competency and accountability can have a profound effect on reducing crashes, injuries, and fatalities. This begins with the factors used to select the driver candidate.

Training is the foundation of all safe practices. The type of course, integration of classroom and applied practice (Figures 10.19a and 10.19b), and instructor qualifications all contribute to the effectiveness of any training.

From the classroom environment to the competency-based training, safety considerations must be at the forefront (Figure 10.20). When conducting driver training courses, make sure of the following.

- Prior to attempting the competency course, the emergency vehicle operator trainee shall successfully complete the classroom instruction and possess a valid driver's license.
- Establish a course safety officer.
  - Vehicle malfunctions must be reported to the safety officer.

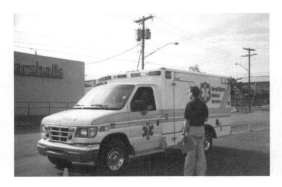

FIGURE 10.20 ◆ Competency course evaluator scoring a student. (*Photo by R. Patrick*)

- Restrict course to authorized personnel.
  - All personnel on the course shall be clearly visible.
  - Any involved personnel may designate the vehicle unsafe.
- An instructor shall accompany emergency vehicle operator in cab of vehicle.
  - All personnel in vehicle shall wear occupant restraints.
  - No food, drink, or smoking permitted in vehicle.
- Only one vehicle may utilize the competency course at any time.
  - Ensure 15 MPH maximum course speed.
  - Vehicles shall operate with headlights on.
  - No vehicle may proceed on course until approved by safety officer.
- The trainee shall follow all applicable traffic laws.

In the opening case study, NIOSH investigators concluded that, to minimize the risk of similar occurrences, fire service organizations should

- Ensure that all personnel being transported, when on-duty, be securely seated and restrained in approved vehicle passenger compartments.

Although it is unclear if a medical or physical condition contributed to this fatal incident, fire departments should consider implementing these safety and health recommendations based on the physical demands and medical requirements of firefighting.

- Provide mandatory preplacement and annual medical evaluations, consistent with NFPA 1582, for all firefighters to determine medical fitness for duty and training exercises.
- Conduct periodic physical capabilities testing to ensure that fire department personnel meet the physical requirements for duty and training exercises.

NIOSH RECOMMENDATIONS/DISCUSSIONS

Recommendation #1. *Fire service organizations should ensure that all personnel being transported, when on-duty, be securely seated and restrained in approved vehicle passenger compartments.*[1,3]

Discussion: NFPA 1500 6.3.1 states that "All persons riding in fire apparatus shall be seated and belted securely by seat belts in approved riding positions." Even though the vehicle in which the victim was riding was not a fire apparatus, prudent safety operations dictate compliance with this requirement for all vehicles used in the course of fire service operations.

Federal standards require that occupant compartments of vehicles be designed to protect occupants during a crash. The cargo area of a pickup truck is not designed to transport people. Statistics from the National Highway Traffic Safety Administration's (NHTSA) Fatality Analysis Reporting System reveal that each year on average, over 200 persons are killed while riding in the cargo area of a pickup truck.

The National Committee on Uniform Traffic Laws and Ordinances (NCUTLO) has developed a Model Occupant Protection Law that states can adopt. The model law addresses riding in nonpassenger areas of motor vehicles. Section five clearly addresses passengers in the cargo area of a pickup truck by stating that no operator shall allow, and no passenger may ride, on or in any portion of a motor vehicle that is not a passenger seating position, including the cargo-carrying areas of a pickup truck. Thirty states (including Tennessee) and the District of Columbia, have addressed the hazard of riding in cargo areas by enacting various laws.

This investigation revealed no specific event or factor that caused the victim to fall from the truck. Many dynamics, including weight of the turnout gear and boots, or possibly weakness from an illness or lack of food that morning, may have contributed to the victim's inability to remain securely seated on the tailgate of the pickup truck. However, had he been seated and restrained in an approved vehicle passenger compartment, the incident would not have occurred.

Although it is unclear if a medical or physical condition contributed to this fatal incident, fire departments should consider implementing these safety and health recommendations based on the physical demands and medical requirements of firefighting.

Recommendation #2. *Fire departments should provide mandatory preplacement and annual medical evaluations, consistent with NFPA 1582, for all firefighters to determine medical fitness for duty and training exercises.*[1,4,5]

Discussion: Guidance regarding the content and frequency of periodic medical evaluations and examinations for firefighters can be found in NFPA 1582, *Standard on Medical Requirements for Firefighters and Information for Fire Department Physicians.* NFPA 1582 §6.1 states that "Medical evaluations of candidates shall be conducted prior to training programs or participation in departmental emergency response activities." Information on medical evaluations can also be found in the report of the International Association of Firefighters/International Association of Fire Chiefs (IAFF/IAFC) wellness/fitness initiative. NFPA 1500, *Standard on Fire Department Occupational Safety and Health Program,* addresses the economic issues raised by implementation of NFPA 1582 and may be reviewed for guidance.

Recommendation #3. *Fire departments should conduct periodic physical capabilities testing to ensure that fire department personnel meet the physical requirements for duty and training exercises.*[1,6]

Discussion: NFPA 1500, *Standard on Fire Department Occupational Safety and Health Program,* requires that fire department members who engage in emergency operations be annually evaluated and certified by the fire department as meeting the physical performance requirements.

It is unknown if the symptoms expressed by the victim the day before the incident were in any way related to a specific illness that is addressed in NFPA 1582, or due to lack of physical conditioning as outlined in NFPA 1500 and defined in 1583. However, the information found in these three standards, along with the IAFF/IAFC wellness/fitness initiative, provides guidance to assist fire departments in early recognition and timely resolution of medical or physical conditions that may affect the firefighter's personal safety and well-being.

Niosh references

1. NFPA. 2002. *NFPA 1500, Standard on fire department occupational safety and health program.* Quincy MA: National Fire Protection Association.
2. NHTSA-FARS. 2002. National Highway Traffic Safety Administration, Fatality Analysis Reporting System [http://www-fars.nhtsa.dot.gov]. Tabular data, 1995–2002: Number of fatal motor vehicle incidents involving riding in the cargo area of pick-up trucks. Date accessed: March 2004.
3. National Committee on Uniform Traffic Laws and Ordinances. 2002. Model occupant protection law. [http://www.ncutlo.org/occprotect02.html]. Date accessed: March 2004.

4. NFPA. 2003. *NFPA 1582: Standard on medical requirements for fire fighters and information for fire department physicians.* Quincy MA: National Fire Protection Association.

5. IAFF/IAFC. 2000. The fire service joint labor management wellness/fitness initiative. Washington, D.C.: International Association of Fire Fighters, International Association of Fire Chiefs.

6. NFPA. 2000. *NFPA 1583: Standard on health-related fitness programs for fire fighters.* Quincy MA: National Fire Protection Association.

Although the preceding report references fire department activities, all ESOs should heed this advice.

CASE STUDY RECAP

Training Program Safety. Safety is second to nothing. Absolutely nothing! To have a safety-related fatality on the training ground is inexcusable. The International Association of Fire Chiefs has referenced these situations as fratricide (the killing of our own). Riding the tailgate of a pickup truck as depicted in the case study, is no different from riding the tail board of a fire truck; it is an unsafe practice. Educators and instructors must set the example by conducting all of their teachings in a safe manner using recognized best practices.

Anywhere ESO Anywhere, Town	Subject		Driving and Use of Personal Vehicles
Administrative **Procedures and** **Guidelines**	**Guideline Number**		
	Adopted		
	Effective Date		
	Revised		
	Due for Revision		
	Pages		2

Purpose: To establish procedures and guidelines for the use and safe operation of all personally owned vehicles during <**ESO NAME**> functions.

Scope: All <**ESO NAME**> personnel.

Responsibility: It is the responsibility of all <**ESO NAME**> personnel who own and operate their own respective vehicles to adhere to this policy for response to and returning from <**ESO NAME**> events.

Policy:

The volunteer or employee responding to or returning from any <**ESO NAME**> event must understand that first and foremost, he or she must arrive at the emergency scene or the station safely in order to be of any help to the public. This policy is intended to assist with such purpose.

A. Valid Pennsylvania Driver's License and Insurance Coverage

No volunteer or employee of <**ESO NAME**> shall operate his or her personally owned vehicle of any kind without the appropriate, valid PA Driver's License and appropriate personal vehicle insurance minimum limits coverage.

<**ESO NAME**> will conduct annual Motor Vehicle Record checks and personal insurance verification on all <**ESO NAME**> personnel.

B. Permission

1. No volunteer or employee shall operate a privately owned vehicle (POV) or private mobile unit of any kind for response to emergency incidents without first receiving permission from an officer authorized to give such permission. The Fire Chief or his or her designee is authorized to give permission to use private vehicles. The operator of the vehicle is responsible for the vehicle and its contents.
2. The use of "Blue" courtesy lights as defined in the Pennsylvania Motor Vehicle Code for the purpose of responding to an emergency station or incident is strictly prohibited. Only designated and approved <**ESO NAME**> Fire Police Officers may utilize such devices during on-scene traffic safety control functions.
3. The driver of any privately owned vehicle being utilized for <**ESO NAME**> purpose when responding to or returning from an emergency, or fire department sponsored event shall abide by all normal motor vehicle laws as any prudent citizen would drive. Such driving includes coming to a complete stop at all intersections controlled by a red traffic signal or stop sign and all railroad crossings. Intersection passage shall occur only upon signaling by a green traffic light or granted right-of-way at a stop sign and railroad crossing.
4. Unauthorized use is any use prohibited by law. Accidents occurring during unauthorized use of vehicles for <**ESO NAME**> incidents will not be covered by <**ESO NAME**>'s insurance program and will result in that volunteer or employee's liability for any property damage/personal injuries or other operating costs associated with that vehicle's use.

C. Seat Belts

Anyone riding in a privately owned vehicle for expressed and approved <**ESO NAME**> purposes must use seat belts at all times.

D. Safety

1. POVs used at <**ESO NAME**> events shall not be backed up without the assistance of a volunteer or employee at the rear of the vehicle directing the driver.
2. Volunteers and employees responding in personal vehicles should never exceed the posted speed limit.
3. Volunteers responding in personal vehicles should always stop at all stop signs and red traffic signals and wait for normal right-of-way before proceeding.
4. Individual volunteers must have personal auto liability insurance with appropriate liability limits that protect not only the volunteer but also the <**ESO NAME**>.
5. The operator's supervising officer or other persons assigned by the Fire Chief shall make investigations of accidents involving a POV conducting <**ESO NAME**> business. The findings of the investigator and the police shall be reviewed by the Fire Chief to determine careless or negligent behavior.
6. In the event a volunteer or employee is involved in an accident while operating or riding in a POV conducting official <**ESO NAME**> activities or injures another person or property, the volunteer or employee shall immediately notify his or her supervising officer in accordance with the township's policy on worker's compensation program. The WC program information is located in the personnel section of the station.

FIGURE 10.21A ◆ Sample SOG for privately owned vehicle operations. (*Courtesy of Richard W. Patrick*)

Figure 10.21b ◆
Sample SOG for pri-
vately owned vehicle
operations. (*Source:
USFA, Emergency Vehi-
cle Safety Initiative*)

Sample POV SOG from Elk Rapids, Michigan

Requirements:

- Must be a member in good standing for one year
- Must be approved by ERTA Chief
- Must have completed the FFTC Emergency Driving Course or equivalent
- Must have completed operator approval/vehicle inspection form on file

Regulations:

1. Lights and sirens will be used within the response area only.
2. Lights and sirens will be used at Antrim County *dispatched incidents only*; personnel who belong to a station outside Elk Rapids response area are not allowed to use this privilege on responses to any other stations, outside the area.
3. For personnel who reside outside the response area, ERTA Chief will determine response status on individual basis.
4. Duty Crew Responding: use of equipment in response area only, responding to *dispatched call* outside the response area—distance unlimited; Backup Crew: use of equipment in response area only to *dispatched calls*.
5. Receiving type radio/pager must be in vehicle and operating whenever the vehicle is in the 10-33 (emergency) response mode; if radio/pager is not available, vehicle will respond 10-40.
6. When responding 10-33 vehicles must keep to road right-of-way only; no passing on the right is allowed.
7. Personnel will obey *State of Michigan P.A. 300* when using this privilege. Lights and an audible signal must be used simultaneously.
8. If a responding personnel comes upon a school bus showing stop signals, personnel will stop until it is given the right-of-way by the school bus.
9. Exemptions to the *Michigan Vehicle Code listed in 257.603* (3) and (4) shall apply as follows: Although (3)(c) allows the driver to "exceed the prima facie speed limits so long as he or she does not endanger life or property," ERTA does not support this.
10. Exemption (3)(b) shall apply as follows: Personnel responding 10-33 will come to a stop, before proceeding through any stop street and proceed only if right-of-way is given by motorists/pedestrians, without endangering life or property.
11. All exemptions shall not, however, protect the driver of POV from consequences of a reckless disregard of the safety of others. If drivers choose to ignore this policy, they do so at their own risk.
12. If POV is used by anyone else other than the personnel, all regulations must be obeyed. If they are not, privilege will be lost for that ERTA person.
13. POV will yield right-of-way to all other emergency vehicles.
14. Lights and sirens are for use in ambulance type work only; not acting in any capacity as police or fire department response.
15. Lights may be used for safety reasons, such as stalled vehicles blocking roadway, etc.
16. All personnel will attend an FFTC Emergency driving course or equivalent according to standard operating procedures.

Discipline:

1. First offense: 90 day loss of light and siren.
2. Second offense: Total loss of light and siren for two years.
3. After two years personnel may seek reinstatement of privilege, not automatically granted.
4. After second offense personnel must requalify on station equipment.
5. Privilege is suspended by ERTA Chief until Review Board's decision on any infractions.

(*continued*)

Review Board:

1. Will consist of ERPD Chief, one Fire Board member, one Township Board member, and the ERTA Chief.
2. All complaints must follow the chain of command.
3. All complaints must be in written form.
4. Any appeals of this Board's decisions will be made to the ERTA Chief.

Selection:

1. ERTA Chief will have the responsibility of issuing lights and sirens (property of ERTA).
2. The ERTA Chief's decision will be standard operating procedure after a review of (a) volunteer application, (b) activity reports (runs etc.), (c) input from ERTA Board Members.
3. ERTA lights and sirens only will be used.
4. If light and siren are lost or damaged, they will be replaced at the member's expense.

Response:

When responding to an emergency with civilian personnel in the vehicle (nonmembers, family members, etc.), lights and sirens will not be used; the responder will not subject the passengers to any undue risk. The POV will be parked a safe distance from the incident and off the roadway, when possible. In no case will the POV be used for a traffic control barrier with civilians inside. Emergency vehicles and POVs not essential to the actual incident shall position themselves out of the traffic lanes.

Lights and siren on a POV are a privilege that is extended to an individual on a need basis by the ERTA Chief. These vehicles will be operated with the limits of the law and department policy.

Exclusions:

Lights and sirens will not be used on the following vehicles: motorcycles, campers, camper-trailers, RV trailers, or utility trailers.

Operator Approval:

| Operator | Inspector |
| Initial | Initial |

Designated inspector to explain the procedure to operator:

> Give member a copy of departmental policies and rules for study.
> Give member "support material" for study and to be returned to department as well as reference books available (Public Act 300).
> Explain that random questions may be asked from the materials.
> Interview the driver and ask random questions from the ERTA department policies manual and in reference to laws on emergency vehicle driving.
> Operator agrees to suspend use of personal (or other municipality owned) equipment according to the parameters of this policy (i.e., under investigation or discipline).

Vehicle Inspection:

| Operator | Inspector |
| Initial | Initial |

> Meets the requirements of Emergency Vehicle inspection.
> Meets the requirements of safety for a motor vehicle inspection (brakes, etc.).
> Understands laws, ordinances, and department policies concerning driving of emergency vehicles.

(*continued*)

Operator to present a valid driver's license and proof of liability insurance.

Operator has completed a probationary period.

Operator has completed FFTC Emergency driving course or equivalent.

Operator has a general understanding of defensive driving concepts.

Operator understands unexpected driving hazards and has a plan for reaction (i.e.: dense fog, headlights fail, wipers fail, off-road recovery, etc.).

Operator understands that complaints of driving techniques will be investigated and may fall under the Enforcement of Discipline policy.

Operator has a general understanding of the psychological effects on the driver when using lights and sirens during an emergency response.

Operator agrees to abide by all ERTA policies and procedures that may apply while driving a POV with emergency lights and sirens equipment.

Signature indicates agreement to all parameters listed in the policy.

Operator   Date
Inspector   Date

AUTHORIZATION OF ADMINISTRATIVE POLICY

ERTA Chief's authorization (ERT Board approval): _____

Date authorized: _____ 10/12/99 _____ Effective Date: 10/12/99

Revised 3/6/01

http://www.elkrapids.info/erta/policy40.htm

SUMMARY

Safety spans every aspect of our lives. Success begins with management's commitment to a universal approach of a safety culture. On the job, personnel need to be provided with a safety atmosphere and the equipment to do the job right—safely. Personnel must also be safety conscious in their every activity. When the alarm activates, safety awareness must go up a notch. Each person is responsible for his or her safety and should also look out for the well-being of the crew. Sound attainable policies allow all personnel to know what is expected and why. Management can provide the tools needed for a safe operation, but the end users—the vehicle drivers—must use the tools correctly. This will permit them to function in a safe manner. Remember, a simple pat on the back for a job safely done goes a long way.

To reduce the possibility of a collision within your organization, follow this recipe: Mix quality drivers with good emergency vehicle driver education and training. Throw in good standard operating procedures and guidelines. Stir in motivation and follow up with concurrent quality assurance. Bake with years of experience and sound, quality leadership. Sprinkle with technological aids, and you'll have a plate to be proud of!

REVIEW QUESTIONS

1. What is the importance of training safety?
2. Discuss safety measures that could avoid injury in the training environment.
3. List the key considerations that place safety as the highest priority.

References

Addario, M., Brown, L., Hogue, T., Hunt, R. C., and Whitney, C. L. 2000. "Do warning lights and sirens reduce ambulance response times?" *Prehospital Emergency Care, 4*(1), 70–74.

Allen, M., Strickland, J., and Adams, A. 1967. As cited in DeLorenzo, R., and Eilers, M. 1991. "Lights and siren: A review of emergency vehicle warning systems." *Annals of Emergency Medicine.*

Clawson, J. J., and Dernocoeur, K. B. 1998. *Principles of emergency medical dispatch,* 2nd vers. 10.3. Priority Press.

Davis, C. C. 1982. *Collisions involving stopped vehicles on freeway shoulders.* Automobile Club of Southern California.

Davis, R. March 21, 2001. "Speeding to the rescue can have deadly results." *USA Today.*

DeLorenzo, R., and Eilers, M. 1991. "Lights and siren: A review of emergency vehicle warning systems." *Annals of Emergency Medicine.*

Federal Signal Corporation. 1992. *Risk reduction in emergency response.*

FEMA. 2004. *Safe operation of tankers.*

FEMA, USFA. (1994–2001). *Fire fighter fatality in the United States.*

Firefighter near-miss reporting. Retrieved October 18, 2005, from http://www.firefighternearmiss.com/home.do.

Harvey, N. May 25, 2003. "Service honors fallen EMS providers." *Roanoke Times.*

Hills, B. L. 1980. As cited in DeLorenzo, R., and Eilers, M. 1991. "Lights and siren: A review of emergency vehicle warning systems." *Annals of Emergency Medicine.*

International Fire Service Training Association (IFSTA). 2002. *Pumping apparatus driver/operator handbook.*

Kahn, C. A., Pirrallo, R. G., and Kuhn, E. M. 2001. "Characteristics of fatal ambulance crashes in the United States: An 11-year retrospective analysis." *Prehospital Emergency Care. 5,* 261–269.

Kupas, D., Dula, D., and Pino, B. 1994. "Patient outcome using Medical protocol to limit 'lights and siren' transport." *Prehospital and Disaster Medicine, 9*(4).

Mitterer, D. M. Spring 2005. "Near misses." *VFIS News.*

National Academy of Emergency Dispatch. http://www.naed.org.

National Association of EMS Physicians; National Association of State EMS Directors. 1994. "Use of warning lights and siren in emergency medical vehicle response and patient transport." Position paper.

National Bureau of Standards. 1978. *Emergency vehicle warning lights: State of the art.* Publication No. 480-16.

NFPA. 1998. *NFPA 1002, Standard for fire apparatus driver/operator professional qualifications.* Quincy, MA: National Fire Protection Association.

NFPA. 2000a. *NFPA 1071, Standard for emergency vehicle technician professional qualifications.* Quincy, MA: National Fire Protection Association.

NFPA. 2000b. *NFPA 1451, Standard for a fire service vehicle operations training program.* Quincy, MA: National Fire Protection Association.

NFPA. 2000c. *NFPA 1915, Standard for fire apparatus preventative maintenance program.* Quincy, MA: National Fire Protection Association.

NFPA. 2000d. *Special analysis based on NFPA's Fire Incident Data Organization (FIDO).* Quincy, MA: National Fire Protection Association, Fire Analysis and Research Division.

NFPA. 2001. *National fire codes: A compilation of NFPA codes, standards, recommended practices, manuals and guides.* Quincy, MA: National Fire Protection Association.

NFPA. 2002a. *NFPA 1041, Standard for fire service instructor professional qualifications.* Quincy, MA: National Fire Protection Association.

NFPA. 2002b. *NFPA 1500, Standard on fire department occupational safety and health program.* Quincy, MA: National Fire Protection Association.

NFPA. 2003. *NFPA 1901: Standard for automotive fire apparatus.* Quincy, MA: National Fire Protection Association.

NIOSH. 2000a. *A captain and a firefighter die from injuries in a tanker rollover— Indiana.* Cincinnati, OH: U.S. Department of Health and Human Services, Public Health Service, Centers for Disease Control and Prevention, National Institute for Occupational Safety and Health, DHHS (NIOSH) Publication No. F2000—10.

NIOSH. 2000b. *Tanker rollover claims life of volunteer fire chief—Missouri*. Cincinnati, OH: U.S. Department of Health and Human Services, Public Health Service, Centers for Disease Control and Prevention, National Institute for Occupational Safety and Health, DHHS (NIOSH) Publication No. F2000–18.

Patrick, Richard W. October 2004. "Emergency vehicle driver training." *24-7 EMS*. www.24-7EMS.com.

Scarano, S. 1981. As cited in DeLorenzo, R., and Eilers, M. 1991. "Lights and siren: A review of emergency vehicle warning systems." *Annals of Emergency Medicine*.

Smith, J. 2005. "Are fire service tanker rollovers preventable?"

Solomon, S. 2002. "The case for amber emergency warning lights." *Firehouse, 27*(2), 100–102.

U.S. Department of Health and Human Services, Centers for Disease Control and Prevention. February 28, 2003. "Ambulance crash-related injuries among emergency medical services workers—United States, 1991–2002." *Morbidity Mortality Weekly Report, 52*(8), 154–156.

U.S. Department of Health and Human Services, National Institute for Occupational Safety and Health. 2001. *26-year-old emergency medical technician dies in multiple fatality ambulance crash—Kentucky*. Pub. No. FACE-2001-11.

VFIS. 2000. *Emergency vehicle driver training program*. Chap. 6.

VFIS. 2001. *Dynamics of emergency vehicle response*.

VFIS. 2005. *Rollover prevention*.

Zagaroli, L., and Taylor, A. January 1, 2003. "Ambulance driver fatigue a danger." *Detroit News*.

Answers to Review Questions

Chapter 1

1. The culture of the leadership is of the highest priority. It is representative of the organization and personnel.
2. Have integrity, display initiative, be authoritative, have insight, maintain interest, accept responsibility, not show favoritism, sustain staff intensity, access and share information.
3. A Theory X leader believes that people are inherently lazy, need to be told what to do, and will work only when threatened. A Theory Y leader tends to believe that providing people with a positive work environment in which the employee accepts responsibility also has the employee seeking additional responsibilities.
4. Supervisors balance personnel needs with the ESO vision. The supervisor must support the risk control efforts through development, education, training, reinforcing, and encouragement of personnel.
5. Driving policies and procedures establish management's intent for safe vehicle operation and to protect both the ESO and its personnel.

Chapter 2

1. Training is the most important aspect of emergency driving.
2. Classroom, competency course, actual road driving, and written test.
3. Knowledge base, skills, ability, and attitude.
4. Initially and preferably on annual basis.
5. Immature, brazen/show-off, laid-back, and comic.
6. Traffic psychology refers to how a driver learns to modify his or her own style of conduct in traffic situations and to monitor the impact of one's own driving behavior on other road users.
7. Fatigue, health, personal problems, age, and habits.
8. (a) Minimize light or wear a sleep mask; (b) use "white noise" such as a fan to block out disruptive noises, turn off the phone, and turn the answering machine volume all the way down; (c) lower room temperature; (d) create an association with sleep by maintaining bedtime routines and using the bedroom for sleep only (OK, sex, too!); (e) post a "day sleeper" sign on the door ; (f) exercise moderately every day (but not within three hours of sleep); (g) do not drink caffeine within five hours of bedtime; (h) get the support of family and friends.
9. Routine, comfort, and confidence.
10. Keep their license up-to-date and valid; report any violation received when driving their personal vehicle; remain physically and mentally fit; and, participate in training when available.
11. Importance of driver training; extent of the problem; personnel selection; SOPs/SOGs; map reading; vehicle positioning; legal aspects of emergency vehicle driving; vehicle dynamics; vehicle inspections and maintenance; vehicle operations/safety; written test
12. Use of mirrors; turning; blind right side and rear positioning; backing; braking and stopping; depth perception (front and rear); height clearance; proper communication.
13. Driving record; personnel file regarding driving-related issues; number of emergency calls driven; length of service as a driver; environment driven in (rural, suburban, urban); actual emergency vehicle driving experience; observed proficiency and supervisory reports compared to performance in the field; length of time since last recertification; introduction of new emergency vehicles; introduction of new technology on existing emergency vehicles.

14. Classes attended (proficiency not verifiable); classes successfully completed (proficiency at time measured via testing or simulation); certification (proficiency measured and certified by the organization).; and licensing (proficiency measured and licensed by the agency).

Chapter 3

1. The four primary exemptions are permission to proceed through a red traffic signal or stop sign, the ability to exceed the posted speed limit, the right to travel against the normal flow of traffic, and park on roadways regardless of traffic flow as long as the law of due regard is exercised.
2. The general difference between rules, regulations, and law is that laws are legislated statutes or ordinances, and rules and regulations, generally developed by the responsible governing body, allow the applicable persons to carry out the intent of the law.
3. True emergency is defined as a situation in which there is a high probability of death or serious injury to an individual or significant property loss.
4. Due regard implies the assurance of general safety of the responders, the public, victim(s), and property. In essence, it implies that no one gets hurt, no damage is caused, and safe passage is assured.
5. Vicarious liability occurs when one person is held responsible for the negligence of another. Typically, this applies in an employment context, wherein the employer (master) is responsible for the negligent acts of the employee (servant) that occur within the context of the employment relationship. For example, an employer may be liable for an accident caused by an employee as the result of the negligent operation of a delivery vehicle.

Chapter 4

1. Policy is a guiding principle or course of action adopted toward an objective or objectives.
2. A procedure prescribes specific ways of doing certain activities in a specific order, whereas a guideline is a statement, indication, or outline of policy by which to determine a course of action, but not necessarily in a specific order or performed the same way every time.
3. An ESO can best obtain buy-in from personnel by involving personnel in the SOP/SOG development process.
4. A policy or SOP/SOG should be taken from circulation if the need has been eliminated or if it does not work.
5. SOP/SOG development and implementation should take a minimum of 45 days.
6. A policy statement provides management's belief and intent on the given subject.
7. The main principle behind how an SOP works is the use of words such as *shall*, *will*, and *must*. SOPs are generally written in a structured order.
8. The main principle behind how an SOG works is the use of words such as *may*, *can*, and *should*. SOGs permit variables.
9. Any of the following are components of a header: numbering system, page numbers, effective date, expiration/review date, title, description of purpose or rationale statement, authority signature(s), scope, general procedures or guidelines, specific procedures or guidelines, and references.
10. It is important to follow safe driving SOP/SOGs to ensure the safety and well-being of the ESO, its personnel, and the public served.
11. Primary SOP/SOG development rests with the chief, director, or administrator of the ESO.

Chapter 5

1. Bumps, mud, potholes, animals, tree limbs, bridges, curves, banking, speed limits, crowns, and water drainage.
2. Concrete to gravel because it is more difficult to control a vehicle on gravel.
3. Another problem a driver will encounter is objects in the road. These could be animals, tree limbs, or dropped debris. Everyone's natural reaction is to swerve to avoid hitting

objects in the road, but this often causes more problems than the object itself. Instead of swerving:

- If it is a small object, hit the object head-on.
- Do not cause a larger collision by swerving into another lane or oncoming traffic.
- If it is a large animal or object, maintain control of the vehicle and attempt to avoid a head-on collision.

4. When it's very hot, the oils used to make asphalt bleed to the surface, making it slick, especially when it rains. An asphalt roadway can also become wavy with heavy use during extremely hot weather. Not only is that very uncomfortable to ride over, but the driver does not have full control of the emergency vehicle because the tires are in contact with the road only half the time.

5. Cornering, braking, accelerating, and maintaining appropriate speed.

6. By training and practice.

7. Total stopping distance consists of perception time, reaction time, and braking time.

8. Drivers want to allow enough room around the emergency vehicle so that they can identify possible hazards, decide on a course of action, and react by either bringing the emergency vehicle to a controlled stop or maneuvering to avoid the hazard. In a road emergency, drivers don't want to get boxed in without an escape route. Maintaining a safety cushion around the emergency vehicle reduces the chances of being involved in a crash. Obviously, the safest position for the emergency vehicle is as far away from any possible collision hazard as possible. It's easy to be involved in a crash with the vehicles in front, beside, and behind.

9. Space management is to observe regularly the vehicles behind the emergency vehicle. Often, curious drivers will either follow the emergency vehicle or use the emergency vehicle to "break" traffic in an effort to move more quickly down the street or highway. In either case, the emergency vehicle driver must be aware of the presence of any vehicles and keep them under observation. Signaling any intent to turn, pass, or stop is extremely important to keep the civilian driver(s) from following too closely or colliding with the emergency vehicle.

10. Emergency units responding along the same route should maintain 300 to 400 feet of distance between them. To make sure the other motorists know there is more than one emergency unit in the area, the driver should use a different siren tone than the vehicle ahead of it. Change tones at intersections and allow the siren to partially wind down prior to the intersection so that both you and the other motorists will be alerted that there are multiple emergency vehicles in the area.

11. The simplest turns are the right and left corners. In a left turn, the driver must cross the near lane before turning into the travel lane. The vehicle is exposed in the intersection longer than when making a right turn. The driver must give oncoming traffic more time.

12. Spotter.

13. Today's emergency vehicles are equipped with power steering. In these vehicles, steering failure occurs whenever the engine quits. It may also occur if all power steering fluid is lost. In either case, the vehicle can still be steered, but it will take more physical strength because the operator has to overcome the failure of the hydraulic system. If steering failure occurs, slow the vehicle and pull off the road. Do not brake heavily in case the vehicle pulls to one side; the driver does not have the strength to overcome this extra force.

Chapter 6

1. Safety is the most important factor when driving to the scene. Drivers must have a route plan if they want to get to the emergency scene quickly and carefully.

2. Route planning involves learning the geographic and local conditions, the individual characteristics of the area, and the organization's procedures to map out the most efficient route to the emergency scene.

3. Everyone in the vehicle must wear a restraint.

4. All equipment should be secure to avoid having equipment become projectile missiles.

5. Unsafe behavior is any behavior that may cause someone harm.

6. The use of emergency warning equipment signals has two basic concepts:
   - They notify other drivers that an approaching emergency vehicle is operating in an emergency mode; and
   - They require other drivers to yield the right-of-way to the emergency vehicle in accordance with state and/or local law.
7. Change the mode of the siren from wail to yelp at least 200 feet from entering an intersection.
8. The driver's vision can be affected in three ways. First, the environment may give the driver problems. Second, the vehicle and the way the driver cares for it may affect the way the driver is able to see things. Finally, the driver's physical condition and preparation for duty will affect his or her eyes' ability to see.
9. Hydroplaning is especially dangerous because the driver loses steering and braking control. As little as one-sixteenth inch of water on the road surface can cause hydroplaning.
10. Slow down before hitting water. This will lessen the splashing and reduce the effects of hydroplaning, giving the driver more control of the vehicle. Gently apply the brakes for a few moments when exiting the deeper puddles to heat the brake shoes and dry them.
11. Crosswinds can blow the vehicle off the road or across the center line, particularly at curves and corners and especially when it's raining, snowing, or icy, and traction with the road is already reduced.
12. There are several things drivers can do to increase their ability to see at night: Don't move immediately from a brightly lit room to a dark vehicle and begin driving. Give your eyes a chance to adjust to the darkness; avoid looking directly into glaring headlights of oncoming vehicles. The human eye takes about 7 seconds to recover fully from being blinded by a bright light. At 60 mph, the vehicle would travel 616 feet in 7 seconds. Don't smoke, and don't wear sunglasses at night.
13. While driving down the road, plan an escape route from every situation around you. The driver should avoid a head-on impact at all costs. Think about how to avoid a crash if it happened in front of you, or to the right or left, or even right behind. Decide which item to hit if a crash is unavoidable. The driver has two choices, but always hit at an angle rather than head-on. Sideswiping a parked car is preferable to colliding with one head-on. Choose to hit items that will absorb the impact rather than solid objects. It is better to hit a utility pole than a concrete bridge abutment.
14. Faced with the certainty of a crash, there are three things a driver can do: brake, accelerate, or turn to avoid it or lessen the impact.

Chapter 7

1. The driver/operator should not be responsible for radio communications, especially when the vehicle is in motion. The driver/operator's main concern is to get from point *A* to point *B* in a safe manner. The driver/operator cannot maintain two hands on the steering wheel as advocated in a safe driving environment, by using one hand to talk on a microphone and the other trying to steer a large vehicle. The potential for the cord from the radio microphone getting wrapped around an object such as the steering wheel is an additional hazard that should be avoided.
2. The three main points relevant to radio etiquette: Confidentiality is essential to patients. Off-the-wall comments are not appropriate at any time, and when transmitted across the radio, everyone with a radio or scanner will hear the comment. Keep conversations to what is necessary and professional. Think about what you are going to say before you say it. Remember to identify your unit designation and whom you are calling. Keep your transmissions brief and to the point. Use plain English and speak distinctly and clearly.
3. Roles technology plays in communication: Certain computerized devices that are installed in the cab allow the dispatch center to generate and send all the pertinent information directly to the responding units. With the development of GPS, units can have a mapping system within their units to get clear and concise directions to the scene of the incident. They can also follow their response on the computer screen and identify potential delays

and other factors that may hamper their response. Cellular phones have become very popular and may be used by your agency. Cellular phones can be monitored by the public if they tune to the frequency you are speaking on. You need to use caution during your conversation and by no means should the driver of the vehicle be utilizing the cellular phone while the vehicle is in motion.

4. A number of times when emergency personnel respond to medical calls they arrive on the scene to find the patient is on the fifth floor of a high-rise or on the other side of a 200,000-square-foot factory. The on-scene time does not adequately reflect when responders reach the patient's side. The "at-patient" time is noted when they actually reach the patient and make contact. When responding to a fire, a key factor to record through communication is water on the fire. These benchmarks and others are important for the emergency responder to communicate and the dispatch center to record for future statistical analysis. Benchmarking is an important concept and component in order for the emergency service industry to progress forward into the twenty-first century.

5. Prior to the start of the call; when you are dispatched on a response; when you arrive at the scene of an incident; at-patient on medical calls or other key trigger points such as water on the fire; incident choreography; when the fire is under control or the patient has been extricated; when transporting patients, notifying dispatch you are en route to your destination; arrival at destination such as a hospital in EMS situations; and when available.

Chapter 8

1. To document any needed maintenance you find; to make sure needed maintenance has been completed before the vehicle is placed in service; and to perform any maintenance for which the organization makes the driver responsible.

2. Inspect the vehicle according to established procedures. Check that all scheduled maintenance has been performed. Check that all needed repairs have been made. If a vehicle is NOT in safe operating condition, the operator has the responsibility to take the vehicle out of service until the problems have been fixed.

3. In August 2000, NFPA 1071, *Standard for Emergency Vehicle Technician Professional Qualifications*, was issued. This standard establishes a set of professional qualifications that can be used to develop educational requirements and corresponding certifications for emergency vehicle technicians and mechanics. In addition, NFPA 1915, *Standard for Fire Apparatus Preventive Maintenance Program*, provides guidance for creating and maintaining a comprehensive maintenance program. Together, these standards can be used to ensure that a department's staff has skills adequate to service and maintain the full spectrum of emergency vehicles. Although NFPA standards are not legally binding unless formally adopted by the authority having jurisdiction (AHJ), many departments, companies servicing emergency equipment, and original equipment manufacturers have adopted NFPA 1071 and NFPA 1915 as part of their internal policies and operating procedures. In an ongoing effort to ensure vehicle safety, the Emergency Vehicle Technician (EVT) Certification Commission was established to write and administer tests that would demonstrate proficiency in established standards. The tests resemble those used by the Automotive Service Excellence (ASE) organization, applying its high "blue seal of excellence" standards to fire equipment. Technicians who receive all of the EVT and ASE certifications are recognized as master certified EVTs. The EVT certification program presently has two certification tracks, one for technicians who service and maintain fire apparatus and another for technicians who service and maintain ambulances.

4. Engine, drive train, cooling system, braking system, electrical system, and environmental control system.

5. The theory on how antilock brakes work is very simple. There is less traction when the vehicle begins to skid. The portion of tire that contacts the road begins sliding on the road surface. A great example of this is when a vehicle slides on ice. Essentially the tire is touching the surface; however, there is virtually no traction. Antilock brakes benefit you in two ways: The vehicle will stop faster and the driver will be able to steer while stopping. The drum brake has

more parts than the disc brake and is typically more difficult to service. The drum brake has two brake shoes and a piston. There is also an adjuster mechanism, an emergency brake mechanism, and a lot of springs. The brakes work when the driver pushes on the brake pedal; then the piston pushes the brake shoes against the drum. The multitude of springs is to create the wedging action that pulls the shoes away from the drum when the brakes are released. The remainder of the springs help hold the brake shoes in place and return the adjuster arm after it actuates. A disc brake works by the brake pad squeezing the rotor, and the force is transmitted hydraulically. The friction between the pads and the disc slows the disc. The most common service required for disc brakes is changing the pads. A disc brake typically has a wear indicator on it. When the material is worn away, the metal wear indicator will contact the disc and make a squealing sound. If a deep score is worn into the brake rotor, it will need to be turned to restore the rotor to a flat, smooth surface. Air brakes are used in many emergency vehicles. These units are drum type. Air enters the chamber when the brakes are applied. The push rod moves out, turning the slack adjuster, which rotates the S cam and forces the shoes into the drum. The biggest factor in favor of the diesel engine is the high torque/displacement factor. The biggest factor against the diesel is its inherent lack of retarding power. Take your foot off the throttle and a diesel virtually free wheels. Add a 6 to 8 percent grade hill to the equation, and the result is overheating brakes, brake fade, and a good chance of a runaway. An exhaust brake traps cylinder compression pressure, creating back pressure.

6. Brake fade occurs when the brake linings get hot. The friction provided by the linings decreases. At this point the linings no longer offer the same resistance to the rotation of the drums and get slick.

7. Tire inflation pressure is the level of air in the tire that provides it with load-carrying capacity and affects the overall performance of the vehicle. The tire inflation pressure is a number that indicates the amount of air pressure—measured in pounds per square inch (psi)—a tire requires to be properly inflated. (You will also find this number on the vehicle information placard expressed in kilopascals [kPa], which is the metric measure used internationally.) Remember, the correct pressure for your tire is what the vehicle manufacturer has listed on the placard, NOT what is listed on the tire itself. Because tires are designed to be used on more than one type of vehicle, tire manufacturers list the maximum permissible inflation pressure on the tire sidewall. This number is the greatest amount of air pressure that should ever be put in the tire under normal driving conditions.

8. See Figure 8.12.

9. Routine maintenance is done on an everyday basis. Scheduled maintenance is done on a regular basis; for example, oil changes every 3,000 miles. Crisis maintenance happens whenever there is a breakdown.

10. There are eight specific areas to be checked during the Quick Check inspection:
    1. Overall appearance
    2. Operator compartment
    3. Exterior: operator's side
    4. Exterior: front
    5. Engine compartment
    6. Exterior: passenger's side
    7. Patient compartment
    8. Exterior: rear

11. An operator might be judged to be negligent with regard to vehicle inspection for two main reasons: (1) failing to inspect a vehicle thoroughly according to the organization's requirements; (2) knowingly operating a vehicle with a problem that should have caused it to be taken out of service.

Chapter 9

1. Highway/roadway safety best practices enhance scene safety by notifying road users of regulations and provide warning and guidance needed for the reasonably safe, uniform, and efficient flow of the traffic stream.

2. Core components of highway/roadway operations include fulfill a need; command attention; convey a clear, simple meaning; command respect from road users; and give adequate time for proper response.

3. The ten best practices to enhance highway/roadway safety follow: There is no substitute for training; multi-agency coordination and communications are a must—a unified incident command is essential; limit your exposure…limit your time; give traffic plenty of warning; protect the scene with apparatus; always work away from the traffic, be prepared to shut down the roadway; be seen and not hurt; dress for the occasion; and accountability matters.

4. Blocking is the positioning of vehicles and apparatus on an angle to the lanes of traffic, creating a physical barrier between upstream traffic and the work area. This can be performed in a block left or block right application.

5. Tapering of cones is the action of merging several lanes of moving traffic into fewer moving lanes.

6. Responders should place cones beyond the most distant operating emergency equipment from the actual incident. The cones should taper in a reverse transition to guide traffic back to normal lane flow.

7. Chapter 6 of the MUTCD specifically addresses temporary traffic control (TTC), which covers emergency scene operations.

8. According to the MUTCD, an advanced warning sign should be placed 4 to 8 times the speed limit in miles per hour (MPH), expressways and freeways at one-half mile, and 8 to 12 times the speed limit in MPH in rural areas. The second advanced warning sign should be placed at 100 feet in low-speed urban areas, 350 feet in high-speed urban areas, 1,500 feet on expressways and freeways, and 500 feet in rural areas.

9. Fluorescent orange-red or fluorescent yellow-green.

10. Signs and cones should be retrieved when the scene is terminated by using a reverse order beginning with the postincident taper of cones backward to the first pre-incident warning sign.

Chapter 10

Preparing to Drive

1. Three components of driver readiness include a walk around the vehicle, adjusting the seat and mirrors, and securing the seat belt.

2. The purpose of route planning is to ensure maximum response safety by choosing the most appropriate and least congested route of travel, having alternative routes, and ensuring a means of egress from current response patterns.

3. Hazards that could interfere with the response include time of day, weather, traffic conditions, and construction zones.

Off-Road Driving

1. Vision and speed are critical components to the safe operation and handling of the vehicle during off-road driving.

2. Any five of the following are best practices:
   a. If equipped, place the vehicle into all-wheel drive prior to proceeding off road.
   b. Always proceed slowly and ensure that the vehicle is under control at all times.
   c. Do not "cut" a new road unless there is no other way to traverse the area.
   d. Have someone on foot scout an unknown route or one with dense underbrush in order to identify hidden hazards.
   e. Go straight up the hill; do not angle across the face of a steep hill.
   f. If the vehicle starts to slide, steer going downhill but do not steer going uphill.
   g. Set the emergency brake if the vehicle stalls on a hill.
   h. Never coast down a hill, always proceed slowly in low gear.
   i. When crossing a ditch or gully, advance slowly and proceed at an angle to avoid "bottoming out" the vehicle.

3. The firefighter could have walked alongside the vehicle with a short hose line, or the fire department could have installed a remote-controlled nozzle from inside the cab.

Rollover
1. The recommended best practices for maintaining vehicle control can include:
   - Always wear your seat belt.
   - Do not panic.
   - Get control of your speed.
   - Maintain control of the steering wheel.
   - Steer straight ahead and slow down.
   - Take your foot off the accelerator, but do not brake.
   - Allow the vehicle to slow down on its own.
   - When you reach a slow, safe speed, turn the steering wheel to the left and gently steer the vehicle back onto the highway.
   - Do not jerk your steering wheel.
2. The five primary components that must be understood to avoid a rollover crash are
   1. The driver's training, experience, physical conditioning, and state of mind.
   2. The vehicle's height, weight, width, and suspension.
   3. Common rollover circumstances—excessive relative speed, soft shoulder drop-off, and uneven surface drop-off and improper recovery.
   4. Physical dynamics of vehicle operations—inertia, momentum, center of gravity, friction, and centrifugal force.
   5. Mechanics of vehicle operations—relative speed; specific road conditions; effects of body roll, center of gravity, and tire sidewall flexibility; effects of weight transfer, understeering, braking, and uneven surfaces; steering angle and tire friction; and liquid slosh effect.
3. Total weight and weight distribution determine the vehicle's center of gravity. The body of a vehicle pivots around the center of gravity side to side. Higher centers of gravity can result in increased rollover potential.
4. Crew movement is dynamic weight. When movement occurs, the weight is shifted and can change the handling characteristics of the vehicle.

Private Vehicle Use
1. This varies by insurer. Check with your personal auto insurance carrier for specific coverages.
2. This varies by insurer. Check with your ESO insurance carrier for specific coverages.
3. Check with your ESO insurance carrier for specific limits.
4. Check with your ESO regarding safe driving policy and supporting SOP/SOGs.
5. Check with your ESO to assure that all SOP/SOGs comply with state emergency vehicle codes.

Vehicle Security
1. Ensure that vehicles in station are secured in such a manner that significantly increases the difficulty of unauthorized access and use and endorses inventory of vehicle keys, routine and random vehicle audits, periodic review of vehicle and station key access logs; and ensures that all vehicles that are off premise are accounted for, especially when not in direct possession of the ESO.
2. Five key components of vehicle security include tracking vehicles that are in service, out of service, on reserve status, in the maintenance garage, and those that are for sale or going for salvage.
3. Vehicle security SOP/SOGs come into play by establishing accountability and tracking processes.

Emergency Dispatch
1. Sound dispatch prioritization systems establish a patient's level of severity, which then allows the determination of the type of vehicle(s) that should respond and the urgency of that response.
2. The vehicle risk control–related component of emergency dispatch protocols is that they can send the right vehicle/equipment/personnel to the right emergency under the right response mode.

3. Practical applications of ED protocol use pertaining to vehicle response encompasses the emergency (L&S) response versus the nonemergency (no L&S) response. In some systems, lights-only response is an option. Use of such determinates can aid in a low-force defensive driving response.

Collision and Near-Miss Investigation

1. Specific procedures can be implemented for reporting unsafe conditions. Examples include written SOP/SOGs addressing
   - Comprehensive apparatus maintenance program
   - Who is authorized to perform maintenance functions
   - How problems are corrected and reported when detected
   - How the process is documented
     - Date and time problem or risk was discovered
     - Description of complaint
     - All actions taken
     - Personnel that discrepancy was reported to
     - Date and time corrective action was taken
2. The investigator collects information on how and why the collision occurred, analyzes the information to determine the cause(s) of the collision, and develops recommendations to prevent the situation from recurring.
3. Provide a safe and healthful work environment for all personnel, identify all collision causes and develop corrective actions to eliminate those causes, implement all recommendations in a timely manner to prevent collision recurrence, and develop safety awareness so that potential unsafe acts and conditions are identified and actions taken to prevent a collision.
4. The definition of near miss can vary by interpretation. For all intended purposes in this text a near miss is an incident that did not incur any physical damage or injury but could be breeding incidents that may result in damage and/or injury.

Training Program Safety

1. Training is the foundation of all safe practices.
2. Assure that training is conducted to recognized and accepted best practices, training is conducted by knowledgeable competent instructors, appropriate PPE is utilized, and safe application of skills is supervised.
3. Through attitude and behavior, organization leaders must reflect the importance of safety in all aspects dealing with vehicles. This attitude must be infused in all organizational policies and training.

Index

Safety—*continued*
  safe driving policy recommendations, 65
  securing equipment and, 117, 118, 125
  sleep and, 18-21
  ten cones of safety, 178-188
  training and, 10-11, 171, 179
  training program safety, 244-252
  unsafe behavior, 118
  unsafe vehicles, 165
  USFA Emergency Vehicle Safety Initiative, 197-199
Samples, of standard operating procedures/standard
    operating guidelines, 45-46, 60, 68, 69, 202-210, 248-252
Scene exposure limitations, ten cones of safety, 181
Scene lighting and marking, roadway operations, 186, 187, 193-195
Scene protection with apparatus, ten cones of safety, 181
Scheduled maintenance, 166
School hours, route planning, 104
Seat belts
  crash avoidance and, 126
  operations and, 54, 117-118, 246-247
Secondary incidents, 170, 172-173
Securing equipment
  crashes and, 125
  safety and, 117, 118, 125
Sedating medications, and drowsy driving, 19
Self-contained breathing apparatus (SCBA), 7
Several liability, 59
Shadow
  positioning apparatus and, 175
  USFA definition, 172
Shall as term, in standard operating procedures/standard
    operating guidelines, 63
Shift workers, driver/operator readiness, 19-21
Shutting down roadways, ten cones of safety, 182
Side mirrors
  backing and, 80
  vision and, 116
Simulator adaptation syndrome (SAS), 34
SIPDE (scan, identify, predict, decide, and execute), 100-101
Sirencide, 234
Siren detectors, 118
Siren modes, 108
Sirens. *See* Emergency sirens
Situational awareness, 89
Size of vehicle, and emergency vehicle driving, 76
Skids, response to, 150
Sleep, driver/operator readiness, 18-21
Sleep apnea syndrome (SAS), 19
Sleep disorders, drowsy driving, 19, 21
Slosh effect, rollovers, 223, 226
Snorkels, 74, 75
Snow, and traction, 113-114
Solomon, Stephen, 75

SOP/SOGs. *See* Standard operating procedures/standard
    operating guidelines (SOP/SOGs)
Sovereign immunity, legal liabilities, 44, 59
Space cushions, crash avoidance, 126
Space management, 79, 126
Special operations. *See also* Emergency vehicle driving;
    Operations; Roadway operations
  collision and near-miss investigations, 238-244
  emergency dispatch and, 233-237
  off-road driving, 218-220
  preparing to drive, 216-218
  privately owned vehicles (POV) and, 226-230
  rollovers and, 221-226
  training program safety and, 244-252
  vehicle security, 230-233
Specific exemptions, 46
Speed limits
  buffer zones and, 183, 184
  on curves, 86
  emergency responses and, 109-110
  emergency vehicle driving and, 79, 86
Speed management
  backing and, 81
  emergency vehicle driving and, 79
  ride quality and, 89
Speed sensors, antilock braking systems (ABS), 151
Spotters. *See also* Flaggers
  and backing up, 80, 126, 199
Squirts, 75
Stall parking, 93
Standard operating procedures/standard operating
    guidelines (SOP/SOGs)
  adoption of, 66
  apparatus placement and, 192-193, 196, 200
  collision and near-miss investigations and, 239, 241
  compliance/enforcement of, 65
  definition of terms and, 61, 62
  examples, 45-46, 60, 68, 69, 202-210, 248-252
  formulation procedure, 63-64
  limitations of, 197
  needs assessments and, 62-63
  NIOSH recommendations/discussions, 61
  periodic reviews of, 64-65
  as reflection of policy, 60
  regional committees and, 195-196
  roadway operations and, 195-197
  samples of, 45-46, 60, 68, 69, 202-210, 248-252
  subject areas of, 66-67, 68, 69
  as training component, 7
  usual components of, 64
Standards
  for controlled intersections, 111-112
  maintenance standards, 146-147
  position statements and, 51, 52
  for safety vests, 185